# **O**rthopedic **R**eview for **P**hysical **T**herapists

# Orthopedic Review for Physical Therapists

TIMOTHY S. LOTH, MD
PHYSICIANS' CLINIC OF IOWA
CEDAR RAPIDS, IOWA

CAROLYN T. WADSWORTH, MS, PT, OCS, CHT
HEARTLAND PHYSICAL THERAPY
CEDAR RAPIDS, IOWA

WITH 181 ILLUSTRATIONS

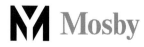

St. Louis  Baltimore  Boston  Carlsbad  Chicago  Naples  New York  Philadelphia  Portland
London  Madrid  Mexico City  Singapore  Sydney  Tokyo  Toronto  Wiesbaden

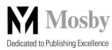

Publisher: Don E. Ladig
Executive Editor: Martha Sasser
Developmental Editor: Kellie F. White
Project Manager: Mark Spann
Production Editor: Julie Eddy
Book Design Manager: Judi Lang
Manufacturing Supervisor: Karen Boehme

Printed in the United States of America
Composition by TSI Graphics
Printing and binding by Maple-Vail Book Mfg. Group

Mosby-Year Book, Inc.
11830 Westline Industrial Drive
St. Louis, MO 63146

**International Standard Book Number 0-8151-2526-7**

98 99 00 01 02 / 9 8 7 6 5 4 3 2 1

# Contributors

William D. Bandy, PhD, PT, SCS, ATC
Associate Professor
The University of Central Arkansas
Department of Physical Therapy
Health Sciences Center, Suite 200
Conway, AR 72035

Paul F. Beattie, PhD, PT, OCS
Assistant Professor
Department of Physical Therapy–Rochester Campus
School of Health Sciences and Human Performance
Ithaca College
300 East River Road, Suite 1-102
Rochester, NY 14623

Robert E. Burdge, MD
Professor and Chairman
Department of Orthopedic Surgery
St. Louis University
3635 Vista Avenue at Grand Blvd.
PO Box 15250
St. Louis, MO 63110-0250

J. Kenneth Burkus, MD
The Hughston Clinic, PC
6262 Hamilton Road
Columbus, GA 31904

Grand A. Dona, MD
Orthopedic Clinic of Monroe
Monroe, LA 71201

Stanley H. Dysart, MD
Marietta Orthopaedics, PA
Marietta, Georgia

Richard C. Fisher, MD
Associate Professor
Department of Orthopedics, University of
   Colorado Health Sciences Center
Denver, Colorado

Keith R. Gabriel, MD
Associate Professor
Department of Orthopaedic Surgery
St. Louis University
Dept. Dir. Pediatric Orthopaedics
Cardinal Glennon Children's Hospital
1465 S. Grand Avenue
St. Louis, MO 63104

Ann Hayes, MHS, PT, OCS
Assistant Professor
Department of Physical Therapy
School of Allied Health Professions
St. Louis University
1504 South Grand Blvd.
St. Louis, MO 63104

LTC D. E. Casey Jones, MD
Deputy Commander
Director, Orthopaedic Residency
Madigan Army Medical Center
Tacoma, WA 98431

Kenneth J. Koval, MD
Chief, Orthopaedic Fracture Service
Hospital for Joint Diseases
Orthopaedic Institute
New York, NY 10003

Timothy S. Loth, MD
Orthopedic Surgery Department
Physicians' Clinic of Iowa
4720 Beaver Avenue, SE
Cedar Rapids, IA 52402

Steven Mardejetko, MD
Orthopedics and Scoliosis
1725 W. Harrison, Suite 440
Chicago, IL 60612

Douglas J. McDonald, MD
Associate Professor
Department of Orthopedic Surgery
St. Louis University School of Medicine
3635 Vista Avenue at Grand Blvd.
PO Box 15250
St. Louis, MO 63110-0250

Michael H. McGuire, MD
Professor and Chairman
Department of Surgery
Creighton University School of Medicine
601 N. 30th Street
Omaha, NE 68131

# Contributors

Deb Nawoczenski, PhD, PT
Associate Professor
Ithaca College
Department of Physical Therapy
300 East River Road, Suite 1-102
Rochester, NY 14632

Garvice Nicholson, MS, PT, OCS
Director, Rehabilitation Services
The Kirklin Clinic at UAB
Associate Professor
Division of Physical Therapy
The University of Alabama at Birmingham
2000 Sixth Avenue South
Birmingham, Alabama 35233

Thomas Otto, MD
Associate Professor
Department of Orthopedic Surgery
St. Louis University
3635 Vista Avenue at Grand Blvd.
PO Box 15250
St. Louis, MO 63110-0250

Robert Pierron, MD
Associate Professor
Department of Orthopedic Surgery
St. Louis University
3635 Vista Avenue at Grand Blvd.
PO Box 15250
St. Louis, MO 63110-0250

Howard M. Place, MD
Associate Professor
Department of Orthopedic Surgery
St. Louis University
3635 Vista Avenue at Grand Blvd.
PO Box 15250
St. Louis, MO 63110-0250

James J. Sferra, MD
Associate Staff
Section of Lower Extremities
Department of Orthopaedic Surgery
The Cleveland Clinic Foundation
9500 Euclid
Cleveland, OH 44195

Michael J. Shereff, MD
Dir. Div. of Foot & Ankle Surgery
Associate Professor
Department of Orthopedic Surgery
Medical College of Wisconsin
8700 Wisconsin Avenue
Box 149
Milwaukee, WI 53226

David W. Strege, MD
Assistant Professor
Department of Orthopedic Surgery
St. Louis University
3635 Vista Avenue at Grand Blvd.
PO Box 15250
St. Louis, MO 63110-0250

Carolyn T. Wadsworth, MS, PT, OCS, CHT
Heartland Physical Therapy, PC
3705 River Ridge Drive, NE
Cedar Rapids, Iowa 52402

Theodore C. Yee, MD
Battle Creek Orthopaedic Clinic, P.C.
Battle Creek, MI

# Dedication

To Grace Thaxton, my grandmother who, at age 106 is still inspiring me! Also to my husband, John and children, Beth and Brian, for their continued support. *CTW*

To my wife Lisa, my children Renée and Karl, and my parents Patricia and Donald, your guidance, patience, and love made this book possible. *TSL*

# Foreword

When Carolyn Wadsworth asked me to write the foreword for a book co-authored by her and Dr. Timothy Loth, I was first of all stunned. Flush with a sense of pride from having just received the Paris Distinguished Service Award by the Orthopaedic Section, APTA, I was eager to support my colleagues. That opportunity presented itself sooner than I had expected—precisely as I was finishing a glass of wine at the reception!

Several months after my conversation with Carolyn, the manuscript arrived. It was an impressive compilation of material. The post-award reception glow had just about worn off, but I was still intrigued by the concept of the book. As I worked my way through the material, I had the recurring thought that this book would be a really great educational tool for both students and clinicians desiring to expand their knowledge of orthopedic physical therapy.

During the time when I was a member of the Orthopaedic Specialty Council, I was frequently asked, "how should I study" and "what should I study" to prepare for specialization. There was always a long answer that included comparing a self-analysis of one's practice, areas of special knowledge, and areas of unique skills with the document then known as the *Orthopaedic Physical Therapy Specialty Competencies*—do this and you would have a study plan. There was also a short answer—study everything. While the self-analysis (especially with the new *Orthopaedic Physical Therapy Description of Advanced Clinical Practice*) is still a very valuable exercise, this book offers a different mode for study. Although it will not replace all other methods of preparation, it does provide a new and invaluable piece of the preparation puzzle. Being able to work with given information and arrive at a clinical decision is the heart and soul of any specialty examination. The process is not a read, remember, and regurgitate exercise by any stretch of the imagination. This book presents a mix of recall, analysis, and synthesis questions that will enhance the reader's clinical reasoning abilities within the broad field of orthopaedic physical therapy.

*Orthopedic Review for Physical Therapists* provides endless possibilities for continuing education. I can see great study group discussions being generated from this text, and a game we used to play— "Question of the Day"—would never be over. And, this undoubtedly could add an exciting element to the next in-service education program. I can't imagine that I am different from most physical therapists in that I love the challenge of problem solving and any time the answer to a question doesn't begin with, "well that depends on . . .", then even better. Certainly, the solutions to the problems we encounter are not always clear, but the format of this book will go a long way toward strengthening the foundation upon which those elusive decisions are made.

I wish to thank the authors for asking me to express these few thoughts. Most of all, I would like to encourage all who are striving to improve their orthopaedic clinical skills, and wish them the best of luck in their studies and in their practices. Our profession is dear to me. There is much speculation about what will be necessary for the survival of our profession in future health care models. I believe that solid clinical practice will be what ensures our place in any health care delivery system, and that Clinical Specialists are the clinician leaders of tomorrow.

**Richard C. Ritter, MA, PT**
Physical Therapist
Bay Area Physical Therapy–Dublin;
Assistant Clinical Professor
University of California–San Francisco;
San Francisco State Graduate Program in Physical Therapy
San Francisco, California

# Preface

The goal of *Orthopedic Review for Physical Therapists* is to broaden and reinforce the reader's understanding of orthopedics. A unique compilation of review questions, written by orthopedic surgeons and physical therapists, provides a stimulating means for reviewing the evaluation, surgery, and therapeutic management of orthopedic pathology.

The recent surge in interest in clinical specialization indicated the need for a comprehensive reference. *Orthopedic Review for Physical Therapists* is an ideal resource for the student or clinician who desires a self-paced, individualized learning experience. We chose an essay question and case study review format to facilitate a more realistic and rigorous preparation than the multiple-choice question format of typical review books. The reader, thereby, can identify his strengths and deficiencies, while reinforcing his understanding of important concepts. This book provides a stimulating alternative way to organize one's study effort, while undertaking the "formidable" task of preparing for specialist certification.

For those not involved in the certification process, this book is more than a study guide. It offers current perspectives on clinical testing, treatment procedures, and rehabilitation protocols that directly enhance patient care. This collection of the most commonly encountered orthopedic clinical problems and their basic science correlations is an excellent learning tool for therapists at any level of training.

We have attempted to discuss popular clinical topics as well as some of the esoteric ones that one might encounter in clinical practice. We attempted to present "accepted" approaches to orthopedic problems and have not sought to present every option for treatment. We have not avoided controversial areas, but instead have identified these, and given short explanations for each advocated approach. All of the questions and answers contained within this text have been verified through multiple author, peer, and editor reviews.

Although physical therapists are a primary audience, other health professionals such as athletic trainers, orthopedic nurses, occupational therapists, primary care physicians, and doctors of chiropractic medicine will find this material useful. It is our hope that *Orthopedic Review for Physical Therapists* will prove intellectually challenging and thereby serve as a stimulus for clinical investigation and excellence in patient care.

# Acknowledgments

The hard work of many individuals contributed to the development of this book. In addition to the gifted contributing authors, we wish to thank the following persons for helping develop and review the text.

Toni Bricker, LPN
Physicians Clinic of Iowa
Cedar Rapids, IA

Dick Evans, PT, OCS
UI Hospitals and Clinics
Iowa City, IA

Kevin Farrell, MS, PT, OCS
St. Ambrose University
Davenport, IA

Gary Kassimir, PT
Private Practice
Reisterstown, MD

Bill Ogard, MS, PT
Assistant Professor, Division of Physical Therapy
University of Alabama, Birmingham
Birmingham, AL

Caryl Rammelsberg
Physicians Clinic of Iowa
Cedar Rapids, IA

Robert Reif, MS, PT, OCS
University of Illinois at Chicago
Chicago, IL

Joseph Threlkeld, PhD, PT
Creighton University
Omaha, NE

Martha Sasser
Executive Editor
Mosby

Kellie F. White
Developmental Editor
Mosby

Lee Ann Uehling
Editorial Manager
TSI Graphics

# Contents

# Chapter 1

# General Orthopedics

TIMOTHY S. LOTH, MD

CAROLYN T. WADSWORTH, MS, PT, OCS, CHT

ANN HAYES, MHS, PT, OCS

RICHARD FISHER, MD

MICHAEL MCGUIRE, MD

DOUGLAS MCDONALD, MD

THEODORE YEE, MD

ROBERT PIERRON, MD

THOMAS OTTO, MD

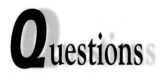

# Questions

1. Describe connective tissue (CT).

2. Compare the cells and matrix of tendon, cartilage, and bone.

3. Describe the development and growth of cartilage.

4. Name the three types of cartilage.

5. Discuss the potential of cartilage to undergo repair.

# 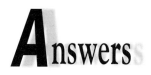nswers

1. Connective tissue is one of the four primary adult tissues. A relatively large amount of intercellular substance (matrix) separates the cells of CT tissue, producing its characteristic appearance. Connective tissue derives from the mesenchymal cells of the mesoderm germ layer that have multiple developmental potentialities. Connective tissues range from irregular, with loosely arranged fibers (adipose, reticular); to regular, which are more fibrous (fascia, ligament, tendon); to highly specialized (cartilage, bone).

2. The fibroblast is the resident cell in nonspecialized CT. It produces the fibers and amorphous components of the matrix. Although relatively inactive in adult life, fibroblasts retain a capacity for growth and regeneration when stimulated, i.e., wound healing. Macrophages are the most numerous of the fluctuating cell populations. Agents of defense, they ingest and destroy particulate matter.

   The fibers in tendon are predominantly collagenous, although reticulin and elastin varieties also occur. The ground substance is a viscous gel with a high proportion of water bound to long-chain carbohydrate molecules and protein–carbohydrate complexes.

   Cartilage contains two types of cells: the young, metabolically active chondroblasts and the chondrocytes. They occupy lacunae and synthesize the matrix components. The fibers in cartilage vary in amount, size, and orientation, contributing the features of three distinct types of cartilage. The ground substance consists of water and dissolved salts in a meshwork of proteoglycans.

   Osteocytes are the major cells of mature bone. They are relatively inactive, but are thought to play a role in bone maintenance. Two other cell types include osteoblasts, associated with bone formation, and osteoclasts, involved with bone resorption. Bone matrix consists of a mineralized ground substance (containing primarily calcium phosphate and calcium carbonate) that is embedded with collagen fibers.

3. In areas where cartilage is to form, the mesenchymal cells proliferate and become closely packed around the fifth week of embryonic life. They elaborate chondroblasts that produce intercellular material, including collagenous fibrils. Cells embedded in the matrix acquire the characteristics of chondrocytes. Continued growth occurs **interstitially** in young cartilage by chondrocytes that retain the ability to divide, proliferate, and lay down matrix. Mature cartilage increases in size through **appositional** growth, in which new layers are added from the inner layer of the perichondrium.

4. Hyaline cartilage, fibrocartilage, and elastic cartilage.

5. Cartilage has limited capabilities to repair itself. Following trauma there is an initial stage of necrosis involving the death of cells and destruction of matrix. An inflammation stage is absent in cartilage because of its avascularity. Without the exudation of reparative cells, the existing chondrocytes must replace the injured tissue. Given their limited metabolic activity, repair is tenuous.

   The location and depth of injury are major determinants of healing capability. Experimental studies on articular cartilage revealed that lacerations deep enough to penetrate the subchondral bone healed more readily than superficial lesions. Defects less than 3 mm wide tended to repair completely, but those greater than 9 mm wide did not. Motion enhances healing of chondral defects by stimulating the differentiation of mesenchymal tissue to hyaline cartilage, although a mixture of fibrocartilage usually accompanies the repair process.

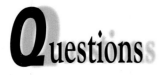
# Questions

6. Describe the two types of embryonic bone development.

7. State three ways in which bone functions as an organ.

8. What are the three phases of fracture healing?

9. Describe key events in the inflammatory phase.

10. Describe the reparative phase.

11. What are the components of fracture callus?

12. Describe the remodeling phase.

13. What are three factors that affect the rate of fracture healing?

14. What are the impediments to normal fracture healing?

15. What are four types of forces that commonly produce fractures?

16. What is a pathologic fracture?

17. What are the components of a fracture management program?

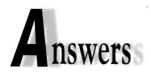

# Answers

6. Bone develops after the seventh embryonic week through intramembranous or intracartilaginous processes. Intramembranous formation produces the cranial vault, mandible, face, clavicles, carpals, and tarsals. Mesenchyme condenses into a bony model, then becomes highly vascularized, stimulating cellular differentiation and proliferation. Osteoblasts and matrix constitute the organic component (osteoid) within which minerals are deposited to produce calcified bone.

   The majority of the skeleton forms through intracartilaginous (endochondral) ossification in which a hyaline cartilage model is transformed to bone. Cartilage cells in the center of the model hypertrophy and die, leaving empty lacunae that calcify. Vascular channels penetrate the model, followed by osteoblasts and osteoclasts that replace the matrix with osteoid that is later mineralized. Secondary ossification centers develop at the ends of long bones, encroaching upon the growth cartilage until the bone reaches its adult size, and the epiphyseal plate fuses.

7. The obvious function of the skeleton is to provide support and structure for the body and protection for the organs. Bone architecture is never static, however, as bone continually remodels in response to stress and functional demands. Another function is provision of blood cells. At birth red, hemopoietic marrow exists throughout the skeleton, but by age 25, it is only found in the flat bones. The skeleton also provides a major storehouse for calcium and phosphorous salts that are constantly being exchanged between the blood and tissue fluids.

8. (1) Inflammatory phase; (2) reparative phase; and (3) remodeling phase.

9. Local necrotic material elicits an immediate and intense acute inflammatory response. Vasodilation and exudation occur. Polymorphonuclear neutrophils (PMNs) enter the region followed by macrophages.

10. The hematoma becomes organized. The pH is acidic. Electronegativity is found in the region of a fresh fracture, which is nonstress generated. Pluripotential mesenchymal cells enter the fracture site with granulation tissue and surrounding vessels. Callus forms. The cartilage in callus is replaced through endochondral ossification. Reabsorption of necrotic bone fragments is performed by osteoclasts.

11. Fibrous tissue, cartilage, and immature fibrous bone.

12. Osteoclastic resorption of poorly organized trabeculae occurs and new bone is laid down in response to lines of force.

13. Blood supply is the major determinant of cell differentiation in a healing fracture. The rate and certainty of healing are directly related to the vascularity of the bone and surrounding tissue. The location of the fracture plays a role in healing; cancellous bone generally heals faster because of its rich blood supply. Fractures heal faster in the young because the periosteum is thicker, stronger, and more osteogenic. Healing is inversely related to the displacement of fracture fragments.

14. The impediments to healing include inadequate immobilization, unsatisfactory reduction, infection, loss of blood supply, interposed soft tissue, and a poor nutritional state.

15. The forces are tension, compression, bending, and torsion.

16. A fracture through bone that is already weakened by tumor or disease.

17. The components include diagnosis, reduction, immobilization, and rehabilitation.

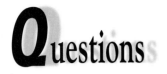

# Questions

18. Why do intraarticular fractures merit special consideration, and what are the two general methods of treatment?

19. What is surgical arthrodesis?

20. Describe the Salter-Harris Classification of epiphyseal plate injuries.

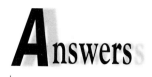

# **A**nswers

18. Intraarticular fractures disrupt the articular cartilage, which has limited healing potential. Residual defects in articular cartilage heal poorly, usually with fibrocartilage. Fibrocartilage is inferior as a joint surface, is more subject to wear and tear, and subsequently results in degenerative changes within the joint. Treatment includes anatomic reduction or early motion.

19. Surgical arthrodesis is fusion of a joint to reduce pain and/or increase stability.

20. Type I involves separation between the epiphyseal plate and the metaphysis. Nondisplaced type I fractures are treated with immobilization. Displaced type I separations are treated with closed reduction and immobilization. The prognosis is good if the blood supply is intact. Type II (the most common) involves separation between the plate and metaphysis and a small metaphyseal fracture with a triangular fragment remaining attached to the plate. Treatment is closed reduction and immobilization, and the prognosis is good, depending on the blood supply. Type III results from intraarticular shearing and is common at the distal tibia. It is an intraarticular injury through the epiphysis and epiphyseal plate. Treatment requires open reduction and immobilization, with the goal of preventing a bony bridge from forming across the plate. The prognosis is satisfactory, depending on the blood supply. Type IV is an intraarticular fracture through the epiphysis, epiphyseal plate, and metaphysis that is usually displaced. Treatment is open reduction and internal fixation (ORIF). The prognosis is variable in terms of future growth. Type V results from axial compression and may be hard to diagnose. The prognosis is poor, and treatment often involves treating the consequences of arrested growth (see Figure 1-1).

**Figure** 1-1

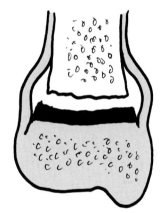

Type I

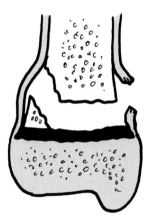

Type II

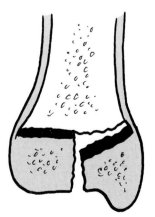

Type III

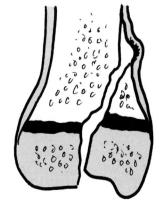

Type IV

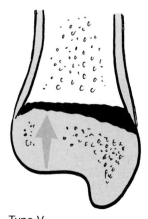

Type V

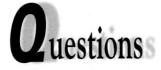

# Questions

21. When are bone changes demonstrated radiographically in osteomyelitis?

22. How much bone substance must be removed to demonstrate radiographic change?

23. What are the clinical features of reflex sympathetic dystrophy (RSD)?

24. Describe the normal hemostatic mechanisms in clot formation.

25. What is the rate of deep vein thrombosis (DVT) in patients with lower extremity joint replacements or fractures?

26. How many of the patients with DVT have pulmonary emboli?

27. What is the most accurate method of detecting a pulmonary embolus?

28. What are the leading causes of mortality in pelvic fractures?

29. What is the most sensitive diagnostic study to evaluate for a possible stress fracture in an extremity that is painful during activity for 2 weeks?

30. What is the most sensitive diagnostic study to evaluate for possible chronic compartment syndrome?

31. How long after the onset of a compartment syndrome does irreversible muscle and nerve damage occur?

32. What is the prime energy source in each of the following? (1) 100-yard dash; (2) intermediate activity (e.g., middle-distance running); and (3) endurance activity (e.g., bicycle riding for 1 hour).

33. What does a myofibril consist of?

34. What is a sarcomere?

35. Draw a sarcomere and the associated bands.

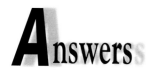

# Answers

21. 10 to 21 days after onset.

22. 40%.

23. Pain, hyperesthesia, and tenderness, usually much greater than expected for the level of injury; swelling; decreased range of motion (ROM); skin color, texture, and temperature changes. Although appearance varies, initially the skin appears pale or cyanotic with associated sweating and coolness. In several weeks, the area becomes reddened, dry, and hot. Much later it again becomes pale and cool, but remains dry.

24. Platelets adhere to the site of injury to form a hemostatic plug. Activation of the coagulation system results in fibrin formation.

25. 50%.

26. 10%.

27. Pulmonary angiography.

28. Blood loss, central nervous system (CNS) injury, and the complications of multiple trauma, e.g., acute respiratory distress syndrome (ARDS).

29. Technetium 99m bone scan.

30. Compartment pressure testing with activity stress. The resting pressure measured both before and after active exercise.

31. Muscle damage occurs in 4 to 12 hours; nerve damage in 12 to 24 hours.

32. (1) Aerobic activity is fueled by the phosphagen system (phosphocreatinine energy source); (2) muscle glycogen is the prime energy source for intermediate activity; and (3) aerobic activity is fueled by muscle glycogen and triglycerides (75%) and fueled by blood-borne fuels (25%).

33. Actin and myosin.

34. The area from one Z line to another.

35.

**Figure** 1-2

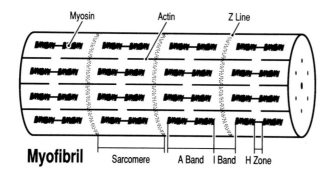

# Questions

36. The I band consists of what protein?

37. What does the A band consist of?

38. What is the H zone?

39. What is a motor unit?

40. Can the ratio of slow-twitch to fast-twitch fibers be altered in an individual by specific training?

41. What are three mechanisms through which organisms can inoculate joints and lead to septic arthritis?

42. In which age groups are infected joints seen most commonly? What percentage of septic joints are monarticular in presentation?

43. Which joint is most commonly infected?

44. What diagnostic procedures should be used to evaluate a suspected septic arthritis?

45. Describe the treatment for septic joints.

46. Describe the clinical characteristics of gonococcal arthritis.

47. Describe tuberculous (TB) arthritis and its treatment.

48. Which viruses can cause polyarticular arthritis?

49. What is the mechanism for arthritis in acute rheumatic fever?

50. What is the prevalence of juvenile rheumatoid arthritis (JRA)?

51. How often is progressive severe joint destruction seen in JRA?

52. What are the associated skeletal anomalies in Sprengel's deformity?

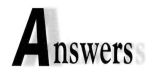

# Answers

36. Actin.

37. Interdigitating fibers of actin and myosin.

38. An area that consists of only myosin fibers.

39. A motor nerve and the muscle fibers it innervates.

40. No, the ratio is genetically determined.

41. (1) Hematogenous spread; (2) extension from preexisting infection in adjacent soft tissue or bone; and (3) direct introduction into the joint through a puncture wound.

42. Infected joints are most common in the very young and the elderly, especially in those with preexisting chronic debilitating disease (e.g., rheumatoid arthritis) or with deficient host defense mechanisms (alcoholics or patients on immunosuppressive drugs). Eighty-three percent are monarticular.

43. The knee.

44. Blood cultures and joint aspiration.

45. Parenteral antibiotics in moderately high doses are given for 1 to 2 weeks. After Staphylococcus aureus infection, oral antibiotic treatment should be continued for another 4 to 6 weeks. The joint is flushed or drained as needed to prevent tense joint swelling. Formal irrigation and drainage, arthroscopy, and serial needle aspirations are options. Physical measures include initial splinting, followed by a program of physical therapy after inflammation subsides.

46. Gonococcal arthritis is found mostly in young women and is often polyarticular (hematogenously spread), with milder joint involvement in contrast to most other types of septic arthritis. Tenosynovitis may be present, as well as macular and vesicular skin lesions on the extremities. The diagnosis is made by isolating the gonococcus from the genitourinary (GU) tract, since it is difficult to isolate from the joint. However, synovial fluid should be analyzed and cultured.

47. TB produces chronic, insidious monarticular arthritis with pain and swelling but often no warmth. X-ray findings are bone and cartilage destruction. The chest film may show signs of TB. Synovial biopsy is often necessary to make the diagnosis that is confirmed by the presence of a granuloma and acid-fast bacteria. Conventional treatment for pulmonary TB is given. The patient often requires surgery for joint reconstruction.

48. Arthritis may be an acute clinical manifestation of rubella, rubella vaccine, mumps, varicella, and infectious mononucleosis, presumably due to invasion of the joint space by the virus.

49. It is thought to be due to an inflammatory or immune response.

50. It is estimated that in the United States 60,000 to 200,000 children are affected. A British study found a prevalence of one case of JRA for every 1500 school-age children.

51. In 5% of patients.

52. Scoliosis; cervical ribs; anomalies of rib and vertebral segmentation (Klippel-Feil syndrome); torticollis; hypoplasia of the pectoralis major (Poland's syndrome), rhomboid, serratus anterior, latissimus dorsi, and (most commonly) the trapezius muscles. Renal anomalies are also seen.

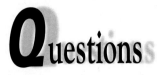

# Questions

53. How should Sprengel's deformity be treated and when?

54. What is the most common birth brachial plexus injury?

55. What muscles are affected in Erb's palsy?

56. What is the second most common birth brachial plexus injury?

57. How should birth brachial plexus injuries be worked up?

58. What is the distribution of weakness in Klumpke's disease?

59. How are brachial plexus injuries treated for the first 18 to 24 months?

60. How should you test for possible neurologic injury associated with shoulder dislocation?

61. How should you evaluate possible neurologic injury in hip dislocation?

62. How should you evaluate possible neurologic injury in distal humeral fractures?

63. Which knee problems are most accurately diagnosed by magnetic resonance imaging (MRI)?

64. What radiologic tests are useful for diagnosing a torn meniscus?

65. What internal derangements of the knee are not well-seen by MRI?

66. What are the advantages and disadvantages of a shoulder arthrogram in evaluating a patient with persistent shoulder pain for a possible rotator cuff tear?

67. What are the advantages and disadvantages of ultrasound in evaluating a patient with persistent shoulder pain for a rotator cuff tear?

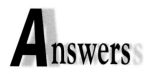

# Answers

53. Only observation is necessary for mild deformities. If operative treatment is indicated, the Woodward procedure is performed between the ages of 3 and 7 years. It involves resection of the supraspinous portion of scapula, release of the vertebral attachments of the muscles, relocation of the scapula inferiorly, and derotation. The vertebral muscles are reattached inferiorly, and an osteotomy of the clavicle is performed to avoid neurovascular problems at the thoracic outlet. Over the age of 8, or when deformity is not severe, excision of the superior angle of the scapula and any vertebral connections can give improved function and cosmesis. This can also be done for patients of any age with minor deformity.

54. Erb's palsy involving the C5-6 nerve roots.

55. The deltoid, biceps, brachialis, supinator, supraspinatus, infraspinatus, and subscapularis muscles are affected.

56. Total plexus involvement producing a limp extremity, loss of tendon reflexes, loss of the Moro reflex, and Horner's syndrome.

57. Radiographs of the neck and both upper extremities should be obtained to rule out a fracture. An electromyogram (EMG) should be performed to document recovery and identify the muscles available for transfer. The usefulness of myelography is controversial. Thermography has been used to evaluate nerve damage also.

58. The wrist and finger flexors and intrinsic muscles are involved.

59. Prevention of contractures and observation for neurologic recovery, ROM exercises, and intermittent static splinting. Some advocate exploration and repair if there has been no improvement after 3 months of observation.

60. Test sensation in the "lateral shoulder patch" area overlying the deltoid muscle. Evaluate for deltoid muscle strength because of the high risk of axillary nerve injury with shoulder dislocation.

61. Evaluate sensation in the lateral calf and dorsal foot and dorsiflexion strength of the foot and toes, since sciatic nerve injury, especially the peroneal branch, is at highest risk in hip dislocation.

62. Check sensation on the dorsoradial hand and evaluate the strength of wrist and finger extension due to the high risk of radial nerve injury.

63. Torn meniscus, avascular necrosis (AVN) about the knee, tumor, and torn cruciate ligament (some false negatives have been reported). MRI does not "see" articular cartilage surfaces well.

64. An MRI shows the highest correlation in diagnosing both medial and lateral meniscus tears, but will show degenerative changes when a full-thickness tear is not present. An arthrogram is not as reliable in diagnosing cruciate tears as MRI.

65. Articular cartilage chondromalacia, plica, and loss of functional integrity of the anterior cruciate ligament; although a complete rupture can usually be diagnosed in a high percentage of cases.

66. An arthrogram best demonstrates a full-thickness rotator cuff tear. Disadvantages are that it shows poor resolution of the glenoid labrum and it is an invasive technique.

67. Ultrasound offers a noninvasive technique, but is somewhat operator-dependent and may miss a full thickness tear that only involves a portion of one musculotendinous unit.

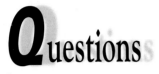
# Questions

68. What are the advantages and disadvantages of MRI in evaluating a patient with persistent shoulder pain for a rotator cuff tear?

69. How can you clinically differentiate acromioclavicular joint pain from other sources of shoulder pain?

70. What are some common sources of referred pain to the shoulder?

71. In athletes with slipping or "dead arm" sensation on overhead throwing, what is the most likely cause of symptoms?

72. What anatomic abnormalities would most likely be present in clinical glenohumeral instability?

73. In athletes who throw, to what is shoulder pain without antecedent trauma due?

74. What nonoperative measures may be helpful in treating an athlete with clinical shoulder instability without dislocation?

75. What problems can be approached for diagnosis and treatment by ankle arthroscopy?

76. What is the most common cause of acute-onset severe flatfoot deformity in adult patients?

77. What is the recommended treatment for a ruptured posterior tibial tendon in adults?

78. A college football player is treated for a hamstring muscle strain and obtains excellent relief. What parameters will you evaluate during rehabilitation to determine an appropriate safe return to competitive-level sports?

79. What clinical findings are indicative of Morton's neuroma?

80. A patient with sacroiliac arthritis and erosive arthritis of the distal interphalangeal joints of both hands with fingernail pitting would likely have what skin changes?

81. A 68-year-old woman with a sudden onset of painful swelling in the knee is found on radiograph to have spur formation, slight narrowing of the medial joint, and fine white specks that seem to outline the menisci. What will joint aspiration likely show on microscopic examination?

82. A 45-year-old man with sudden painful swelling of the knee reports no trauma. He has also had a sudden onset of swelling, redness, and pain in his foot twice in the last 6 months that spontaneously resolved over 2 to 3 days. He started medical treatment for hypertension a month before his first episode. What would knee aspiration likely show?

83. A 60-year-old woman has painful burning of both feet. Vibratory sense is decreased in the toes but intact at the knees. Pulses are present at the dorsalis pedis and posterior tibial arteries. What is the most likely abnormality on screening blood chemistry?

84. What is the best treatment for flexible pes planovalgus in a 3-year-old child?

85. You are consulted on an infant in the newborn nursery who is found to have talipes equinovarus. What treatment do you recommend for the foot deformity?

86. What is the best treatment for internal tibial torsion in a 12-month-old infant?

87. What treatment should be offered to a 6-week-old infant with a subluxable hip and no other abnormalities?

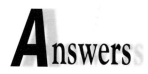

# Answers

68. MRI offers a noninvasive technique that will demonstrate both tendinitis and partial rotator cuff tears. It is very reliable in evaluating complete tears of muscle tendon groups and may see other pathologic changes such as tears of the glenoid labrum. There may be false positives or difficulty in evaluating the "thickness" of partial tears.

69. By localized tenderness, reproduction of pain by anteroposterior stress on the clavicle, horizontal adduction of the arm, pain in the last 30° of abduction, and by a trial of local anesthetic block of the joint.

70. The cervical spine (radiculopathy), heart (myocardial infarction), lung (pneumonia, pancoast tumor), gallbladder, and periscapular muscle spasm (tension fibrositis).

71. Instability of the glenohumeral joint.

72. Anterior glenoid labrum detachment from prior dislocation and a lax anterior capsule associated with straight anterior or multidirectional instability.

73. Tendinitis, instability, or poor training techniques.

74. Strengthening exercises for the rotator cuff, especially the anterior rotator cuff; flexibility exercises for the shoulder, especially the posterior rotator cuff; modification of the training program emphasizing a warm-up period, proper follow-through in throwing mechanics, and incorporation of a gradual progression of force in throwing.

75. Osteochondral fracture of the talus, persistent postsprained ankle joint pain, synovitis, and posttraumatic ankle arthritis.

76. A ruptured posterior tibial tendon.

77. Reconstruction with the flexor digitorum or flexor hallucis longus tendon.

78. Hamstring strength, especially the quadriceps–hamstring ratio, should match his uninvolved extremity. The patient should be advised of the importance of maintaining balanced strength and flexibility when he returns to competitive sports.

79. Tenderness in the third web space of the foot, pain with medialateral compression of the metatarsals, a history of pain with activity during shoe wear (typically improved by removing the shoes and rubbing the foot), and a history of snapping or intermittent numbness of the third and fourth toes.

80. Psoriasis.

81. Calcium pyrophosphate crystals that are associated with pseudogout.

82. Uric acid crystals.

83. Increased blood glucose. The patient's symptoms suggest polyneuropathy, and diabetes would be the most common cause.

84. Observation. Anticipate spontaneous improvement over the next 3 years.

85. Refer to an orthopedic surgeon for manipulation and casting immediately.

86. Observation. Anticipate spontaneous improvement over the next 6 to 12 months.

87. Abduction splint such as a Pavlik harness.

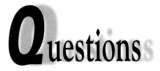

88. A 4-year-old child whose feet were normal since birth is brought for evaluation of intoeing. The clinical exam reveals inversion of both feet with high arches. The examination findings are normal except for a small hair patch over the lumbar spine. What should further evaluation include?

89. You evaluate a 7-year-old girl who reports "tripping and clumsiness." Clinical examination shows inversion of the left foot and decreased dorsiflexion of the ankle compared to the right ankle. When the patient runs, she "postures" the left arm with flexion of the elbow. What is the most likely cause of her problems?

90. You evaluate a 12-year-old boy for a limp. He rubs his anterolateral thigh while describing intermittent right "leg" pain. Upon clinical examination, he is overweight and although he has full knee ROM, the right lower extremity does not externally rotate as far as the left during hip and knee flexion. What further diagnostic studies are indicated?

91. You evaluate a 5-year-old boy for a limp. He gives no history of pain but the clinical exam shows decreased abduction of the left hip compared to the right. His parents give no history of current or recent illness. He is afebrile and shows no other abnormalities during examination. What will an AP pelvis film likely show?

92. A 2-year-old child has refused to walk and has become progressively more fussy in the last 24 hours. Upon examination, any attempt to move the left hip from a flexed and externally rotated position causes the child to cry more loudly. What tests should be ordered at this time?

93. Aspiration of the hip of the child in question 92 is easily accomplished and 2 cc of purulent material is sent for Gram stain and culture. What treatment should now be administered?

94. What are the indications for surgical treatment of a herniated lumbar disc?

95. What are the contraindications to lumbar disc excision by percutaneous techniques?

96. An 11-year-old female gymnast has been having increasing low back pain for 6 weeks. Clinical examination is normal except for slight tightness in the hamstring muscles in an otherwise very flexible, athletic preadolescent girl. AP and lateral radiographs are normal. What further tests should be done prior to medical clearance for competitive gymnastics?

97. Radiographs in this girl show elongation and a fracture line in the L5 pars interarticularis. The bone scan is positive at the same area. What should the treatment be?

98. A 64-year-old patient, 8 years status post lumbar disc excision, shows lumbar spondylosis on plain radiographs. Clinical symptoms include radicular pain and decreased extensor hallucis longus muscle strength. What is her differential diagnosis?

99. What radiographic studies should be ordered for this patient?

100. Which imaging technique has greater sensitivity for detection of disc herniation—CT or myelogram?

101. What imaging technique is the best diagnostic procedure for suspected spinal neoplastic lesions causing myelopathy (both extradural and intramedullary)?

102. What is biomechanics?

103. What is the Systeme International d'Unites (SI units)?

104. What are the four basic SI units used in the study of biomechanics?

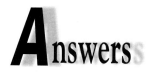

# 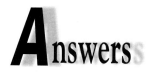nswers

88. A radiograph of the lumbar spine to evaluate for spinal dysraphism and MRI of the spine, especially to look for a tethered spinal cord or diastematomyelia.

89. Cerebral palsy due to perinatal distress.

90. An anteroposterior (AP) film of the pelvis and a lateral film of the right hip to evaluate for slipped capital femoral epiphysis.

91. AVN due to Legg-Calve-Perthes disease.

92. A complete blood count with white blood cell (WBC) differential, sedimentation rate, blood culture, radiograph, and aspiration of left hip for suspected infection.

93. Parenteral antibiotics and an open decompression and irrigation of the hip joint.

94. Urgent surgery if cauda equina syndrome develops; elective surgery if persistent pain or a neurologic deficit correlating with a radiographically proven herniated disc is unresponsive to nonsurgical treatment for greater than 6 weeks.

95. Absence of indications for surgical intervention; an extruded or sequestered disc fragment demonstrated by radiographic studies; and/or coexistent spinal abnormalities such as facet arthritis, severe spondylosis, or spinal stenosis (relative).

96. Oblique films to evaluate for elongation or fracture of the pars interarticularis and a bone scan with oblique lumbar imaging to determine activity of possible stress reaction or spondylolysis.

97. Restriction of activities to decrease impact load and hyperextension of the lumbar spine. If pain persists, the patient should be placed in a body shell back brace such as a Boston brace molded to decrease lumbar extension.

98. (1) Spinal stenosis; (2) nerve root entrapment by facet hypertrophic arthropathy; (3) herniated nucleus pulposus, recurrent or new; (4) referred pain of degenerative spondylosis; and (5) a residual neurologic deficit from previous herniated nucleus pulposus.

99. A computerized tomography (CT) scan will identify bone changes or significant disc herniation, either new or recurrent. Also consider IV enhancement to differentiate the scar from recurrent disc herniation or myelogram or CT to evaluate spinal stenosis or nerve root encroachment.

100. CT.

101. MRI.

102. Biomechanics is the study of mechanical motion as it relates to biological systems.

103. The SI is the modernized metric system adopted by the General Conference of Weights and Measures in 1960. It is the international language of mechanics and biomechanics.

104. The meter (m), the kilogram (kg), the second (s), and the kelvin (K).

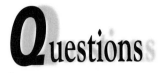

# Questions

105. What is a pascal (Pa)?

106. What is a joule (J)?

107. What is abiotrophy?

108. What is density?

109. What is the Donnan osmotic pressure?

110. What is dynamics?

111. As it applies to implant materials or bone, what is strength?

112. As it applies to implant materials or bone, what is rigidity?

113. What are the two systemic effects of orthopedic implant materials?

114. What are the two biomechanical requirements of a fracture fixation device?

115. What two mechanical terms are used to describe the performance of an implant?

116. Describe a load-sharing system.

117. What does doubling the thickness of a bone plate do to its bending strength?

118. What does doubling the width of a bone plate do to its bending strength?

119. Compare the torsional stiffness of a slotted and an unslotted intramedullary rod.

120. One of the requirements of a successful total hip arthroplasty is to obtain load transfer from the prosthesis to the femur. What are the three mechanisms by which this occurs?

121. What is a surface load transfer system?

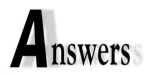

# Answers

105. A pascal is the pressure that is produced by a force of 1 newton applied over an area of 1 square meter, i.e., 1 Pa = 1 N/m². A pascal is the international unit of pressure and stress.

106. A joule is the unit of work done by the force of 1 newton moving an object through a distance of 1 meter in the direction of the force; i.e., 1 J = 1 Nm.

107. Abiotrophy is a degeneration or failure of the microscopic or macroscopic structure of a body tissue or part. This term may also refer to conditions that result from some inborn defect that is not evident until sometime after birth. Huntington's chorea, for example, is an abiotrophic disease process.

108. Density is the mass per unit volume.

109. The Donnan osmotic pressure is the pressure that is generated across a semipermeable membrane from a solution of lesser solute concentration to one of greater solute concentration.

110. Dynamics is the study of forces acting on a body in motion.

111. Strength is the resistance of a material to an applied load.

112. Rigidity is the resistance of a material to deformation, i.e., rigidity = load/deformation.

113. Toxicity and allergic reaction. Allergic reactions to cobalt chrome and nickel have been reported.

114. First, that it maintain the alignment and apposition of the fractured bone. Second, that it be able to transmit forces through the device or bone fragments to optimize fracture healing.

115. Strength and stiffness of the implant. Strength is a function of the yield strength. Stiffness is a function of the elastic modulus multiplied by the cross-sectional area of the implant.

116. Load sharing is the equal or unequal distribution of load through two adjacent materials. An example is a fractured radius internally fixed with a compression bone plate. The compressive load is shared by both the radius and the bone plate. When an axial compressive load is applied to the bone plate system, the bone and the plate share the load in a manner proportional to the relative stiffness of the two materials.

117. Bending strength is proportional to the thickness of a plate squared. Therefore, doubling the thickness increases bend strength by a factor of 4.

118. Bending strength is directly proportional to the width of a plate. Therefore, doubling the width increases the bending strength by a factor of 2.

119. Torsional stiffness is greater for an unslotted intramedullary rod.

120. First, it is possible to apply a direct load to the femoral neck area by the use of a collar. Second, by use of a tapered femoral stem, it is possible to create a compressive load between the stem–cement or stem–bone interface. Third, adhesions between the prosthesis and bone or prosthesis–cement or cement–bone interfaces will allow transfer through shear mechanisms. This is an intramedullary load transfer system.

121. A surface load transfer system is a joint arthroplasty or portion thereof in which the load is transferred directly from the prosthetic system to the underlying cancellous or cortical bone. The femoral component of a total knee, the tibial component of a total knee, and the acetabular component of a total hip all represent surface load transfer systems.

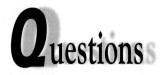

**122.** What is Young's modulus?

**123.** What is ductility?

**124.** What is the yield strength of a material?

Use the following diagram (Figure 1-3) to answer questions 125 through 128.

**125.** In the stress–strain curve, compare the stiffness of materials X and Y.

**126.** What does point A refer to?

**127.** What does point B refer to?

**128.** Assuming X and Y represent orthopedic biometals, which metal would share the load more evenly with bone?

**Figure** 1-3

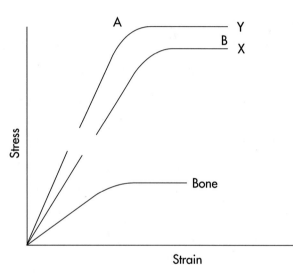

**129.** What is the instantaneous center of rotation or "motion"?

**130.** What is strain?

**131.** What is stress?

**132.** What is the endurance limit?

**133.** At what age does lamellar bone begin to form?

**134.** At what age has lamellar bone fully matured?

**135.** What is the biomechanical function of lamellar bone?

**136.** Compare the relative stiffness of cancellous bone to cortical bone.

**137.** What biomechanical factors govern the shape of a fracture of human bone?

**138.** Load applied in torque results in what type of fracture?

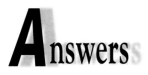

# Answers

122. Young's modulus is the ratio of stress to strain at any point in the elastic region of a load deformation curve. This is also known as the modulus of elasticity and is an expression of a material's stiffness.

123. Ductility is that quality of a material that allows deformity prior to failure under load.

124. Yield strength is the stress at which a material takes on permanent deformity on a stress–strain curve.

125. The modulus of elasticity for material Y is greater. Therefore, it is stiffer than material X.

126. Point A is the yield point, i.e., the point at which a material can no longer retain its elasticity and undergoes plastic deformation.

127. Point B is the failure point, i.e., the point at which the material fractures.

128. Metal X. The modulus of elasticity is smaller for metal X than for metal Y and therefore better suited for load sharing.

129. The instantaneous center of motion is the point in space existing at an instant in time when all other points on the object rotate.

130. Strain is a measure of deformation, or potential energy, or the amount of work a deformed body is capable of doing in returning to its undeformed state. The unit is a change in size or shape of a body.

131. Stress is the intensity or load per unit area that develops at a point in response to an externally applied force. The unit used to describe stress is force per unit area.

132. The endurance limit is the maximum stress level under which no fracture will occur, regardless of the number of loading cycles applied.

133. Lamellar bone begins to form at about 1 year of age.

134. Lamellar bone does not fully develop and mature until the third decade of life.

135. Lamellar bone increases the stiffness (modulus of elasticity) and the yield strength of bone. There is a corresponding increase in the brittleness.

136. Cancellous bone is one fifth to one tenth of the stiffness of cortical bone in axial compression.

137. The shape of a fracture depends upon the inherent qualities of the bone fractured, the externally applied load, and the amount of energy released. Therefore, fractures of immature bone, cancellous bone, and cortical bone will vary with similar exogenous loads.

138. Spiral fractures.

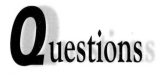

# Questions

139. Load applied in tension results in what type of fracture?

140. Load applied in bending creates what type of fracture?

141. Load applied in axial compression results in what type of fracture?

142. What biomechanical function do flexor tendon pulleys perform?

143. What biomechanical effect takes place with loss of the flexor pulley system?

144. Prehensile kinetics refers to movements of the hand in which objects are brought or held within the arches of the hand. What are the two types of prehensile movement?

145. Efficient prehensile function depends on what basic hand qualities?

146. How does the relative strength of extrinsic finger flexion compare with extrinsic finger extension?

147. Functional wrist motion requires a flexion and extension arc of how many degrees?

148. What is the biomechanical function of articular cartilage in a typical diarthrodial joint?

149. Articular cartilage has been described as a biphasic material. What is meant by that term?

150. What is the biomechanical effect of immobilization on ligament tensile strength?

151. What are the effects of maturation and of aging on the tensile strength of tendon and ligament?

152. What is the rate of growth of regenerating nerve fibers?

153. What are the effects of stretching a muscle tendon complex as a part of physical training?

154. What is the fundamental chemical change during muscle fatigue?

155. What are the three main muscle fiber types?

156. Endurance training is associated with a relative increase in what fiber types?

157. What is the mean ROM of the tibiofemoral joint in the sagittal plane during normal walking?

158. What is considered a minimum ROM at the tibiofemoral joint for normal activities of daily living?

159. What is meant by the "screw home" mechanism of tibiofemoral motion?

160. What are the three types of knee joint surface motion?

# **A**nswers

**139.** Tension typically causes an avulsion or transverse fracture.

**140.** Typically, a bending load causes a short oblique fracture.

**141.** An impaction fracture.

**142.** In combination, the five annular (A) and three cruciate (C) pulleys hold the flexor tendon close to the skeletal plane of the finger ray, therefore maintaining a relatively constant moment arm.

**143.** Loss of the pulleys creates a bowstring effect during flexion of the finger, increasing the moment arm and therefore increasing the tendon excursion requirement. From a practical standpoint, this creates a weakness in flexion of one or more joints in the finger ray.

**144.** Power grip and precision grip.

**145.** (1) Relatively mobile first carpometacarpal and fourth and fifth metacarpophalangeal joints, and relatively rigid second and third carpometacarpal joints; (2) well-balanced extrinsic and intrinsic muscle function; and (3) adequate sensory function.

**146.** Extrinsic finger flexion generates more than twice the force of extrinsic finger extension.

**147.** 65°.

**148.** Articular cartilage increases the area of load distribution and provides a wear-resistant surface by reducing friction.

**149.** The biphasic nature of articular cartilage consists of a 25% collagen proteoglycan solid matrix and a 75% interstitial fluid component. The complex chemical interaction of the matrix and fluid portions allows for significant mobility and permeability of the fluid, rendering unique properties to articular cartilage.

**150.** Immobilization has been found to decrease the tensile strength of ligaments.

**151.** Maturation, i.e., growth up to the age of 20 years, is associated with a gradual increase in the quantity and quality of collage molecule cross-links that is associated with a gradual increase in tensile strength. Aging is associated with a decrease in the tensile strength of collagen.

**152.** The maximum rate of growth is 1 mm/day.

**153.** Stretching increases muscle and tendon flexibility and elasticity. It has also been shown to allow the musculotendinous unit to store more energy.

**154.** Muscle fatigue occurs when adenosine triphosphate (ATP) breakdown exceeds ATP synthesis.

**155.** Type 1, or slow-twitch muscle fibers; type 2A, fast-twitch oxidative muscle fibers; and type 2B, fast-twitch glycolytic muscle fibers.

**156.** Type 1 and type 2 A fibers.

**157.** The mean range is 0° to 67°.

**158.** The ROM should be from full extension to at least 117°.

**159.** As the knee moves from flexion to full extension, the tibia externally rotates. This "screw home" mechanism appears to increase the stability of the knee joint in full extension.

**160.** Rotation, rolling, and gliding (translational) motion.

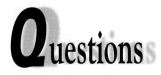

161. What is the biomechanical function of the patella?

162. What properties of bone are important in determining whether it fractures?

163. What is fatigue failure?

164. Bone has resistance to both compression and tension stress. What components of bone are responsible for each of these properties?

165. Use the following diagram (Figure 1-4) for this question. If total body weight is equal to 50 kg, distance a = 15 cm, and distance b = 3 cm, calculate the value of P (patellar tendon force) during single limb stance.

**Figure** 1-4

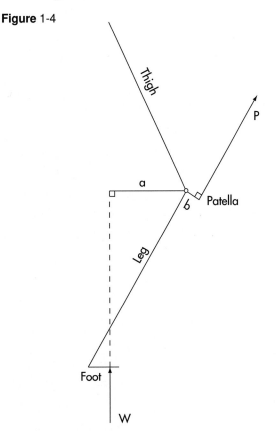

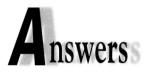

# Answers

161. The patella allows for a wider distribution of forces on the distal femur. In addition, it effectively lengthens the lever arm of the quadriceps muscle through knee ROM. It also prevents tendon–joint contact in flexion.

162. Energy-absorbing capacity, modulus of elasticity, fatigue strength, and density.

163. A fracture that occurs when a material is subjected to repeated or cyclic stresses that are lower than the ultimate tensile strength of the material, but lead to material failure.

164. Collagen resists tension forces. Mineral matrix resists compression. (Bone is a viscoelastic material.)

165. P = 250 kg.

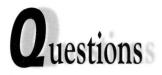

Use the following diagram (Figure 1-5) for questions 166 through 168.

**166.** Given the following values, calculate the value for M (force produced through elbow flexors): W (gravitational force of forearm) = 20 N; P (force produced by weight held in hand) = 10 N.

**167.** Calculate the joint reaction force (J) given the same values.

**168.** What is value of J when P is increased to 30 N?

**Figure** 1-5

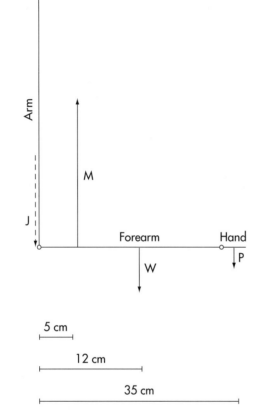

**169.** What are some of the advantages of utilizing a rigid dressing with pylon following a traumatic transtibial amputation of a lower limb?

**170.** A typical gait deviation for an individual with a transfemoral amputation is lateral bending of the trunk over the involved extremity. What are the most common prosthetic and amputee causes for this deviation?

**171.** What are the upper extremity (UE) motions needed to open the terminal device of an above-elbow prosthesis so that a person can pick up a fork from the table where she is sitting?

**172.** Describe the importance of having as long a residual limb as possible with a lower extremity (LE) prosthesis.

**173.** Where are the pressure-tolerant areas on the residual limb of an individual with a transtibial amputation?

**174.** What lower extremity contractures are common in individuals who have sustained a transfemoral amputation?

# Answers

166. M = 118 N. This is calculated by using the equilibrium equation for moments (M): $\sum M = 0$.

167. J = 88 N. The joint reaction force is calculated by using the equilibrium equation for forces (F): $\sum F = 0$.

168. J = 208 N.

169. The advantages are: (1) Improved wound healing secondary to the closed environment; (2) edema control of the residual limb due to the constant sustained pressure; (3) prosthetic shaping of the residual limb; (4) residual limb protection; (5) early partial weight bearing on the residual limb that prepares it for using a permanent prosthesis in ADL and gait; and (6) decreased gait deviations since the individual can continue to ambulate with a bilateral reciprocal gait.

170. Prosthetic causes include: (1) The medial wall of the prosthesis is too high, causing discomfort in the groin area; (2) the prosthesis is too short, so the individual must lean over it during stance phase in order to clear the opposite swing limb; (3) the lateral wall of the prosthesis is insufficient in its support for the hip abductor muscle function, so the individual leans over it during stance phase to move his center of gravity (COG) laterally. This reduces the hip adductor moment at the hip joint axis of rotation and subsequently causes a reduction in the amount of torque that the hip abductor muscle must supply in order to counterbalance the hip adductor moment; (4) the prosthesis is aligned in too much abduction; and (5) inadequate lateral distal pressure relief.

   The amputee causes include: (1) Weak or absent hip abductor muscle strength; (2) abduction contracture of the residual limb; (3) poor balance reactions; (4) previous habit; (5) sensitive residual limb; and (6) an extremely short residual limb that is insufficient as a lever arm for maneuvering the prosthesis.

171. Since the prosthesis is being held close to the body, biscapular abduction would be the UE motion that would open the terminal device. If the person wanted to open the terminal device away from her body, she could use shoulder flexion on the prosthetic side.

172. A longer LE residual limb is analogous to a longer lever arm around a joint axis of rotation. Torque that is produced at a joint is the result of force multiplied by the lever arm length. If a longer lever arm is available, a greater amount of torque can be produced at that joint with the same amount of force. In addition, a longer residual limb has a greater area over which to disperse the force/pressure from the prosthesis onto the limb.

173. (1) The patellar ligament (tendon); (2) the pretibial muscle mass found between the tibial crest and the fibula; (3) the lateral fibular surface between the fibular head and the distal end; (4) the inferior surface of the medial tibial condyle; (5) the popliteal fossa; and (6) the soft tissue area that is found distally and posteriorly on the residual limb.

174. Hip flexion, lateral rotation, and abduction contractures are common.

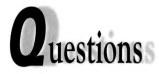
# Questions

175. Explain the importance of maintaining flexion of the anatomic knee during the stance phase of gait on the prosthetic side of an individual wearing a patellar tendon bearing (PTB) prosthesis.

176. After a period of guarded gait training with a patient utilizing a PTB prosthesis, you remove the prosthesis and note a reddened area on the skin at the anterodistal tibia. What are the common prosthetic causes of this problem?

177. Explain the two concepts that are the basis for the mechanics of a body-powered upper extremity prosthesis.

178. Describe the advantages and disadvantages of suction suspension on a prosthesis for a transfemoral amputation.

179. Describe the differences between phantom limb sensation and phantom pain.

180. What are the advantages of a flexible transfemoral socket?

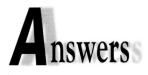
# Answers

**175.** Maintaining anatomic knee flexion during the stance phase of gait utilizing a PTB prosthesis increases the posterior lever arm of the prosthetic foot, which causes the floor reaction line to remain behind the anatomic knee joint during stance. This leads to a flexion moment during the entire stance phase of gait. When flexion occurs at the anatomic knee joint, it increases the weight-bearing area of the residual limb. In addition, knee flexion places the quadriceps muscle of the residual limb on a slight stretch, which encourages it to work more effectively, especially during the loading response of gait and the early part of midstance.

**176.** (1) The prosthesis was improperly donned, causing the anatomic structures that are normally relieved of pressure to receive pressure; (2) the prosthetic foot is outset too far on the socket; (3) there are inadequate relief areas within the socket itself; (4) there are an inadequate number of plys of prosthetic socks, so the residual limb is sinking too deeply into the socket; and (5) there is pistoning of the residual limb within the prosthetic socket due to either: (a) the socket diameter being too large in relation to the residual limb, or (b) an improper suspension system.

**177.** The first relates to the length–tension relationship. The harness system not only suspends the artificial limb on the body, but it assists in the function of the prosthesis through the cable system attached to it. If the harness/cable system is not the correct length, the gross motor activities that power the prosthesis will place inadequate tension on the cables and therefore limit the resulting motions of the elbow and hand/hook. The second concept relates to force. The individual must learn to produce the correct amount of muscular force in order to produce the desired prosthetic action. In summary, if a body-powered upper extremity prosthesis is going to work successfully, the harness/cable system must be the proper length and the individual must generate adequate muscular force.

**178.** The advantages include: (1) It does not require a prosthetic sock; (2) it is cosmetically acceptable; (3) it is more comfortable to wear than other forms of suspension; (4) it produces a more natural gait; (5) it reduces pistoning between the residual limb and prosthesis; (6) it is psychologically more acceptable to some individuals; and (7) since individuals use more of their remaining muscles with this type of suspension, the muscles hypertrophy rather than atrophy and circulation improves.

The disadvantages include: (1) It requires a relatively long limb length; (2) it requires fairly good skin condition (skin grafts can limit the ability to use with some patients); (3) it requires good strength and cardiovascular condition in order to don the prosthesis; (4) it can lose suction for a number of reasons and cause the prosthesis to fall off; (5) it cannot be used with volumetrically unstable limbs or unstable body weights; (6) it increases perspiration and skin irritation; and (7) it can be noisy.

**179.** Phantom limb sensation is typically described as the sensation of a limb that is no longer there. It is quite normal to feel phantom limb sensation after an amputation. It is usually present upon awakening from surgery and can be felt as the sensation of the entire limb or just the distal portion of it. It can be described as a tingling, numbness, or pressure sensation and usually decays with time, although it can be present throughout life. Phantom limb sensation rarely interferes with sleep or the rehabilitation process.

Phantom pain is a relatively rare occurrence after amputation surgery. It is not usually present upon awakening from surgery and is described as a cramping, choking, or burning sensation. Phantom pain, which can be constant or intermittent, is overwhelming and preoccupying to the patient. It can be temporarily relieved by narcotics, but requires a higher dosage when it eventually returns. Phantom pain is believed to be related to preoperative limb pain in location and intensity.

**180.** The flexible transfemoral socket is more comfortable in sitting and dissipates heat better than rigid transfemoral sockets. There is improved proprioception and better muscle accommodation in flexible sockets; and in most instances, they weigh less than rigid sockets.

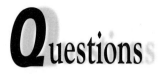# **Q**uestions

181. Describe the differences between quadrilateral and ischial containment sockets for the patient with a transfemoral amputation.

182. State the three ways that knee stability is achieved in a prosthesis for a patient with a transfemoral amputation.

183. What are the advantages and disadvantages of the pneumatic knee mechanism that is used in a transfemoral prosthesis?

184. State the common prosthetic causes of excessive knee extension in the stance phase of gait in a patient wearing a PTB prosthesis.

185. When is it appropriate to use resistance against the residual limb when attempting to strengthen it?

186. Can a transfemoral prosthesis accommodate any amount of hip flexion contracture?

187. A 65-year-old woman suffered a right cerebrovascular accident (CVA) 4 months ago. At present, she can ambulate for about 15 feet, at which time she fatigues. She has difficulty advancing her left LE during swing, which is exhibited by decreased hip flexion, weakness, and 0° dorsiflexion. She does have fair knee control during stance. Describe the LE orthotic that would be appropriate for her.

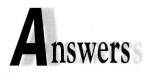
# Answers

181. The ischial tuberosity is contained within the ischial containment socket; the ischial tuberosity sits on the posterior wall of the quadrilateral socket. The quadrilateral socket appears more successful if used with patients who have longer and firmer residual limbs; the ischial containment socket appears more successful with patients who have shorter and fleshier residual limbs. The quadrilateral socket's weight-bearing areas are primarily the ischial tuberosity and the gluteal muscles; the ischial containment sockets include the ischial tuberosity, the pubic rami, and the soft tissue in the area. The ischial containment socket has a smaller medial–lateral socket dimension than the quadrilateral socket, whose anterior–posterior dimensions are more narrow. Both sockets attempt to encourage medial lateral stability during gait. The quadrilateral socket is less successful at this due to the fact that it has no bony lock to maintain hip adduction while ambulating. Both sockets also incorporate the adductor longus tendon and the greater trochanter within the socket.

182. (1) The amount of knee stability can be inherent in the knee component chosen for the prosthesis; (2) knee stability can be attained through the alignment of the socket; and (3) the patient can utilize remaining muscle power on his residual limb to encourage knee stability while using the prosthesis.

183. The advantages include: (1) The pneumatic knee is cadence-responsive; and (2) the prosthetist can usually repair it without having to ship it to the manufacturer.

    The disadvantages include: (1) It is heavier and more expensive than some of the simpler knees; and (2) it requires more maintenance than some of the simpler knees.

184. The prosthetic foot component has a heel that is too soft. This allows the ground reaction force to remain anterior to the knee joint axis of rotation causing knee extension.

    The socket is aligned posterior to the prosthetic foot component, causing an increase in the length of the forefoot keel and a decrease in the heel lever arm. This also allows the ground reaction force to remain anterior to the knee joint axis of rotation, causing knee extension. Insufficient flexion of the socket itself, similar to having the prosthetic foot actually set in plantarflexion, causes the ground reaction force to pass anterior to the knee joint axis between the loading response and terminal stance, creating knee extension.

185. The healing of the incision, the amount of postoperative pain, and the type of postoperative dressing covering the incision all determine when resistive exercises for the residual limb can be attempted.

186. A prosthesis for a transfemoral amputation has 5° of flexion built into it in addition to the amount of a hip flexion contracture, if present. If the patient has no hip flexion contracture, the socket is built with the minimal 5° of flexion. A hip flexion contracture of 15° or less is usually easily accommodated within the prosthesis; however, each situation must be evaluated independently. Whether the contracture can be accommodated depends on the severity of the contracture and the length of the residual limb. The longer the residual limb, the harder it is to accommodate the contracture within the socket.

187. Any of the following would be appropriate for this woman: a plastic prefabricated ankle foot orthosis (AFO), a piano wire orthosis, or a custom-molded AFO set in neutral. These orthotics would be appropriate since they assist dorsiflexion in swing, which the patient needs, but do not affect plantarflexion by any appreciable degree, which the patient does not have difficulty with. In addition, since her knee is stable in stance, it is not necessary to stabilize it by bracing the ankle. Any type of a single- or double-channel adjustable AFO would not be appropriate since it would be too heavy for the patient, who fatigues after 15 feet of ambulation.

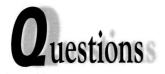

**188.** State the benefits of using lower extremity orthotics with a pediatric population.

**189.** What are the advantages and disadvantages of using a bony contact cervical orthosis for stabilization of the cervical spine?

**190.** What are three reasons for prescribing an upper extremity orthotic?

**191.** State three biomechanical principles that you should follow when prescribing orthotics or prosthetics.

**192.** How will ankle motion be affected by placing a spring in the posterior chamber and a pin in the anterior chamber of a double-channel adjustable ankle foot orthosis?

**193.** Describe the advantages and disadvantages of the Thoracolumbosacral Flexion Control (Anterior Hyperextension) brace.

**194.** What effect does Vitamin D have on serum calcium (Ca) and phosphate ($PO_4$)?

**195.** What effect does calcitonin have on serum calcium and phosphate?

**196.** What stimulates and suppresses calcitonin release?

**197.** Where is calcitonin secreted?

**198.** Which causes osteoporosis, hyperthyroidism or hypothyroidism?

**199.** What are the causes of osteomalacia?

**200.** What is the basic pathologic disturbance in rickets?

**201.** What are the clinical findings in rickets?

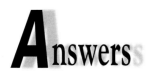
**Answers**

188. Orthotics can increase the sensory input a child receives since they assist her in relating to and exploring the world. They can also improve the child's ability to interact with others and limit complications that can interfere with ADL. Weight-bearing orthotics can help to encourage increased bone density.

189. The advantages include: (1) It gives rigid fixation with an improved rate of fracture union; (2) it allows for early mobilization of the patient; and (3) it applies an increased amount of force for stabilization without much skin breakdown.

    The disadvantages include: (1) It requires a knowledgeable person to apply it; (2) there is increased risk of infection at the pinhole sites; and (3) it is heavy.

190. (1) Upper extremity orthotics can substitute for absent motor power and/or they can assist weak segments of the upper extremity; (2) they can support segments that require positioning or immobilization; and (3) they can be used as a base for the attachment of a device.

191. (1) When applying force, attempt to utilize as long a lever as possible; (2) when applying force, attempt to distribute it over as large an area as possible, so the pressure is dispersed; and (3) in dealing with orthotic and prosthetic joints, try to align the mechanical joint as close to the anatomical position as possible.

192. Dorsiflexion will be assisted through a limited ROM.

193. The advantages include: (1) It is the only lightweight spinal appliance that relies solely on a three-point pressure system to serve its purpose; (2) it is relatively comfortable for the patient to wear and is fairly easy to don; and (3) it is effective in limiting flexion of the spine and maintaining the patient in spinal lordosis.

    The disadvantages include: (1) The potential for excessive force applied to the patient's skin and sternum and the pubis through the three-point pressure system; (2) skin breakdown and pressure sores; and (3) it is not very effective in limiting frontal plane motion.

194. Vitamin D increases serum Ca and $PO_4$ through increased bone release, intestinal absorption, and kidney Ca and $PO_4$ absorption.

195. Calcitonin decreases serum Ca and $PO_4$ through inhibiting bone and intestinal resorption and increasing kidney excretion.

196. Calcitonin release is suppressed by hypocalcemia and stimulated by hypercalcemia.

197. C cells in the perifollicular area of the thyroid.

198. Hyperthyroidism.

199. Deficiency of Vitamin D (postgastrectomy), primary biliary cirrhosis, pancreatic insufficiency, Vitamin-D-resistant rickets, hypophosphatasia, drug-induced osteomalacia (phenytoin, phosphate-binding antacids, etc.), intestinal malabsorption, and acquired and hereditary renal disorders (Fanconi's syndrome).

200. Failure of mineralization of osteoid.

201. Decreased height and weight; muscular weakness; lethargy and hypotonia; craniotabes (softening and thinning of the skull) and persistent fontanelles; rachitic rosary; thickening of the ankles, knees, and wrists with bone tenderness; bending of the soft bones of the lower extremity with weight bearing, producing tibial varus or valgus deformity and coxa varus; hepatomegaly; and poor dentition.

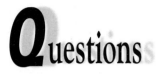
# Questions

202. What is the major skeletal manifestation of Cushing's disease?

203. What effect does PTH (parathormone) have on serum calcium and phosphate?

204. Name the most common etiologic factors associated with avascular necrosis of the femoral head.

205. A 60-year-old woman consults her physician about the value of a bone mineral density study. She asks if bone mineral density measurement is predictive of her chances of having a hip fracture in the future. How should she be advised?

206. How does fracture risk increase with decreasing bone mass?

207. Which of the current methods for measuring bone mineral density is associated with the lowest dosage of radiation?

208. List the major indications for performing bone mineral density measurements.

209. A 42-year-old woman with severe asthma has been on and off corticosteroids for many years. Her current dosage is 60 mg of prednisone per day, but she assures you that the dose is being tapered and she should be off the drug soon. What would you expect her bone mineral density to show?

210. What are the effects of prednisone on bone that account for this change?

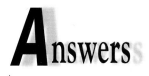

# Answers

202. Osteoporosis.

203. PTH increases serum Ca and decreases serum $PO_4$ through bone release of Ca by osteoclastic activity, intestinal Ca absorption, and increased kidney Ca absorption and $PO_4$ excretion.

204. High-dose steroids, Caisson disease, sickle cell disease, excessive alcohol intake, lupus, fractures of the femoral neck, hip dislocations, and radiation exposure.

205. Studies indicate that hip fracture risk is proportional to femoral bone mineral density and to the age of the patient. Bone mineral density measurement is useful in assessing the overall fracture risk, but will not give a definitive individual prognosis. The other major risk factor for fractured hips in the elderly is the propensity to fall.

206. The risk increases 1.5 to 2 times for each standard deviation decrease in the bone mineral measurement.

207. Dual energy X-ray absorptiometry. The highest dosage is from quantitative CT followed by single photon absorptiometry. The latter involves somewhat less than 15 mrem of radiation per examination. Dual photon and energy absorptiometry are associated with the lowest radiation dosages. The dual energy X-ray film absorptiometry is the most common method in use at this time.

208. (1) Estrogen deficiency, if used as an assessment for the need of estrogen replacement therapy; (2) X-ray film evidence of decreased bone mineral density, especially that seen on spinal X-ray films; (3) initiation of glucocorticoid therapy; and (4) patients with proven primary hyperparathyroidism, if treatment decisions need to be evaluated.

209. A marked decrease for her age.

210. Corticosteroids cause an increase in urinary calcium loss, a decrease in intestinal absorption of calcium, a decrease in osteoblast function, and an increase in the bone resorption rate. All of these adversely affect the bone's ability to maintain its normal architecture and mineral content.

211. A 57-year-old man came to the emergency department with pain in his right leg after a fall from a height of one step while at work. He denied previous symptoms in his lower extremities and stated that he had been in good general health. Initial X-ray films and a bone scan are shown (Figure 1-6, A, B, and C). What is his likely diagnosis?

**Figure** 1-6

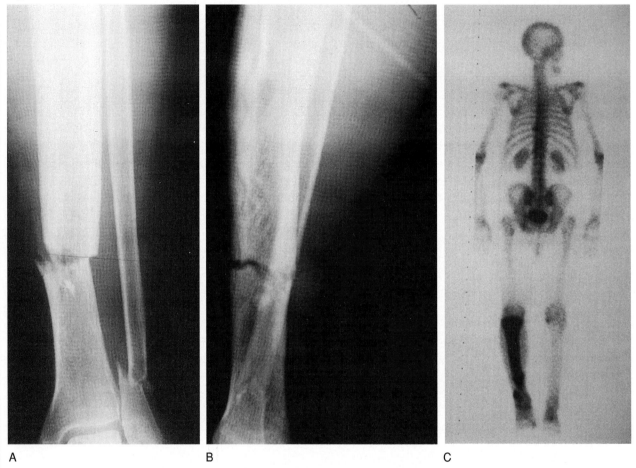

A                                       B                                       C

212. Name the most common sites of fracture with Paget's disease.

213. List the major complications of Paget's disease.

214. Describe the pathologic disturbances and characteristics of Ehlers-Danlos syndrome.

215. Describe the orthopedic management of Ehlers-Danlos syndrome.

216. Describe the clinical features of Marfan's syndrome.

217. Describe the primary defect found in achondroplasia.

218. Describe the primary deformity seen in achondroplasia in the first year of life that demonstrates a tendency to resolution.

219. List the spinal regions where stenosis is frequently encountered in achondroplasia.

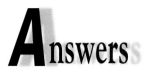

# Answers

**211.** The fracture appears to be pathologic, and the bone changes are compatible with Paget's disease. X-ray film changes are usually pathognomonic for Paget's disease, showing a coarse trabecular pattern, general enlargement of the involved bone, and lytic and sclerotic changes. Occasionally, tumors are associated with the Pagetic process (prostatic carcinoma is the most common nonskeletal tumor). The incidence of sarcoma developing within Pagetic bone is about 1%.

**212.** The spine, tibia, humerus, and femur. In the femur, subtrochanteric fractures are the most difficult to treat. These fractures usually require surgical stabilization and have a high incidence of nonunion.

**213.** Skeletal complications are: fracture, deformity, secondary osteoarthritis, and sarcoma. Other complications are: high-output cardiac failure, hearing loss, headache, mental status change, and hypercalcemia.

**214.** Ehlers-Danlos syndrome is a heritable disorder of CT involving collagen and elastin metabolism. There are seven subtypes with variable inheritance patterns, the most common being autosomal dominant. The syndrome is characterized by skin that is hyperlax, thin, fragile, bruisable, and pseudotumors that form over knees and elbows. Joint hypermobility, hernia, scoliosis, genu recurvatum, and recurrent dislocations of hips, patella, and shoulders also occur. Traumatic joint effusions and hemarthrosis can occur secondary to hypermobility.

**215.** The most common problems are scoliosis and joint dislocation. Scoliosis is managed as idiopathic scoliosis. Joint dislocations (most commonly the patellofemoral and shoulder joints) are managed conservatively.

**216.** Marfan's syndrome affects the skeleton, heart, and lens of the eye. Affected persons have tall stature, disproportionate growth of extremities in comparison to the trunk, arachnodactyly, scoliosis, pectus excavatum, protrusio acetabuli, pes valgus, and genu recurvatum; the eye lens may be superiorly dislocated; cardiovascular defects include heart valve abnormalities, aortic dilation, and aneurysm.

**217.** Abnormal endochondral bone formation.

**218.** Thoracolumbar kyphosis.

**219.** At the level of the foramen magnum in the first year of life, and in the lumbar spine where symptomatic spinal stenosis develops in the third decade of life.

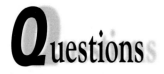

220. Describe the clinical features of arthrogryposis.

221. Describe the orthopaedic management of an acute hemarthrosis in a hemophiliac patient.

222. What are the orthopaedic manifestations of hemophilia?

223. Describe the radiographic changes noted in a knee affected by hemophilic arthropathy.

224. What two joints are most frequently involved with hemophilic arthropathy?

225. A patient with hemophilia presents with a right hip flexion contracture, numbness along the anteromedial aspect of the right leg, and a quadriceps paresis with muscle power of 3/5. Attempts to extend the hip cause increasing pain with radiation down the anterior thigh and into the anteromedial leg. What is the most likely diagnosis in this patient?

226. How common are bone tumors?

227. How do patients with neoplasms of bone or soft tissue present?

228. What are other ways new patients present with skeletal neoplasms?

229. What is the role of trauma in the development of tumors?

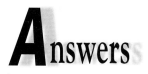

220. Arthrogryposis is a nonprogressive syndrome of joint contractures and varying degrees of fibrosis of muscles that is present at birth. The upper limbs are internally rotated, the shoulders and elbows are stiff, and there are severe peripheral contractures. The lower limbs are externally rotated, the hips and knees are stiff, and clubfoot is common. Intelligence is normal.

221. The patient and family should self-administer appropriate factor replacements; splint the joint in a compressive dressing for several days; aspirate if the joint is markedly distended; and in 3 to 7 days begin physical therapy for ROM.

222. Hemarthrosis, soft tissue bleeding, and the sequelae of these hemorrhages; nerve palsy, pseudotumor, myositis ossificans, chronic hemophilic arthropathy, and subacute hemophilic arthropathy.

223. Widening of the distal femoral epiphysis, squaring of the inferior pole of the patella, flattening of the distal femoral condyles, and widening of the intercondylar notch.

224. The knee and the ankle.

225. Spontaneous hemorrhage into the iliopsoas muscle with secondary femoral nerve compression. The most appropriate treatment includes factor replacement and rest followed by mobilization of the hip and knee. Complete resolution of the femoral nerve deficit is anticipated.

226. Primary benign and malignant tumors of the skeleton are very uncommon and make up less than 1% of the benign and malignant lesions of the body.

227. The clinical presentation varies depending on the location, but up to 90% of patients will present with pain or a mass.

228. Occasionally, pathologic fracture may be the first sign of a tumor, particularly in patients with metastatic disease. Lesions near the axial skeleton may present primarily with neurological dysfunction, and occasionally patients will present with a deformity.

229. There is no good evidence to suggest that trauma is a direct cause of tumors, although many patients will link the onset of their symptoms to a traumatic event. It seems more likely that a traumatic event draws attention to a preexisting lesion, perhaps making it symptomatic at an earlier point in time.

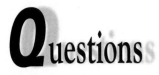

# Questions

**230.** Does the duration of a patient's symptoms give any clue to the diagnosis?

**231.** How is the pain from a neoplasm usually described?

**232.** What physical finding is probably the most helpful in evaluating a neoplasm?

**233.** What two clinical features are most helpful in establishing a diagnosis?

**234.** How is the location of the lesion helpful in establishing the diagnosis?

**235.** The radiographic evaluation of a patient with skeletal neoplasm involves what four modalities?

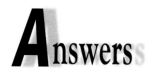**A**nswers

**230.** It is generally not that helpful. Certainly a lesion that has been present for many years is more likely to be benign, but this is not universal. The symptom progression in a chondrosarcoma, for example, may be very indolent and in certain soft tissue lesions (particularly synovial sarcoma), the patient may notice a mass for years prior to diagnosis. For most aggressive benign and malignant neoplasms, symptoms will develop over a few months and usually within a year. Extremely rapid development of pain or a mass in the range of days to weeks suggests an acute inflammatory process.

**231.** Most patients describe their pain as deep, aching, or boring, often accentuated at night. Importantly, the pain is usually slowly progressive.

**232.** The presence of a soft tissue mass in association with a bone lesion is helpful as it generally denotes an aggressive and probably malignant tumor.

**233.** The age of the patient and location of the lesion. Many lesions of bone and soft tissue tend to occur in well-recognized age groups. For example, solitary bone cysts, aneurysmal bone cysts, osteochondromas, and Ewing's sarcomas are examples of lesions that occur almost exclusively in young persons, usually prior to skeletal maturity. Osteosarcoma generally occurs in the second or third decade of life. Giant cell tumors are rare prior to skeletal maturity. Chondrosarcoma and malignant fibrous histiocytoma are lesions of adulthood, and metastatic carcinoma and myeloma are rare before age 45.

**234.** Although many lesions are metaphyseal in origin in long bones, some lesions (particularly giant cell tumors and chondroblastoma) almost always involve the epiphyseal region and subchondral bone. Ewing sarcoma and adamantinoma have a predilection for the diaphyseal portion of bone, and some lesions (such as enchondroma) have a distinct distribution to the small bones of the hands and feet.

**235.** Plain radiograph, CT, MRI, and technetium 99m bone scanning are the most helpful imaging modalities. Other modalities such as ultrasound, angiography, myelography, and other radionucleotide studies such as gallium scanning, have limited roles and are only used in specific circumstances.

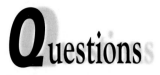

# Questions

**236.** Of the primary imaging techniques, which gives the most information with regard to the character of a lesion?

**237.** For further evaluation of a lesion, which is better, CT or MRI?

**238.** What are the strengths of CT?

**239.** What are the advantages of MRI?

**240.** What role does technetium 99m Tc bone scanning have in the evaluation of bone lesions?

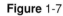 **nswers**

**236.** The plain radiograph. For many lesions of bone, it may be diagnostic and, if not, will usually establish a reasonable differential diagnosis (see Figure 1-7). For primary soft tissue lesions, it will usually confirm the absence of any bone involvement.

Figure 1-7 is an AP radiograph of the distal femur in a 15-year-old girl. There is an obvious destructive lesion present with areas of sclerosis and lysis. In this age and location, the most likely diagnosis is osteosarcoma.

**Figure** 1-7

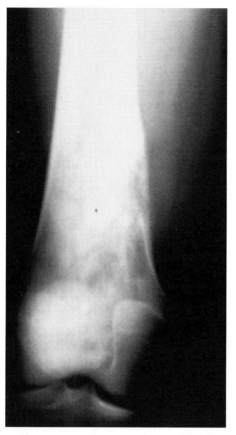

**237.** This is an unfair question, since each has strengths and weaknesses and they are used to gain different information. It should be remembered that on the whole, the CT and MRI are competitive exams and not complementary. It is unusual that the evaluation of a lesion will require both.

**238.** CT is superior to MRI in demonstrating calcification, periosteal reaction, and endosteal thinning.

**239.** MRI is superior to CT in determining the interosseous and extraosseous extent of a lesion, but gives less information with regard to the character or histologic diagnosis. MRI is also superior in illustrating soft tissue lesions.

**240.** Prior to MRI, bone scanning was helpful in determining the local extent of a lesion. However, since the MRI is now superior in this regard, bone scanning is used primarily to determine whether the lesion is solitary or whether there are other bony lesions. Another use of the bone scan may be to gain some appreciation of a lesion's biological activity. Lesions that radiographically appear nonaggressive and have a completely negative bone scan are most assuredly benign and probably asymptomatic.

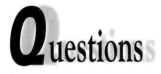

# Questions

241. How are tumors of bone and soft tissue classified?

242. Which is more common, primary tumors of bone or metastatic tumors?

243. What is the most common primary malignancy of bone?

244. Of the primary benign bone lesions, which occurs most frequently?

245. What are the common sites of osteosarcoma occurrence?

246. How can you differentiate a benign from a malignant lesion by viewing the radiographs?

247. What is the most common metastatic tumor in women?

248. What is the most common metastatic tumor in men?

249. What are the most common sites for metastatic spread in the skeleton?

250. The patient is a 63-year-old man with a sudden onset of severe low back pain following a fall at home. A radiograph and biopsy specimen are shown (Figure 1-8, A and B). What is your diagnosis?

**Figure** 1-8

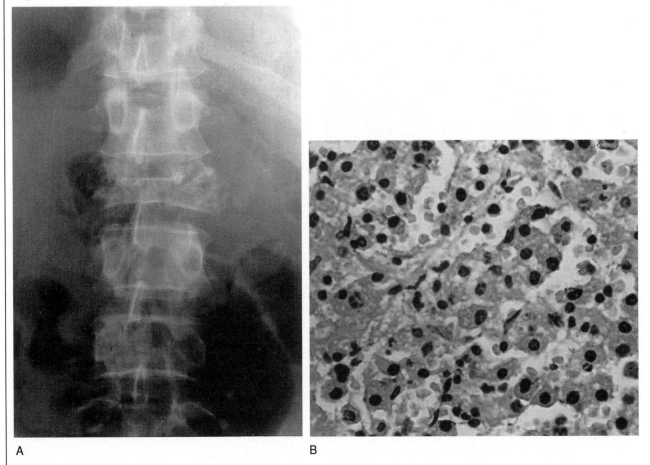

A        B

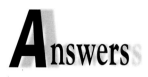
# Answers

241. Tumors are first characterized as being either primary lesions of bone or soft tissue, or metastatic. Primary tumors are then classified based upon their presumed cell of origin or differentiation and their malignant potential.

242. Metastatic lesions are far more common than primary tumors.

243. Overall, myeloma is the most common, with osteosarcoma being the second most common primary bone malignancy.

244. As a group, the benign cartilage lesions are the most common with osteochondromas making up a majority of the lesions.

245. Like many bony tumors, they tend to be metaphyseal in origin and generally occur at sites of most rapid skeletal growth. Approximately one half of all lesions will occur around the knee with the distal femur by far being the most common site. Other relatively common sites include the proximal femur, proximal humerus, and para-acetabular areas of the ilium. The lesions are particularly rare distal to the wrist and ankle.

246. Conventional radiographs reveal distinguishing features of benign and malignant lesions. In a benign process, the host bone responds by developing a rim of reactive bone around the neoplasm. This development results in a sharp margin between the lesion and the surrounding bone. Malignant lesions, however, have a broad zone of transition and cause permeative destruction of bone with little or no host bone response. Periosteal new bone, when solid and dense, suggests a benign lesion. An expansile appearance with elevated periosteal new bone, as in a Codman's triangle, is suggestive of a more aggressive or malignant lesion.

247. Breast, followed by lung, thyroid gland, and kidney.

248. Prostate, followed by lung, thyroid gland, and kidney.

249. The spine, followed by the ribs, pelvis, proximal ends of long bones, sternum, and skull.

250. Multiple myeloma. This is the most common primary malignant lesion of the skeletal system. As a solitary lesion, it is known as a plasmacytoma. Radiographs show radiolucent, punched out lesions with no surrounding bony reaction. Occasionally the lesions show a more diffuse permeative pattern of bone loss. The plasma cell is the proliferating cell in myeloma. Multiple myeloma has a peak incidence in the sixth and seventh decades of life and is rare before the fifth decade.

**251.** A 21-year-old man presents with a 2-month history of left thigh pain and a mass. His radiograph is shown (Figure 1-9, A). The histopathology is also shown (Figure 1-9, B). What is your diagnosis?

**Figure** 1-9

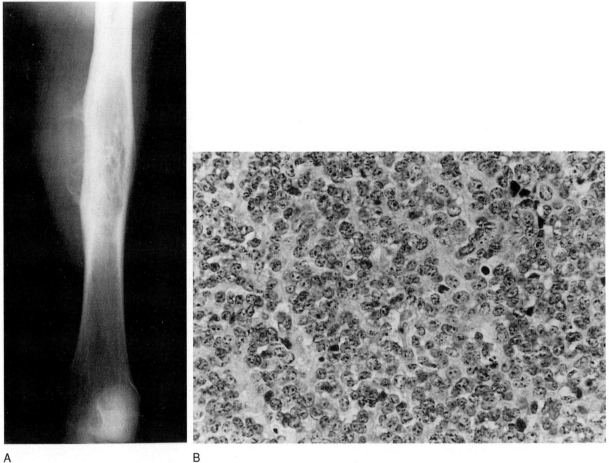

A              B

**252.** How is this lesion treated?

**253.** What is the overall 5-year survival rate for these patients?

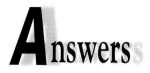
# Answers

**251.** Ewing's sarcoma. Radiographically, the lesion has a permeative pattern with cortical disruption. Ninety percent of these lesions occur prior to 21 years of age. The tumor usually originates in the medullary cavity of the bone in the metaphyseal and diaphyseal regions of long bones. Many of the lesions arise in the pelvis and escape early detection. Histologically there are homogenous populations of densely packed cells. The origin of these cells is unknown but it is thought to be the pluripotent mesenchymal stem cell. Most cells stain positive for glycogen on periodic acid Schiff (PAS) tests.

**252.** Ewing's sarcoma is generally considered a radiosensitive tumor and often requires the combination of surgery, chemotherapy, and radiotherapy. The traditional approach to treatment has consisted of radiation for the primary lesion and chemotherapy as systemic treatment. The addition of surgical excision (with a wide surgical margin) of the primary lesion leads to improved local control and improved survival.

**253.** The current overall survival prognosis for patients with Ewing's sarcoma is 50%. In favorable sites where surgical resection is possible, the 5-year survival rate is 60% to 80%. In unfavorable sites, the rate is 20% to 30%.

254. The patient is a 50-year-old woman who has had a painful mass in her right shoulder for the last 8 months (see Figure 1-10, A and B). What is your diagnosis?

**Figure** 1-10    A

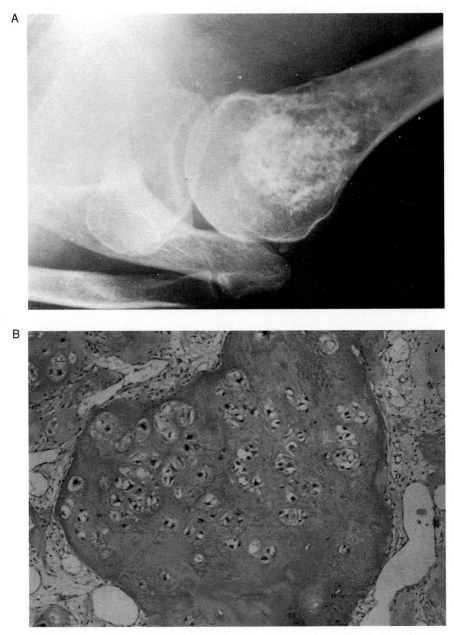

B

255. How do chondrosarcomas differ from osteosarcomas in terms of their age distribution and localization?

256. What is the recommended treatment for this lesion?

257. Does chemotherapy or radiation contribute to the treatment of chondrosarcoma?

258. What is the survival rate for chondrosarcomas?

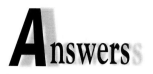

# Answers

254. Chondrosarcoma. The punctate, mottled densities attributable to calcification of a chondroid matrix are a characteristic finding. This pattern of mineralization with endosteal erosion, cortical thickening, and expansion suggests malignancy.

255. Chondrosarcomas are tumors of adulthood and advanced age with a peak distribution in the fifth and sixth decades. Osteosarcoma has a peak distribution in the second decade. Most osteosarcomas occur around the knee, whereas chondrosarcomas frequently occur in the proximal limb girdles, including the pelvis and proximal femur. Chondrosarcomas also occur around the shoulder, both in the proximal humerus and the scapula.

256. Complete surgical removal with a wide surgical margin. This can be done either through amputation or limb-sparing resection.

257. No. Chondrosarcomas are relatively chemo-resistant and radio-resistant.

258. This is dependent on the grade of the lesion. With high-grade lesions, the overall survival rate may be as low as 40%. This may be attributable, in part, to the ineffectiveness of current chemotherapy. For lower-grade lesions, the survival rate may be closer to 80%. The dedifferentiated chondrosarcoma carries a very poor prognosis with a 5-year survival rate of less than 20%. Another variant with a poor prognosis is mesenchymal chondrosarcoma.

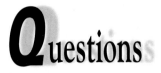

**259.** The patient is a 45-year-old man with massive swelling in his left shoulder, minimal pain, and multiple sores over both hands. From the radiograph (see Figure 1-11), what is your diagnosis?

**Figure** 1-11

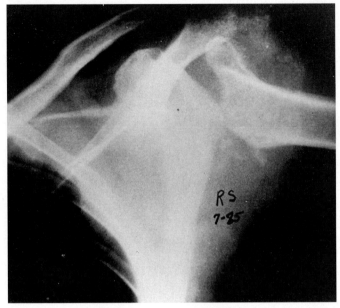

**260.** What disease entities can give rise to a Charcot joint?

**261.** What would be the most appropriate treatment for this patient?

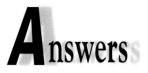

**259.** Neuropathic (Charcot) joint. The gross destruction of the glenohumeral joint with bone fragmentation in a patient with minimal pain suggests a Charcot joint arthropathy. The multiple sores on both hands suggest a loss of sensation. This patient was found to have cervical syringomyelia.

**260.** Charcot arthropathy is due to loss of joint sensation. Alcoholism, congenital indifference to pain, diabetes, syphilis, myelomeningocele, syringomyelia, and leprosy can all give rise to neuropathic arthropathy. In the upper extremity, syringomyelia is the most common cause of a neuropathic joint.

**261.** Nonoperative care of the joint would be the treatment of choice. Joint arthroplasty is contraindicated in Charcot joint arthropathy.

# Chapter 2

# Pediatric Orthopedics

KEITH GABRIEL, MD

TIMOTHY S. LOTH, MD

STEVEN MARDJETKO, MD

# Questions

1. Describe the diagnostic anatomical feature of congenital vertical talus (CVT).

2. What is the expected age range for Legg-Calve-Perthes disease (LCP)?

3. What is the expected sex ratio for LCP?

4. How often is LCP bilateral?

5. In cases of bilateral symmetrical LCP, what other radiographs should be obtained?

6. What other entities might present initially as bilateral LCP?

7. What constitutes the classic presentation of LCP?

8. What are the four stages of LCP?

9. Describe four radiographic findings that may be seen during the initial stage of LCP.

10. What is the "crescent sign"?

11. Describe Salter's proposed sequence in the development of clinical LCP.

12. How long does it usually take for a patient to progress through the LCP sequence?

13. How long does it take for a hip to progress from clinical presentation to the fragmentation stage?

14. What is the most important single factor determining outcome in LCP?

15. What is the first treatment goal for the newly diagnosed LCP patient?

16. How may hip motion be reestablished?

17. Once motion is regained, what is the usual treatment concept?

18. Suggest nonsurgical methods of containment in LCP.

19. When should nonsurgical containment devices be discontinued?

20. Suggest surgical methods for containment in LCP.

21. What radiographic criteria are useful to predict long-term prognosis in healed LCP?

22. Describe a system for predicting long-term function that considers the relative contours of both the femoral head and acetabulum after healing of LCP.

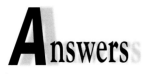

# Answers

1. Dorsal dislocation of the tarsal navicular with respect to the head of the talus.

2. Ages 2 to 12 years, although most cases occur between 4 and 8 years.

3. Male : female, about 4 : 1.

4. In 10% to 12% of cases.

5. Other epiphyseal areas should be evaluated. Radiographs of the wrists, knees, lateral skull, and lateral spine are helpful.

6. Multiple epiphyseal dysplasia; spondyloepiphyseal dysplasia; endocrine disorders such as hypothyroidism; and various problems, such as sickle cell, that cause avascular necrosis.

7. A painless limp (externally rotated) in a 4- to 8-year-old boy. Unexplained anterior knee pain is another very typical presentation.

8. (1) Initial (avascular); (2) fragmentation; (3) reossification (regrowth, regeneration); and (4) healed (residual).

9. (1) Ossific nucleus fails to grow and therefore looks smaller; (2) the surrounding bone may become osteopenic, and therefore the ossific nucleus looks more dense; (3) cartilage of the femoral head continues to grow, and therefore the medial joint space looks widened; and (4) a "crescent sign" (Caffey's sign) may be seen.

10. A radiolucent line in the superior lateral periphery of the ossific nucleus. It represents a stress fracture or compression fracture in the subchondral bone.

11. One or more vascular insults occur, causing an avascular necrosis of the ossific nucleus. Without additional trauma, this remains subclinical. Superimposed trauma or repetitive microtrauma creates a stress or compression fracture of the avascular subchondral bone, which we see as the "crescent sign." The repair processes thus set in motion constitute clinical LCP.

12. This varies widely, but 18 to 24 months is a useful estimate.

13. This varies widely, but 6 to 8 months is a useful estimate.

14. Patient age. Eight years seems to be a watershed, with a much poorer prognosis for older children irrespective of the extent of head involvement.

15. Reestablish a normal range of hip motion.

16. Traction with physical therapy or serial broomstick (Petrie) casts. Occasionally surgical release of the adductor longus muscle is needed.

17. Containment of the involved portion of the femoral head within the acetabulum by nonsurgical or surgical means.

18. Petrie casts; orthoses such as the Newington brace or the Scottish rite brace.

19. When the lateral column of the femoral head reossifies.

20. Varus osteotomy of the proximal femur or innominate (Salter) osteotomy of the pelvis.

21. Sphericity of the femoral head and congruency of the head within the acetabulum.

22. Spherical congruence—no arthritis develops; aspherical congruence—mild to moderate arthritis develops late in life; aspherical incongruence—severe arthritis before age 50 (Stuhlberg, Cooperman, Wallensten, 1981).

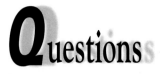

23. List some of the recognized orthopedic disorders associated with neurofibromatosis (NF).

24. Describe the findings at the hindfoot in the physical examination of clubfoot.

25. Describe the findings at the midfoot in the physical examination of clubfoot.

26. Describe the findings at the forefoot in the physical examination of clubfoot.

27. What is the deformity of the talus in clubfoot?

28. Describe the tibiotalar (ankle) joint in clubfoot.

29. Describe the subtalar joint in clubfoot.

30. What displacement occurs at the talonavicular joint in clubfoot?

31. What deformity may be seen at the calcaneocuboid joint in clubfoot?

32. What is the relative relationship of the medial and lateral columns of the clubfoot?

33. Briefly list several of the theories proposed to explain the etiology of clubfoot.

34. What are common findings on the lateral radiograph in clubfoot?

35. What are common findings on the AP radiograph in clubfoot?

36. Discuss the initial management of clubfoot.

37. What may forcible dorsiflexion during the conservative treatment of clubfoot create?

38. What is the "nutcracker mechanism"?

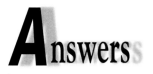

23. Scoliosis, pseudarthrosis of the tibia, pseudarthrosis of other long bones (e.g., radius, ulna, fibula), disorders of bone growth (e.g., gigantism), erosive defects from contiguous tumors, multiple fibrous cortical defects, and subperiosteal calcifying hematoma.

24. The hindfoot is positioned in equinus and varus. This causes the heel to appear foreshortened, and often what appears to be the heel is only the fat pad. The tuberosity of the calcaneus is actually more proximal, directly behind the ankle joint. The heel has been described as "keel-shaped."

25. There is no palpable gap between the medial malleolus and tarsal navicular. The head of the talus presents as a prominence on the dorsolateral midfoot.

26. The forefoot is in adduction. Even considering the hindfoot varus deformity, the forefoot is in additional supination. This brings the medial aspect of the first ray into close approximation to the distal medial tibia.

27. The neck of the talus is foreshortened and thickened. The head and neck are deviated medially and plantarward compared to the normal declination. Many believe that this is the primary deformity in clubfoot.

28. Abnormal equinus causes the dome of the talus to extrude anteriorly, i.e., the entire talus is displaced forward in the mortise. There is unresolved controversy as to whether the talus might also rotate medially or laterally in a horizontal plane within the mortise.

29. Displacements occur in three planes. Horizontal rotation brings the anterior process of the calcaneus beneath the head and neck of the talus while simultaneously moving the tuberosity laterally toward the fibular malleolus. The calcaneus is also in varus and equinus with respect to the talus.

30. The navicular is displaced medially onto the neck of the talus. The navicular may actually abut the inferior tip of the medial malleolus, forming an abnormal articular facet.

31. The cuboid is displaced medially and slightly proximally. The articular surface of the anterior calcaneus becomes slanted (angulated) medially.

32. Medial side shorter, the lateral side longer.

33. Germ plasm defect, arrested fetal development, intrauterine positioning, myofibroblast contraction at the medial foot, neuromuscular defect, and circulatory defect, among others.

34. "Parallelism" of the calcaneus and talus is key. This is recognized as a decrease in the lateral talocalcaneal angle (normal 30° to 50°), which does not increase on the maximum dorsiflexion lateral view. Talus and calcaneus are together in equinus.

35. Parallelism of the talus and calcaneus is recognized by a decreased AP talocalcaneal (Kite's) angle (normal 20° to 40°). A line projected along the lateral border of the calcaneus is not continuous with the cuboid due to medial displacement. Forefoot adductus is recognized by an increase in the talus-first metatarsal angle (normal 0° to 20°, with a positive value indicating forefoot adductus).

36. Repeated manipulations and the use of some type of holding device. Casts are the most common holding device, although taping and bracing may be effective.

37. An iatrogenic "rocker-bottom foot" or the "flat-topped talus."

38. The talus is anteriorly displaced in the ankle mortise, and normal tibiotalar motion is prevented by the contracted capsule and ligaments. With forcible dorsiflexion during manipulation, the talus is compressed between the calcaneus and tibia.

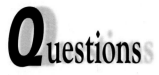

# Questions

39. Suggest important concerns prior to initiating treatment of a cavus foot.

40. Suggest a theory of the pathogenesis of cavus foot.

41. Describe pes cavovarus.

42. Describe a test for determination of the flexibility of the hindfoot in pes cavovarus.

43. What is the most common skeletal deformity seen in myelomeningocele?

44. Suggest a role for orthotic management in (paralytic or developmental) myelomeningocele scoliosis.

45. Suggest problems that may be anticipated with spinal orthosis wear.

46. Suggest realistic goals for lower extremity management in thoracic-level myelomeningocele.

47. Suggest a reasonable orthopedic goal for management of the knee in myelomeningocele.

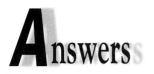 **nswers**

39. A cavus foot is almost always a manifestation of neurologic disease. A comprehensive history and physical examination are needed. Radiographs of the spine are basic, and other imaging studies may be indicated. Consultation with a neurologist should be considered.

40. If the anterior tibialis muscle is relatively weak, or the peroneus longus muscle relatively strong, the first ray becomes plantar flexed. The long toe extensor muscles are simultaneously used to substitute for the anterior tibialis muscle, causing clawing of the toes and secondary depression of the distal metatarsals. This is called the "windlass" mechanism. Alternatively, primary paralysis of the intrinsic muscles prevents proper extension of the interphalangeal joints. Again, the clawing of the toes causes secondary depression of the metatarsal heads.

41. The first ray (and sometimes the second) is more plantar flexed than the lateral rays. This relative pronation of the forefoot causes the entire foot to be inverted, with heel varus and elevation of the medial arch.

42. The Coleman block test is performed by placing a block under the affected heel and lateral two rays. The medial rays of the forefoot are allowed to droop toward the floor. The hindfoot position is then assessed visually from behind, or by means of special radiographs (see Figure 2-1).

 **Figure** 2-1

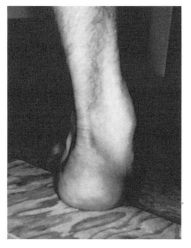

43. Scoliosis (in over 50% of patients) related to neurologic levels. The prognosis is worsened by the presence of congenital spinal deformity.

44. Bracing is not definitive management. It may be used as a temporary measure to permit additional growth or when other medical or social concerns are predominant. A congenital deformity cannot be braced.

45. Insensate skin may break down; growing ribs may deform and further decrease chest capacity; and abdominal pressure may interfere with breathing and eating.

46. Prevention of fixed contractures is paramount to facilitate sitting and use of braces. In the absence of muscle function, this can usually be accomplished by physical therapy, positioning, and orthoses.

47. Prevent fixed contractures. Tendon lengthenings are most often employed; tendon transfer is rarely indicated.

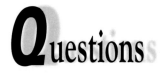

48. Suggest an orthopedic goal for the foot in myelomeningocele.

49. What clinical parameter helps in the decision between observation and active treatment of metatarsus varus?

50. Suggest nonoperative treatment for relatively rigid metatarsus varus in a prewalker.

51. Suggest a criticism of simply reversing shoes, or of the "swung-out" reverse lasted shoe when used to treat metatarsus adductus.

52. When teaching parents to perform stretching exercises for the child's metatarsus adductus, what cautions should be observed concerning heel position?

53. Suggest several clinical presentations of tarsal coalition.

54. Describe nonoperative treatment for tarsal coalition.

55. What are the major complications associated with treatment of slipped capital femoral epiphysis (SCFE)?

56. What are the treatment goals in SCFE?

57. What is the most common hip disorder in adolescents?

58. Is there a racial difference in the incidence of SCFE?

59. Is there a sex difference in the incidence of SCFE?

60. Describe the body habitus of the typical SCFE patient.

61. Describe the typical presentation of chronic SCFE.

62. How does Kline's line help in the diagnosis of SCFE?

# Answers

48. A plantigrade foot that can be braced. Only with a defect at the sacral level can patients be made brace-free.

49. The relative rigidity of the foot. If the foot cannot be easily overcorrected by gentle passive manipulation, some active treatment is indicated.

50. Most practitioners recommend serial manipulation and casting.

51. These may accentuate heel valgus, creating or exacerbating a skewfoot. Most practitioners do not think that shoes will correct the metatarsus adductus deformity.

52. The heel must be supported in neutral or slight varus. Allowing the heel to move into valgus may create or exacerbate a skewfoot.

53. Repetitive ankle sprains in an adolescent; peroneal spastic flatfoot; and activity-related pain in the subtalar or midtarsal area.

54. Oral nonsteroidal antiinflammatory drugs (NSAIDs); activity modification; and various arch supports, pads, and orthotics. In acute or severe cases, a short period (e.g., 3 weeks) of cast immobilization may be tried.

55. Chondrolysis and avascular necrosis.

56. Prevention of further slipping and avoidance of complications.

57. Slipped capital femoral epiphysis.

58. Yes, the condition is more common in African-Americans.

59. Yes, the condition is more common in males.

60. The obese, hypogonadal individual would be most typical. One theory suggests that these patients have a subclinical hormonal imbalance, such as relatively low sex hormones. Some patients, by contrast, are tall and thin. Perhaps they have relatively high levels of growth hormones. However, actual hormonal imbalance has not been confirmed in these "typical" patient types.

61. Variable pain in the groin, often radiating to the anteromedial thigh or knee. The affected limb may be shortened 1 to 2 cm. Abduction, internal rotation, and flexion are limited. There may be disuse atrophy of the thigh. The resulting limp is usually a combination of these factors, but the external rotation may be the most obvious change in the gait.

62. In both the AP and the lateral radiograph, a line projected along the superior margin of the femoral neck should intersect a portion of the femoral head. In SCFE, the line either misses the head entirely or intersects less of the head when compared with the unaffected side.

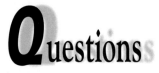

# Questions

63. Describe the Southwick method of measuring the femoral head-shaft angle.

64. Suggest appropriate steps to take immediately when SCFE is diagnosed.

65. What might be a method of nonoperative treatment?

66. Suggest criticisms of cast management of SCFE.

67. Describe usual surgical treatment options for SCFE.

68. What are possible criticisms of pin fixation of SCFE?

69. Suggest criticisms of open bone graft epiphysiodesis.

70. What advantages may there be to open bone graft epiphysiodesis?

71. Discuss the role of reduction in management of SCFE.

# Answers

**63.** On a lateral radiograph, a line is drawn connecting the corners of the femoral capital epiphysis, and a perpendicular to that line is constructed. A third line is projected parallel to the femoral shaft. The angle is measured between the perpendicular and the femoral shaft lines. The normal angle is 0° +/– 10° (see Figure 2-2).

**Figure** 2-2

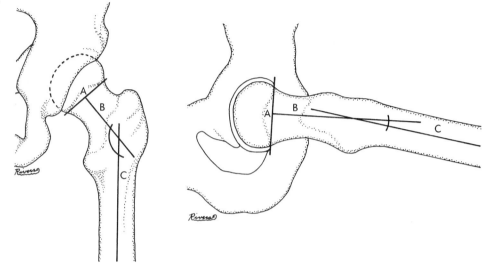

**64.** The patient must not be allowed to bear weight on the affected extremity. Definitive treatment should be begun urgently in order to prevent further displacement.

**65.** Spica cast immobilization for 12 weeks has been recommended by at least one practitioner (Steele). However, operative management is currently the standard of care in most areas.

**66.** Some series show an increased incidence of chondrolysis with casting. Additional displacement can occur if the cast is discontinued too soon.

**67.** These may consist of internal fixation with pins or open bone graft epiphysiodesis.

**68.** Unrecognized penetration of the pins into the joint has been associated with complications such as chondrolysis. "Nesting" of the tips of several pins may result in avascular necrosis (AVN). Entry holes in the lateral cortex can act as stress risers, especially if located distal to the level of the lesser trochanter. Physeal closure may not be rapid, and overgrowth off the pins can occur. Pin removal is a second operation.

**69.** The magnitude of the operation is greater than pinning, and the technique may be unfamiliar to many. Curettage of the physis may actually destabilize the slip further, risking additional displacement. Postoperative casting may be indicated, especially in acute cases.

**70.** Most series show extremely low rates of chondrolysis or AVN—much lower than most series of pinning. Physeal closure after an operation may be more rapid. There is no second operation for hardware removal.

**71.** Reduction of chronic slips is contraindicated because of high AVN rates. Reduction of acute slips is controversial for that same reason. Some slips present so acutely that they may more properly fit into a category of type I physeal fractures; reduction is probably indicated in this small subset.

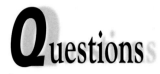

# Questions

72. Discuss the role of traction in reduction of the acute portion of an acute or chronic SCFE.

73. Suggest three categories of osteotomy that may be considered in dealing with displacement of the proximal femur in SCFE.

74. Why are proximal osteotomies (adjacent to the physis) not more popular?

75. What is the criticism of osteotomy at the base of the femoral neck?

76. Suggest a criticism of intertrochanteric or subtrochanteric osteotomy.

77. What happens to hip motion when SCFE is successfully stabilized in situ?

78. What happens to bony deformity when SCFE is successfully stabilized in situ?

79. How do weight training and weight lifting differ?

80. Discuss some effects of weight training on prepubescent children.

81. What about the safety of strength training for prepubescent children?

82. Discuss "Little Leaguer's shoulder."

83. Describe "Little Leaguer's elbow."

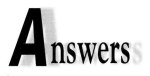
# Answers

72. Some series suggest that traction, including internal rotation, may effect a "gentle" reduction of the acute portion of the slip. Traction is also sometimes used to decrease symptoms of synovitis prior to surgical intervention.

73. Osteotomy may be performed in the proximal femoral neck adjacent to the physis, at the base of the femoral neck, or more distally in the intertrochanteric or subtrochanteric region.

74. Although osteotomy at this level (Dunn, Fish) more directly restores the anatomy, the AVN rates have been prohibitive in most series.

75. Once again, osteotomy at this level (Kramer) places the vascular supply of the femoral head at risk.

76. These compensatory operations (Southwick) improve the femoral head-to-acetabulum relationship by actually creating another deformity at the level of the trochanters. This may complicate later reconstructive surgery such as total hip arthroplasty.

77. Motion may never return to normal, but there is significant improvement and restoration of motion within the first 6 months.

78. There is a documented tendency toward improvement. The anterolateral "hump" of the femoral neck is resorbed as some reactive new bone is laid down at the inferomedial neck. Trochanteric overgrowth may increase, as may limb length discrepancy, depending on growth remaining.

79. The different terms are meant to distinguish the training technique from the competitive sport. Weight training implies that progressive resistance exercise techniques, whether with free weights or machines, are used in a controlled program designed to enhance one's strength, size, and power. Power lifting or Olympic weight lifting refers to competition, usually on the basis of single repetition for maximal load.

80. These children can increase strength, but this increase is thought to be due to recruitment and synchronization of muscle fibers. Actual hypertrophy of motor units does not occur, probably owing to the lack of circulating androgens in this age group.

81. Policy statements from the major concerned medical groups, such as the American Academy of Pediatrics, all stress the use of submaximal resistance in a controlled, supervised setting. In this type of setting, physeal fractures and stress fractures may occur, but are uncommon. The common injuries are muscle pulls and tendinitis. There does not seem to be any direct harm to the physeal plate from the controlled use of submaximal loads.

82. This typically presents as an insidious, progressive, and deep pain in the dominant shoulder of a Little League pitcher. Repetitive stress can cause an epiphysiolysis of the proximal humerus. The physical examination may be very nondescript, but the radiograph shows widening and irregularity of the proximal humeral physis. The treatment is rest, stretching to reestablish full range of motion (ROM), and strengthening to assure muscle balance. Attention must be directed to correcting the mechanics of pitching. If recognized and treated, there are no known sequelae.

83. Elbow problems in Little League pitchers are almost always repetitive stress injuries due to valgus forces. This particular condition is due to tension stress at the medial epicondylar apophysis. The symptom is pain at the medial side of the elbow. The physical findings are local swelling, sometimes with ulnar nerve dysfunction. Radiographically, the epicondyle may be enlarged, sclerotic, or even fragmented, with widening of the physeal plate.

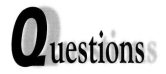

# Questions

84. What is "swimmer's shoulder"?

85. A 12-year-old female gymnast complains of pain at the distal radius. What might be seen on a radiograph?

86. Suggest the repetitive stress mechanism that causes popliteus tendinitis.

87. How does femoral version differ from femoral torsion?

88. What is the mean femoral anteversion at birth and at skeletal maturation?

89. What is the normal tibial lateral rotation noted at birth and at maturity?

90. What physiologic contractures are noted in the newborn?

91. True or False? In the management of lower extremity rotational deformities, all of the following treatment methods have been proven effective: (1) twister cables; (2) shoe modifications; and (3) Dennis-Browne bar.

92. What is the most common cause for intoeing in the second year of life?

93. What is the most common cause for intoeing after the age of 3 years?

94. True or False? The natural history of flexible pes planus is favorably altered by the use of arch supports and UCB heel cups.

95. Describe the presently accepted thinking on the etiology of Blount's disease.

96. Lateral patellar dislocation is associated with what lower extremity deformities?

97. Recurrent patellar subluxation in adolescents frequently has a number of predisposing factors. List them.

98. The "miserable malalignment syndrome" is a common cause of persisting lateral patellar subluxation. Describe the rotational profile of these children.

99. Describe the pathologic changes associated with osteochondritis dissecans in the adolescent.

100. Describe the most common location of osteochondritis dissecans in the knee.

101. Which radiographic view most often identifies osteochondritis dissecans?

102. What is the best management for nondisplaced osteochondritis dissecans of the medial femoral condyle identified in a skeletally immature male?

103. What is the appropriate management of loose fragments of osteochondritis dissecans in the skeletally mature adolescent?

104. Describe the pathologic changes in Osgood-Schlatter disease.

105. At what age is Osgood-Schlatter disease most common?

106. What is the natural history of Osgood-Schlatter disease?

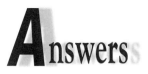
# Answers

84. This repetitive stress injury is an impingement syndrome of the shoulder, which occurs in many overhead sports, most typically freestyle swimming.

85. The repetitive stress syndrome that occurs in this situation is an epiphysiolysis at the distal radius. The physeal plate may be widened and irregular with lucent defects in the adjacent metaphysis. The process responds to rest.

86. This is caused by excessive internal rotation of the tibia during running or similar activity. Excessive pronation of the forefoot, running on banked surfaces, and running on hills have all been implicated.

87. Version describes rotation within normal ranges. Torsion describes abnormal rotation deviating from the mean by 2 standard deviations or more.

88. At birth, femoral anteversion averages 40° and decreases to 15° at skeletal maturation.

89. Lateral rotation at birth is approximately 5° and at maturity averages 15°.

90. Mild hip flexion and lateral rotation contractures maintain the infant's lower extremities in a position of lateral rotation throughout the first year of life.

91. False.

92. Medial tibial torsion.

93. Femoral anteversion.

94. False. The natural history of treated and untreated children is identical.

95. Blount's disease is thought to be an osteochondrosis secondary to excessive mechanical stress, which converts a physiologic bowing into tibia vara in a susceptible individual.

96. External tibial rotation, genu valgum, and knee flexion contracture.

97. Generalized joint laxity, genu valgum, increased Q-angle, patella alta, incongruence of the patellofemoral joint, hypoplasia of the vastus medialis muscle, lateral retinacular contracture, and lateral condylar hypoplasia.

98. Femoral antetorsion with external tibial torsion.

99. Periarticular osseous necrosis with overlying cartilage softening, occasionally associated with fragment displacement.

100. The lateral aspect of the medial femoral condyle.

101. Tunnel view of the knee.

102. Activity modification and a short period of immobilization supplemented with isometric strengthening exercises of the knee.

103. If the fragment is less than 5 mm, simple excision. If the fragment is larger, placement into the recipient bed and internal fixation is suggested.

104. Apophysitis secondary to repetitive microtrauma results in inflammation and new bone formation at the tendon–bone junction.

105. In boys, age 13 to 14 years. In girls, age 10 to 11 years.

106. In the majority of cases, complete resolution in 1 to 2 years of onset.

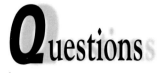

# Questions

**107.** In the presentation of Osgood-Schlatter disease, what study is mandatory to rule out other possible pathologies such as tumors?

**108.** Which of the following treatment modalities are contra-indicated in Osgood-Schlatter disease? (1) Rest and immobilization; (2) isometric knee exercises; (3) knee pads; or (4) steroid injections.

**109.** Sinding-Larsen-Johansson syndrome, also known as "juvenile jumper's knee," is associated with what pathology?

**110.** Describe the most common etiology and location of Baker's cyst in childhood.

**111.** Describe the natural history of Baker's cyst in childhood.

**112.** What is the most common cause for the discrepancy between apparent leg length as measured from the umbilicus to the medial malleolus and true leg length as measured from the anterior superior iliac spine to the medial malleolus?

**113.** Which electrodiagnostic study can be used to differentiate a myopathic from a neuropathic process?

**114.** Which hereditary muscle disorder is characterized by difficulty in postcontraction relaxation and has a characteristic EMG finding suggestive of rapid repetitive discharges?

**115.** True or False? Nerve conduction velocities will remain normal in patients with anterior horn cell disease, spinal nerve root injury, and myopathy.

**116.** True or False? Type IIB muscle fibers are characterized by fast-twitch potential, high glycolytic and adenosine triphosphatase (ATPase) activity, and low oxidative metabolism activity.

**117.** What is the normal ratio of type I to type II muscle fibers in skeletal muscle?

**118.** Describe the typical histologic changes of muscle tissue in myopathy.

**119.** What is the key factor in deterioration of gait in a child with Duchenne's muscular dystrophy?

**120.** What is the clinical significance of Maryon's sign?

**121.** True or False? Calf muscle enlargement of Duchenne's muscular dystrophy occurs in an attempt to compensate for weak proximal musculature.

**122.** The development of scoliosis occurs in nearly all children with muscular dystrophy. Rapid progression is frequently noted once the child becomes confined to a wheelchair, usually between ages 10 and 12. These curves do not respond to bracing. Should surgery be considered, which technique provides the most consistent results?

**123.** What is the most likely diagnosis in a child who develops a pattern of muscular weakness similar to Duchenne's muscular dystrophy, but whose symptoms started after the age of 8 years and who continues to ambulate beyond the age of 20 years?

**124.** A 4-day-old infant has left hip dysplasia characterized by positive Ortolani and positive Barlow signs. The right hip appears stable. A Pavlik harness is chosen as a means of obtaining initial reduction. Describe the accepted optimal hip position to achieve reduction.

**125.** This infant has now been treated with the harness for 4 weeks but the left hip remains unstable upon examination with positive Ortolani and positive Barlow signs. What should the next course of action be?

# Answers

107. AP and lateral radiograph of the knee.

108. Steroid injections, because they can induce weakening of the patellar tendon and subcutaneous fat necrosis.

109. Traction apophysitis of the distal pole of the patella secondary to repetitive stress.

110. Synovial popliteal cysts that arise between the semimembranosus and gastrocnemius tendons. They are most often idiopathic in origin.

111. Spontaneous resolution within 2 to 5 years.

112. Pelvic obliquity (which may be secondary to suprapelvic or intrapelvic causes).

113. Electromyogram (EMG). Neuropathic changes are seen as fibrillation potentials, which are characterized by prolonged polyphasic high-voltage action potentials. Myopathic disorders show low-voltage polyphasic action potentials.

114. Myotonia dystrophica.

115. True. Nerve conduction velocities should not be affected by spinal cord, nerve root, or muscle disorders.

116. True. Type I fibers are characterized by slow-twitch, high oxidative capacity and low ATPase level. Type IIA fibers appear to have characteristics intermediate between types I and IIB.

117. 1:2.

118. Type I fiber predominance, muscle cell phagocytosis, low-grade inflammatory reaction, and replacement fibrosis.

119. Development of quadriceps weakness with loss of muscle power below 3/5.

120. This sign, which represents a tendency for a child to slip through the examiner's arms with both arms going into full abduction, suggests shoulder girdle weakness.

121. False. Calf pseudohypertrophy is associated with progressive clinical weakness of the ankle plantar flexors and development of heel cord contracture.

122. In general, children with curves over 40° are best managed by stabilization using Luque rods and sublaminar wires and the Galveston technique. The goal should be to operate on these children while their curve is flexible and their forced vital capacity remains over 30%.

123. Becker's muscular dystrophy.

124. 90° to 100° of flexion achieved by tightening the anterior straps, 45° to 50° of hip abduction maintained by placement of the anterior straps along the anterior axillary line. The posterior straps serve as tethers to prevent adduction beyond 20°. Rotation of the limbs should be essentially neutral and the anterior straps should pass across the axis of the knee.

125. Abandon Pavlik harness treatment and proceed with alternatives such as spica cast application.

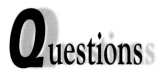

126. Following a 2-month period of hip spica casting, the left hip stabilizes. The spica cast is removed and an abduction splint is used at night and nap times. At 1 year of age, concentric reduction with an acetabular index equal to the uninvolved side is noted. Physical examination is perfectly normal. At this point, what do you recommend?

127. A 10-year-old girl is brought to your office with complaints of increasingly high arches. Her parents state that she seems to be walking on the outside edges of her feet. What might be included in your initial differential diagnosis?

128. What specific information would you seek in the family history?

129. What skin findings will you seek when performing the spinal examination?

130. The family of the patient in question 127 reports that she has had an increasingly clumsy, "staggering" gait over the past year. Your lower extremity examination finds diminished deep tendon reflexes and bilateral up-going Babinski responses. You should be especially aware of what spinal condition in this patient?

131. Your diagnostic suspicions from question 130 are confirmed. A radiograph shows the patient to have a 20° right dorsal curve. What are your thoughts regarding management of the scoliosis?

132. A family has recently immigrated from Southeast Asia. Their 10-year-old child has unilateral atrophy of the calf musculature and a cavus foot. The foot is remarkable in that the heel is in extreme calcaneus: it almost looks to you like a pistol grip. The patient's foot was previously normal, and the deformity developed after a severe febrile illness. What is your diagnosis?

133. You are asked to see an infant in the nursery who has a foot deformity. The dorsum of the foot is lying nearly against the anterolateral distal tibia, yet the heel seems to be rigidly in an equinus posture (see Figure 2-3). What do you suspect?

**Figure** 2-3

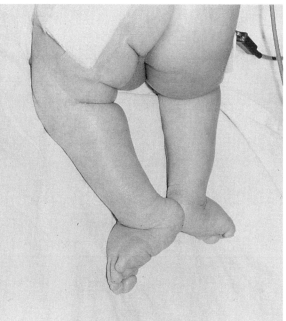

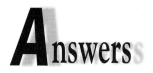

**126.** Continued follow-up through maturity. Approximately 20% of treated children with apparently stabilized, normal hips at 1 or 2 years of age develop late and significant acetabular dysplasia.

**127.** This may be a developing cavus, or cavovarus, foot. Think of a possible neurologic etiology: neuropathy, such as Charcot-Marie-Tooth disease; spinal cerebellar degeneration such as Friedreich's ataxia; or structural spine problems such as diastematomyelia.

**128.** Many of the peripheral neuropathies are inherited. You need to know whether there have been other family members with such neurologic disorders. You also need to know whether other family members have similar foot deformities (i.e., a cavus foot) or suggestive hand deformities, such as wasting of the intrinsic muscles.

**129.** A hairy patch or skin dimple over the spine or hyperpigmented midline nevus. These may be associated with occult spinal dysraphism.

**130.** The description suggests Friedreich's ataxia. Most of these patients develop scoliosis.

**131.** Bracing is poorly tolerated and not effective for the control of scoliosis in Friedreich's ataxia. If this curve progresses, surgery may be necessary. Eagerness to treat must be tempered by the reality that Friedreich's ataxia is a progressive neurologic disorder with death usually occurring before age 40 years.

**132.** Polio. Worldwide, polio is the most common cause of a calcaneocavus foot deformity.

**133.** Congenital vertical talus (CVT), also known as rocker bottom foot, Persian slipper foot, or congenital convex pes valgus.

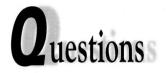

**134.** As you continue your examination, you carefully but persistently massage and manipulate the foot. Will you be able to reduce the position to neutral?

**135.** The nursery staff have already obtained a "clubfoot series." Are these radiographs helpful?

**136.** What do you plan to tell the parents about the success of nonsurgical treatment?

**137.** An infant in the nursery has a foot deformity in which the dorsum of the foot is lying nearly against the anterolateral distal tibia, and the heel is quite prominently in calcaneus posture. What do you suspect?

**138.** Will you be able to reduce this foot deformity to the neutral position by gentle manipulation as you perform the physical examination?

**139.** An infant in the nursery has a unilateral foot deformity with the heel in equinus and varus and the midfoot in adductus. The foot is not supple. What is the initial treatment?

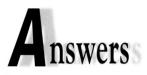

# Answers

134. Probably not. CVT is almost always rigid. In fact, if you can reduce the foot to a true neutral position, you are probably not dealing with CVT.

135. Minimally. A clubfoot is usually evaluated with a maximum dorsiflexion lateral radiograph. For CVT, a maximum plantar flexion lateral view is preferred (see Figure 2-4). In CVT, a line projected through the talus will extend plantarward of the navicular, even with the foot held in maximum plantar flexion. Because the navicular is not ossified in the newborn, the line projected through the talus may be referenced to the cuboid; in CVT this line will be plantarward.

**Figure** 2-4

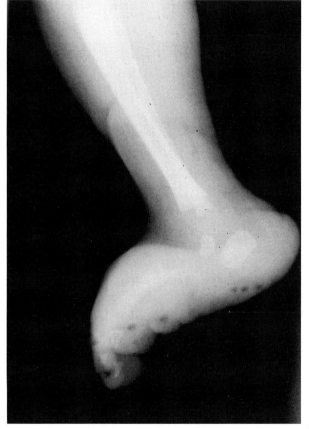

136. Passive stretching and sequential casting may help stretch soft tissues, but this is almost never sufficient treatment. A true CVT will virtually always require surgical correction.

137. Calcaneovalgus foot deformity. The key is that the heel is in calcaneus, actually aligned with the forefoot. The entire foot has dorsiflexed through the ankle. There is no midfoot breach as would be seen with a CVT.

138. At least to neutral, although perhaps not into plantar flexion at the ankle. The ability to correct the hindfoot to neutral is an important discriminator when assessing the severity of a foot deformity.

139. This description sounds as though the child has a clubfoot (talipes equinovarus). Initial management should begin as soon as possible, and should include sequential passive manipulation and application of a holding device. Taping or casting are the usual holding devices, although some braces have been described.

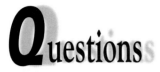

**140.** Can you speculate about the sex of the child and the side of the deformity in question 139?

**141.** A family is interested in overseas adoption. A photograph shows a child with apparent unilateral quadriceps muscle atrophy and a mild ipsilateral hip flexion contracture. Medical records have not yet been translated. The agency spokesperson says that the child was ill approximately 2 years ago and now walks by pushing the involved knee with the hand. What do you suspect?

**142.** As an adult, what systemic symptoms might this patient develop?

**143.** A 12-year-old girl is referred because of repeated ankle sprains. The referring physician has already obtained routine ankle radiographs and stress films of the ankle, all of which are normal for this age. What do you suspect?

**144.** You evaluate a 6-year-old boy with a painless limp, which has been noticed by the parents for the last 3 months. You characterize the limp as a gluteus medius lurch. Which condition is first in your differential diagnosis?

**145.** An obese 12-year-old girl is brought to your office because her mother has noticed that the patient has been walking with a limp for the past 3 months. You observe a gluteus medius lurch and an outward foot progression angle on the affected side. What do you suspect?

**146.** An obese 14-year-old boy presents with unilateral "knee pain." You check ROM of the knees and hips and suspect SCFE. What findings lead you to that diagnosis?

**147.** The father of the patient in question 146 is a mechanic. He asks you why SCFE should cause a change in hip ROM.

**148.** A 3-year-old girl is sent for evaluation of a painless limp. Her mother says the patient has "always walked that way," and cannot understand why her new pediatrician insisted on referral. On the girl's left, you notice the combination of a gluteus medius lurch with short leg "bobbing." Which condition is first in your differential diagnosis?

**149.** An 11-year-old boy falls from his bicycle, sustaining a knee injury with immediate effusion. The anterior drawer test is positive. What do you suspect?

**150.** A 9-year-old boy sustains a twisting injury to the knee. He describes repeated buckling, which is associated with brief sharp pain. Upon examination, you can reproduce the pain by extending the knee from a fully flexed position with the tibia internally rotated. A similar test, but with the tibia externally rotated, does not cause pain. What do you suspect?

# **A**nswers

140. Clubfoot is more common in boys and more common on the right.

141. Polio. Quadriceps weakness is a classic sequelae.

142. Postpolio syndrome with early fatigue, new weakness in either previously affected or unaffected muscles, new atrophy, cold intolerance, and muscle and joint pain.

143. Tarsal coalition. Repeated ankle sprains in an adolescent is a classic presentation.

144. This is a classic presentation for Legg-Calve-Perthes (LCP) disease.

145. Slipped capital femoral epiphysis (SCFE).

146. Knee examination will be unremarkable, with full ROM. The hip on the affected side will have decreased internal rotation and decreased flexion, compared to the unaffected hip. You should specifically see decreased internal rotation of the affected hip in flexion compared to extension; that is, there will often be an obligatory external rotation of the hip as you passively move it from extension toward flexion.

147. You explain that the capital femoral epiphysis has remained in the acetabulum, but that the femoral metaphysis (neck) has moved anteriorly and superiorly. As you attempt to flex the hip, the edge of the metaphysis impinges on the anterior lip of the acetabulum. By external rotation of the thigh, the impingement is relieved so that further flexion is possible.

148. Hip dysplasia. Despite various screening programs, late diagnosis of a congenitally or developmentally dislocated hip is still a problem.

149. This history is absolutely classic for tibial spine avulsion. This is the childhood equivalent of an anterior cruciate ligament rupture. No one knows why so many of these injuries happen with a fall from a bicycle.

150. This positive Wilson's test is suggestive of an osteochondritis dissecans lesion.

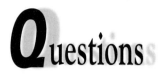

**151.** A 10-year-old soccer player sustains knee trauma with immediate effusion. Upon examination, you find an extensor lag; available active extension is weak. The radiograph is shown (see Figure 2-5). What is this injury?

**Figure** 2-5

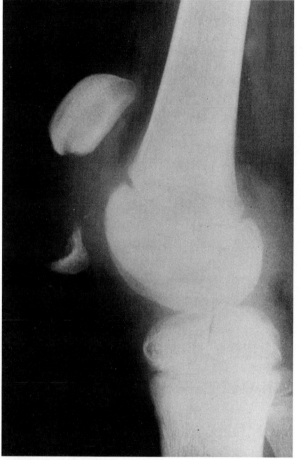

**152.** An 8-year-old sustains an inversion injury to the ankle. The patient complains of lateral foot pain. What do you suspect?

**153.** Suppose the patient from question 152 were complaining of lateral ankle pain?

**154.** A 4-year-old boy, first child for this family, is evaluated because of a new difficulty walking up stairs; his parents say that he "hangs on the bannister." His preschool teacher has reported that he is now the slowest runner in the class, but last year, he was usually in the middle of the group. What do you suspect?

**155.** As you interviewed this patient's parents, the boy was playing on the examination room floor. You ask him to "stand up" for examination. What do you watch for?

**156.** Your suspicions are increased as you complete the physical examination. The parents ask if there is a blood test you could order to diagnose the problem.

**157.** The blood test confirms your suspicions. The child's neurologist now requests a specimen of another tissue. What changes might you see on that sample?

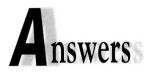

# Answers

**151.** A patellar "sleeve" fracture. The patellar ligament (tendon) avulses a sleeve of cartilage with a small rim of subchondral bone. During surgery, the amount of cartilage avulsed is often surprisingly large.

**152.** Avulsion of the base of the fifth metatarsal (MT) or an actual fracture of the fifth MT.

**153.** In this age group, a Salter I separation of the physis of the distal fibula would be more common than an "ankle sprain." The exact location of the tenderness should be your guide, even if the radiograph is unremarkable. Treatment should include immobilization with a cast. Because physeal injuries, especially if nondisplaced, heal rapidly, 3 weeks of immobilization with a short leg walking cast is usually sufficient.

**154.** Progressive neuromuscular disorders, such as muscular dystrophy or spinal muscular atrophy.

**155.** Gower's sign (or maneuver), indicating pelvic girdle muscle weakness. A positive Gower's sign is if the child cannot rise to the standing position without using his hands, but instead must use his upper extremities to push or "climb" his legs to stand.

**156.** Yes, major elevation of the creatine phosphokinase (CPK) level is very suggestive of a muscular dystrophy. Acutely, this enzyme may be elevated to 200 times laboratory normal.

**157.** A muscle biopsy is frequently requested. If the child has a primary muscle disorder, presumably muscular dystrophy, classic findings would include fiber size variation, fiber type disproportion, branching of fibers, necrosis of fibers or groups of fibers, phagocytosis, and replacement of muscle fibers by fat.

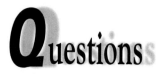

**158.** Four years pass. Despite physical therapy and bracing, the boy from question 154 has developed contractures at the ankle and hip that are interfering with walking. What should be done next?

**159.** The patient from question 154 has spinal muscular atrophy. At age 10, he uses a wheelchair as his primary means of ambulation. He has developed a long, sweeping scoliosis measuring 30°. What is the prognosis for this scoliotic curve?

**160.** You are called to the nursery to see an infant who is not spontaneously moving her right upper extremity. As you wait for the elevator, what do you think to include in a differential diagnosis?

**161.** The baby in question 160 has normal radiographs. As you observe her, you see that she does, in fact, move her fingers into flexion and extension. She does not abduct or externally rotate the shoulder and does not flex her elbow. What problem does she have?

**162.** You meet the parents of the infant in question 161. What should be your treatment recommendation at this point?

**163.** The parents of the infant in question 161 ask about the chances for recovery. What do you tell them?

**164.** Consider a situation as in question 160. However, as you examine the infant, you see that she seems perhaps a bit cross-eyed, her right pupil is small, and her right eyelid is lower than the left. What does this tell you about the prognosis?

**165.** A 6-year-old patient who has trisomy 21 presents for evaluation of neck pain. What studies are appropriate? Why?

**166.** The patient from question 165 has 7 mm of atlantoaxial motion documented on the flexion and extension radiographs. Is this normal?

**167.** A 4-year-old patient who has trisomy 21 comes to you with presenting symptoms that include an increasing limp, intermittent refusal to walk, and a frequent audible "pop" at the left groin. What do you suspect?

**168.** A 1-month-old girl has held her face turned toward the right since birth. There has been no trauma. She has not been systemically ill. You notice her facial asymmetry. In addition to limited motion (rotation), what do you expect to find as you examine her neck?

**169.** On which side is the affected muscle located?

**170.** You are called to the phone before you finish examining this child. The family leaves the office. Because of unfortunate social situations, the patient from question 168 is not evaluated again until age 3 years. She still holds her head with the face turned toward the right. What is the recommended treatment at this point?

**171.** As you evaluate the child from question 170, you find that she walks with a painless limp. The bench examination confirms asymmetry of the thighs and unilateral limitation of hip abduction. What do you suspect?

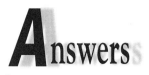

**158.** Patients having muscular dystrophy frequently develop ankle equinus contractures. Tendo Achilles lengthening is usually considered. Because of relative preservation of the tibialis posterior muscle, some practitioners have advocated rerouting that tendon through the interosseus membrane to the dorsum of the foot. At the hip, contracture of the tensor fasciae latae iliotibial band creates flexion and abduction. Percutaneous release of the origin of the tensor fasciae latae muscle, along with percutaneous section of the iliotibial (IT) band distally, can relieve the contracture. Percutaneous technique is preferable to formal open Ober and Yount procedures, because the patient must be rapidly mobilized—SAME DAY!—after surgery to prevent loss of strength.

**159.** Once the patient becomes confined to a wheelchair, progression of the scoliosis is essentially inevitable. The primary disease also causes a decline in respiratory function. Bracing may be used to delay surgery but is not effective as definitive management of the scoliosis. Spinal fusion should be considered relatively early, before the concomitant deterioration in pulmonary function poses an unacceptably high surgical risk.

**160.** Brachial plexus palsy and various birth fractures, such as those involving the clavicle or humerus.

**161.** Erb's palsy (upper brachial plexus palsy).

**162.** Passive exercises to maintain the ROM of all right upper extremity joints. Prolonged splinting in abduction and external rotation is not favored because of possible secondary shoulder dislocation.

**163.** The majority of brachial plexus palsies (approximately 80%) will resolve spontaneously. The majority of the recovery will take place in the first 3 to 6 months, although continued spontaneous improvement may be seen up to 18 months.

**164.** Horner's syndrome implies a very proximal (root level) nerve injury, with poor prognosis for spontaneous recovery. Phrenic nerve paralysis is similarly a poor prognostic sign.

**165.** It will be necessary to obtain cervical spine radiographs, specifically to include lateral views in maximum flexion and maximum extension. Between 15% and 20% of patients having Down's syndrome may have C1-C2 instability. Additionally, occipitoatlantal instability has been described in the Down's syndrome population.

**166.** No, normal motion should be 4 mm or less. Most practitioners would consider C1-C2 fusion if motion is 10 mm or more, even in asymptomatic patients. Between 5 and 9 mm seems to be a "gray area," and asymptomatic sedentary patients may be observed. Because the patient from question 165 has symptoms of neck pain, fusion should be offered at 7 mm of motion.

**167.** Spontaneous, or "habitual," subluxation of the hip. Some Down's syndrome patients (perhaps 4% or 5%) can truly dislocate the hip, presumably due to generalized ligamentous laxity.

**168.** A localized firm mass (the "olive") in the substance of the sternocleidomastoid muscle.

**169.** If the patient's face is turned toward the right, then the left sternocleidomastoid muscle is expected to be abnormal.

**170.** Surgical release or lengthening of the left sternocleidomastoid muscle. Nonoperative methods generally do not work in this age group.

**171.** A hip dislocation. About 20% of infants with congenital muscular torticollis will also have hip dysplasia.

172. A high school football player is evaluated for persistent anterior thigh pain several weeks after an especially violent tackle. His radiograph is shown (Figure 2-6). Should this lesion be biopsied?

**Figure** 2-6

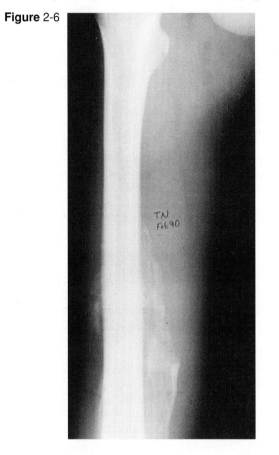

173. Three months later, the patient can still feel the mass in his thigh and occasionally complains of local pain. He requests excision. What do you advise?

174. How are closed fractures of the distal end of the clavicle treated in children?

175. At which cervical levels do most children's cervical spine injuries occur?

176. How is posttraumatic C1-2 instability treated in children?

177. What is the incidence of progressive spinal deformity in immature children (girls less than 12 years old, boys less than 14 years old) with paraplegia or quadriplegia?

178. When does spondylolysis occur in children?

179. What problems are encountered in pelvic fractures in children? What problems are associated with hip fractures in this age group?

180. Describe the treatment of a traumatic dislocation of the hip in a child.

181. Describe treatment of femoral shaft fractures in infants, 2- to 10-year-old children, 10- to 15-year-old children, and children older than 15 years.

182. What is the most common location for stress fractures in children?

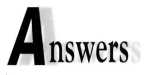
# Answers

172. This is a very typical history and typical radiograph for posttraumatic myositis ossificans. One typical finding is that the outer circumference of the mass is radiographically more mature than the center. A biopsy is not necessary and, in fact, might be mistaken for a malignancy.

173. Excision at this point might simply lead to a recurrence of the process. These lesions typically require nearly a year to mature sufficiently to permit successful excision. Activity seen on a technetium 99m bone scan is a good guide; the area of myositis should show no greater uptake than the adjacent normal bone.

174. Excellent results can be expected with closed treatment regardless of displacement. A figure-eight bandage, sling, or collar and cuff are applied. Anticipate remodeling up to the age of 16 years.

175. Most occur between the occiput and C3 or C4. This is the reverse of adult cervical spine injuries, most of which occur at C4 or below.

176. Extension reduction and surgical stabilization followed by 8 to 12 weeks in a halo or Minerva jacket.

177. 86% to 100%.

178. After walking age—most commonly by 7 to 8 years of age.

179. Pelvic fractures are associated with severe trauma with short-term risks to life and limb. In the long term, however, most do well. Hip fractures, on the other hand, are associated with many complications (nonunion, coxa vara, avascular necrosis) and necessitate early aggressive treatment.

180. Emergent closed reduction, then skin traction for 1 week followed by nonweight-bearing crutch ambulation for 3 weeks.

181. Infants are treated in an immediate spica cast. In children 2 to 10 years old, if on resting radiograph there is less than 2 cm shortening, then a spica cast is applied. If there is more than 2 cm shortening, treatment is split Russell traction. In children aged 10 to 15 years, treatment is 90/90 traction and a spica cast when sticky. Children 15 years or older are treated like adults (internal fixation or distal tibial traction followed by a femoral cast brace).

182. The tibia.

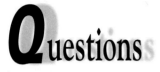

# Questions

183. How do you treat children with tibial stress fractures?

184. How should you treat ankle ligament tears in children?

185. Describe the treatment of very symptomatic Osgood-Schlatter disease.

186. What are some average healing times for closed and open displaced tibiofibular fractures in children?

187. Which fat pad can be normally seen in an elbow?

188. What is the mechanism of injury for most supracondylar fractures of the humerus in children?

189. What is the most common nerve injury in children with supracondylar fractures?

190. What is "Little Leaguer's elbow"?

191. How should posterior elbow dislocation in children be treated?

192. You return home after the physical therapy departmental Christmas party to find that your 4-year-old son is crying and lying in bed watching TV. He complains of pain in the right elbow. The babysitter admits to no history of trauma. He developed elbow pain after being swung around by the arms, while playing. Physical examination reveals no bony deformity. The elbow is held in a mildly flexed position. The olecranon is in normal relationship to the lateral and medial epicondyles. Most of the tenderness is localized to the radial aspect of the joint. ROM is limited by pain. What is the most likely diagnosis?

193. How are subluxations of the radial head reduced?

194. In what direction does the radial head dislocate in Monteggia fractures?

195. True or False? Injuries in children that are suspicious for child abuse need to be reported to the appropriate state authority.

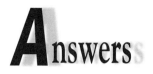
# Answers

183. Rest. For an active, noncompliant child: a long leg cast for 4 to 6 weeks.

184. Complete tears of the entire medial or lateral ligamentous complex warrant repair. Partial tears are best treated through early weight bearing with external support (cast brace, Ace wrap, pneumatic splint).

185. Quadriceps muscle strengthening, hamstring muscle stretching, and activity modification. If symptoms persist, a cylinder cast is applied with the knee in extension for 3 to 4 weeks. Rarely, excision of ossicles after closure of the growth plate may be necessary.

186. Closed fractures heal in 5 to 13 weeks, open fractures 3 to 5 months.

187. The anterior fat pad. The posterior fat pad is not seen unless displaced from the olecranon fossa by an elbow effusion.

188. Elbow hyperextension, which allows the olecranon to impact posteriorly producing an extension-type supracondylar fracture.

189. Radial nerve injury.

190. A medial epicondyle stress fracture.

191. By closed reduction. Supinate or hypersupinate the forearm to unlock the radius and ulna from the humerus; then reduce. The elbow is placed in a cast 90° of flexion, midpronation for 5 to 7 days, then the cast is removed and active ROM exercises are begun.

192. "Nursemaid's elbow," also known as subluxation of the radial head.

193. By full supination. If the radial head is not reduced, proceed to full flexion of elbow. If recurrent, (three episodes or more) apply a cast for 3 weeks. Usually no immobilization is needed.

194. In the same direction as the apex of the ulnar fracture in all cases.

195. True. State and federal laws on child abuse make reporting mandatory and places the onus of reporting on the treating physician.

uestions

**196.** A 5-year-old right-hand-dominant girl fell while riding her bicycle, sustaining a closed supracondylar humerus fracture seen on radiograph. The radial and ulnar pulses are not palpable. How should this patient be treated? (See Figure 2-7.)

igure 2-7

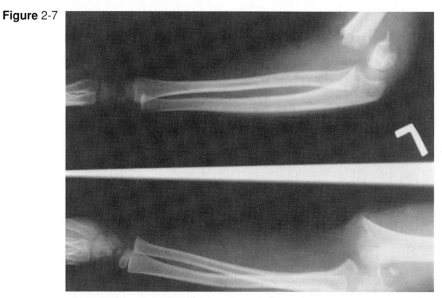

**197.** Before reaching the operating room, it is noted that the patient has lost her ability to flex the thumb interphalangeal (IP) joint as well as the index finger distal interphalangeal (DIP) joint. No sensory changes are noted. Passive flexion and extension of the digits does not produce any excessive pain. What is causing this problem?

**198.** What is the treatment of choice for anterior interosseous nerve palsy associated with a displaced supracondylar fracture?

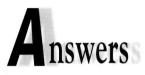

# Answers

**196.** A supracondylar fracture with a pulseless hand should be expeditiously reduced. The loss of pulse may be indicative of either arterial spasm secondary to stretch, direct trauma, arterial thrombosis, or arterial severance. If after reduction of the fracture the extremity remains pulseless, surgical exploration of the brachial artery should be performed. Waiting an hour after the reduction for resolution of the spasm is reasonable. However, because patients are usually taken to the operating room for closed reduction with percutaneous pinning or open reduction and internal fixation of this type of supracondylar fracture, most surgeons would immediately explore and repair any damage to the artery if the pulse did not rapidly return after reduction. Traction and reduction of the displaced supracondylar fracture have also been advocated with close monitoring for return of pulse. If the pulse has not been restored within an hour of the institution of traction, then exploration of the artery is advised.

**197.** The patient most likely has a neuropraxia of the anterior interosseous nerve.

**198.** In this particular case, while exploring the brachial artery, you should also evaluate the median nerve and the anterior interosseous branch for damage. In most cases of closed supracondylar fracture without vascular impairment following open or closed reduction of the fracture, the patient should be followed-up clinically. The vast majority of these palsy cases should resolve spontaneously over the course of several months.

# Chapter 3

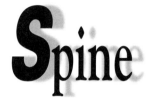

## Spine

KENNETH BURKUS, MD

HOWARD M. PLACE, MD

PAUL F. BEATTIE, PhD, PT, OCS

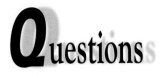

# Questions

1. What joints comprise the craniovertebral complex?

2. What ligaments are responsible for maintaining the stability of the craniovertebral joint complex?

3. In what disorders would you suspect instability of the craniovertebral joint system?

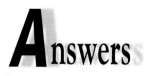

# Answers

1. The craniovertebral joint complex consists of five synovial articulations. The occipital-atlanto (O-A) joints are formed by the occipital condyles and superior articular processes (facets) of the atlas (C1). The atlanto-axial (A-A) joints are formed by the inferior articular processes of C1 and the superior articular processes of the axis (C2). The atlanto-odontoid joint is a pivot type of articulation that moves in a closed chain with the A-A joint. It is formed by the odontoid process (dens) articulating with the posterior surface of the anterior mass of the atlas and the transverse ligament.

2. There are two main ligament systems stabilizing the craniovertebral joint complex. The first system surrounds the entire motion segment, and the second system stabilizes the atlanto-odontoid complex. Stabilizing the O-A joint is the strong atlanto-occipital membrane, which is reinforced anteriorly by the anterior longitudinal ligament and posteriorly by the ligamentum nuchae. The facet joints of O-A and A-A are stabilized by joint capsules.

   The atlanto-odontoid joint is spanned posteriorly by the very strong tectorial membrane, which blends into the periosteum on the inner surface of the foramen magnum and continues inferiorly from C2 as the posterior longitudinal ligament. Deep to this membrane is a series of fibers collectively known as the cruciate (cross-like) ligament system. Vertical fibers from this system run from the odontoid process to the foramen magnum superiorly and to C2 inferiorly. The apical ligament also connects the dens with the foramen magnum. Transverse fibers span between the left and right anterior-lateral portions of C1 covering the odontoid process and acting to prevent anterior translation of C1 on C2. Arising from the superior-lateral tips of the odontoid process and traveling to the foramen magnum are the paired alar ligaments. These structures prevent excessive rotation and side bending between the occiput and C2 (see Figure 3-1).

**Figure** 3-1

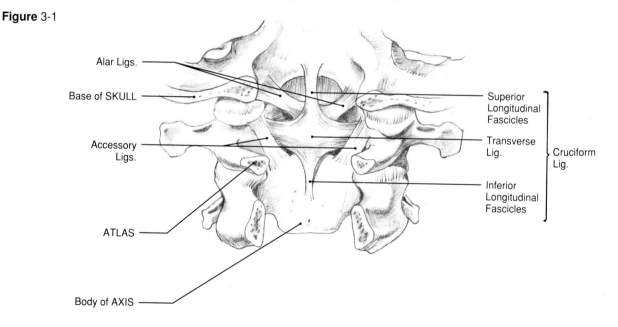

3. There are many conditions that result in instability of the craniovertebral joint system. Individuals who are at increased risk to develop this problem include those with Down's syndrome, synoviolytic diseases such as rheumatoid arthritis, and most spondyloarthropathies. You should also suspect instability in patients who have collagen disorders such as Ehlers-Danlos syndrome that result in diffuse hypermobility.

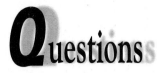

**4.** What findings obtained in a patient's history may alert the examiner to the potential presence of craniovertebral instability?

**5.** What region of the spine is most commonly involved in juvenile rheumatoid arthritis?

**6.** How much rotation occurs at the A-A joint in comparison to the rest of the cervical spine?

**7.** Which test in the physical examination demonstrates excessive laxity of the transverse ligament of the atlas?

**8.** Which test in the physical examination demonstrates excessive laxity of the alar ligaments?

**9.** A 50-year-old woman with severe rheumatoid arthritis is evaluated with a routine screening lateral radiographic film of her cervical spine. This shows an 8-mm anterior atlanto-dens interval that completely reduces with extension. The patient has no complaint of neck pain and no neurologic signs or symptoms. What is the most appropriate treatment for this patient at the present time?

**10.** What is the etiology of this patient's cervical instability?

**11.** What ligamentous structures have been rendered incompetent when the anterior atlanto-dens interval has increased to 12 mm?

**12.** How can stress view radiographs assist the identification of instability of the craniovertebral joint complex?

**13.** Identify the structures on Figure 3-2.

**Figure** 3-2

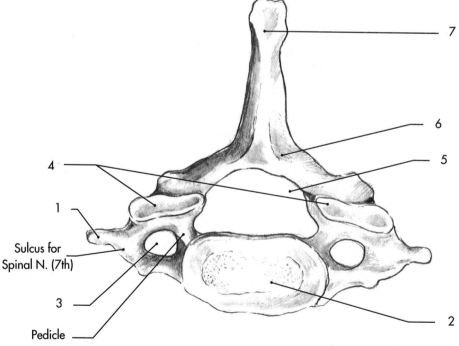

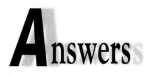

**4.** In addition to the disorders mentioned above, an examiner should consider the presence of craniovertebral instability in any patient who has sustained trauma to this area. This is especially important when the mechanism of injury involved forced flexion, extension, or compression.

Because of the high density of motor, sensory, and sympathetic fibers in this area, as well as the vertebral artery, a wide variety of symptoms may be present with craniovertebral instability. Any individual who reports transient or sustained dysesthesia of the face (trigeminal nerve), neck (cervical plexus), occiput (greater occipital nerve), or more than one extremity (cervical spinal cord) may have instability of the craniovertebral area. This is especially a concern if these symptoms are increased during neck flexion. Patients may complain of a heaviness of the head or an inability to hold the head up against gravity. Other common complaints include vertigo, syncope, nystagmus, diplopia, and nausea.

**5.** The cervical spine; the thoracic and lumbar spine are rarely involved.

**6.** Approximately 50%.

**7.** The transverse ligament test is performed by gently attempting to anteriorly translate both transverse processes of C1 in the supine patient. A positive response would be any of the symptoms listed in question 4. Additionally, some examiners claim to be able to detect an excessive amount of anterior translation at C1. (There appears, however, to be no data which describes the reliability of this finding.)

**8.** The alar ligament test is performed with the examiner standing behind the seated patient. The examiner pinches the spinous process of C2 between his thumb and index finger, then gently bends the patient's head to the right and then to the left. With an intact alar ligament, the examiner should palpate the spinous process of C2 moving in the direction opposite that of the side bending; i.e., the spinous process will rotate to the right when the examiner tilts the head to the left. A positive response would be a reproduction of the symptoms listed in question 4 as well as the failure of the spinous process to rotate during side bending.

**9.** The natural history of cervical spine disease in rheumatoid arthritis is unpredictable. The course can vary considerably. At this time, the patient has no symptoms related to her cervical instability. Not all patients with this degree of A-A instability will show definite progression. Orthopedically, she should be treated with continued observation. Aggressive medical management of her rheumatoid arthritis is recommended to address the underlying etiology of her cervical instability.

**10.** The dens articulates in two synovial joints; one is located anteriorly between the ring of C1 and the anterior aspect of the dens, and the other is located posteriorly between the posterior aspect of the dens and the transverse ligament. In this patient, the transverse ligament has been rendered incompetent by the aggressive destructive process related to her rheumatoid arthritis.

**11.** When the anterior atlanto-dens interval has progressed to greater than 10 mm, the alar, apical, and transverse ligaments are no longer functional.

**12.** Subtle degrees of instability may not be apparent on plain films. However, during cervical flexion you may observe an increased atlanto-odontoid interval. In adults if this distance is greater than 3 mm, you should consider the presence of instability.

**13.** (1) Posterior tubercle; (2) vertebral body; (3) transverse foramen; (4) superior articular facets; (5) vertebral canal; (6) lamina; and (7) spinous process.

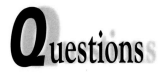

14. What are the joints of Luschka?

15. A patient with a C6-7 unilateral disc herniation will demonstrate weakness in which muscle groups?

16. A patient with a C4-5 unilateral disc herniation will demonstrate weakness in which muscle groups?

17. A patient with a C4-5 unilateral disc herniation will demonstrate dysesthesia in what part of the upper extremity?

18. A patient with a C6 radiculopathy will demonstrate weakness in which muscle groups?

19. A patient with a C6 radiculopathy will demonstrate sensory changes in what part of the upper extremity?

20. On palpation of the neck, the cricoid cartilage is at what level of the cervical spine?

21. A 38-year-old woman presents with a 6-month history of burning pain in the lateral brachium. She has no complaint of upper extremity weakness. Her symptoms arose following a motor vehicle accident. Radiographs obtained at that time revealed mild DJD of the cervical spine but no other abnormalities. What is the most likely segmental level of her symptoms?

22. The patient in question 21 states that her symptoms are increased noticeably when she attempts to bend her neck forward. What is the most likely cause of this problem?

23. When examining the patient in question 21, she complains of increased symptoms with all neck movements and decreased symptoms with manual traction. What is the most appropriate initial treatment?

24. What are the physical findings associated with thoracic disc herniations?

25. What other disease processes can mimic the signs and symptoms of thoracic disc herniations?

26. What are the treatment options for thoracic disc herniations?

27. What is the inheritance pattern for idiopathic adolescent scoliosis?

28. Adolescent idiopathic scoliosis is associated with what risk factors for progression?

29. What is the prevalence of adolescent idiopathic scoliosis in the United States?

30. A 10-year-old girl is referred by a local school nurse for evaluation of a spinal deformity (Tanner stage I). A radiograph demonstrates a 26° right thoracic scoliosis. She has had no prior spinal radiographs. How should she be treated?

31. An 11-year-old (Tanner stage II) boy is referred for evaluation of a spinal deformity. He has had no prior radiographs. A radiograph on the day of the clinic visit demonstrates a 31° thoracic scoliosis. How should he be treated?

32. A 14-year-old girl with 34° left lumbar scoliosis (Tanner stage IV) is referred. She is 18 months postmenarche. The spinal radiographs shows that she has a Risser stage IV curvature. How should she be treated?

33. Underarm thoracolumbosacral orthoses (TLSOs) are best used for which curve patterns in adolescent idiopathic scoliosis?

34. When is a patient weaned from a brace for adolescent idiopathic scoliosis?

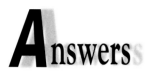
# Answers

14. The uncovertebral joints of Luschka are the articulations in the cervical spine between the uncus (an osseous prominence along the lateral margin of the cephalad vertebral end plate) and the caudal surface of the adjacent vertebral body.

15. A C7 radiculopathy produces weakness in the triceps and extensor digitorum communis muscles.

16. A C5 radiculopathy produces weakness in the deltoid and biceps muscles.

17. A C5 radiculopathy produces dysesthesia along the lateral border of the brachium.

18. The biceps, brachioradialis, and wrist extensor muscles are affected.

19. A C6 radiculopathy produces dysesthesia in the thumb and index finger.

20. The cricoid cartilage is at the C6 level.

21. These symptoms correspond to the C5 dermatome. C4 is primarily in the supraclavicular region, and C6 typically involves the thumb and lateral hand.

22. Limited cervical flexion with unilateral upper extremity radiculopathy in a 38-year-old person is strongly suggestive of a symptom-producing intervertebral disc herniation.

23. Considering the diagnosis and extrapolating from the effects of movement on pain, the appropriate initial treatment would be cervical traction.

24. Neurologic deficits vary and depend on the level of the herniation; the size of the spinal canal; and the size, position, and composition of the disc. Approximately half of these patients have lower extremity weakness. Long track signs including spasticity, hyperreflexia, and an abnormal Babinski response are commonly found. Approximately one third of patients will have some bladder or bowel dysfunction.

25. Demyelinating diseases (multiple sclerosis, amyotrophic lateral sclerosis), spinal cord tumors or infarction, transverse myelitis, angina pectoris, intercostal neuritis, and pleuritis.

26. Observation, posterior transpedicular decompression, posterolateral costotransversectomy decompression, anterior transthoracic decompression, and fusion.

27. There are at least three recessive autosomal alleles in the inheritance pattern for adolescent idiopathic scoliosis.

28. Age, maturity, sex, magnitude of the curve, and curve pattern are the associated risk factors.

29. In the U.S. population, 2% to 4% have curves of 10° or more.

30. Only 1 out of 4 patients with a scoliosis curvature between 25° and 30° will progress. The patient should be followed closely at 4-month intervals for curvature progression. If the curvature progresses 5° or more, the girl should be braced.

31. Skeletally immature patients with a curvature in the 30° range should be treated with a brace immediately. Without treatment, the majority of these patients will demonstrate progression of their curvature patterns.

32. The patient should be followed-up in approximately 6 months. She is not a candidate for bracing. Only patients with at least 9 months of growth remaining should be started in a bracing program.

33. TLSOs are best used for curves with an apex at or below T8.

34. When there has been no increase in height for a 4-month period and the Risser sign is at least 4, the patient can be weaned from the brace.

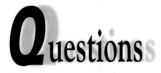
# Questions

35. Has electrical surface stimulation been shown to be an effective treatment to control the progression of adolescent idiopathic scoliosis?

36. What percentage of patients with Duchenne's muscular dystrophy will develop scoliosis?

37. When does the scoliosis curve pattern progress in patients with Duchenne's muscular dystrophy?

38. A 10-year-old girl is seen with a 21° left thoracic scoliosis. She has had no prior radiographs. How should she be treated?

39. A 6-year-old girl with a myelomeningocele at the L1 level has a 25° thoracolumbar scoliosis. Over a 2-month period, her curvature has increased to 55°. How should she be treated?

40. A 3-year-old boy is seen in clinic with an isolated anterior vertebral failure of formation at a single level and a kyphosis that has progressed from 38° to 45° over a 6-month period of observation. How should he be treated?

41. By what mechanism does the upper extremity receive its sympathetic innervation?

42. What are the major anatomical features of the lumbar spine?

43. What is the primary function of the annulus fibrosus?

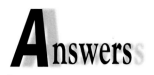
# Answers

**35.** No.

**36.** Eighty percent of patients with Duchenne's muscular dystrophy will develop scoliosis.

**37.** When the patient stops walking and becomes wheelchair bound, the scoliosis curve progresses.

**38.** Magnetic resonance imaging (MRI) of the entire spinal cord should be performed. Left thoracic scoliosis is associated with occult neuromuscular etiology such as spinal cord tumors and fistulas.

**39.** The patient needs to be evaluated for hydrocephalus, syringomyelia, and a tethered cord syndrome. An acute increase in scoliosis curvatures in myelodysplastic patients has been associated with ventricular shunt malfunction and hydrocephalus. If no hydrocephalus is present, syringomyelia or spinal cord tethering should be ruled out.

**40.** Bracing is ineffective in cases of congenital kyphosis secondary to failures of formation. Patients with less than 55° of kyphosis and less than 5 years old respond well to posterior spinal fusion without instrumentation.

**41.** Preganglionic sympathetic fibers exit the upper thoracic spinal cord, traveling with the ventral roots to the ventral rami where they enter the paravertebral sympathetic ganglion via the white rami communicantes. These fibers travel superiorly to synapse in the inferior and middle cervical sympathetic ganglia. Via the gray rami communicantes, the middle cervical sympathetic ganglion supplies C5-6, and the lower (Stellate) cervical ganglion supplies C7-T1.

**42.** The vertebral bodies are connected by the intervertebral discs and the neural arches are joined by the facet joints. Each vertebra has three functional components: (1) the vertebral body, designed to bear weight; (2) the neural arch, designed to protect the neural elements; and (3) the bony processes (spinous and transverse), designed as outriggers to increase the efficiency of muscle action. The disc surface of the vertebral body demonstrates, on its periphery, a ring of cortical bone. This ring acts as the anchoring site for the attachment of the fibers of the annulus. The cartilaginous end plate lies within the confines of the ring.

Intervertebral discs are complicated structures both anatomically and physiologically. They are constructed in a manner similar to a car tire, with a fibrous outer casing—the annulus, containing a gelatinous inner tube—the nucleus pulposus. Fibers of the annulus are divided into three main groups consisting of concentric fibrous rings surrounding the nucleus pulposus. The anterior fibers of the annulus are strongly reinforced by the powerful anterior longitudinal ligament. The posterior longitudinal ligament only gives weak reinforcement to the posterior fibers of the annulus; this weakness may contribute to posterior disc herniations.

**43.** The annulus serves to stabilize the spine, preventing abnormal translation of one vertebral body relative to another. It also serves in a shock-absorbing capacity through the loading of the fibers transmitted largely through the nucleus pulposus. This function of the annulus is compared to the hoops around a barrel.

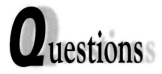

# Questions

44. What are the types of lumbar disc herniations?

45. What are the differences between protruded (prolapsed), extruded, and sequestrated intervertebral disc herniations?

46. What are the common radiographic findings of degenerative disc disease?

47. Does degenerative disc disease cause low back pain (LBP)?

48. What are the radiographic signs of segmental instability due to disc degeneration?

# **A**nswers

**44.** (1) Normal disc; (2) radial bulging (intact annulus); (3) disc protrusion (intact posterior longitudinal ligament [PPL]); (4) disc extrusion (ruptured PLL); and (5) disc sequestration (migration away from disc space). (See Figure 3-3.)

**Figure** 3-3

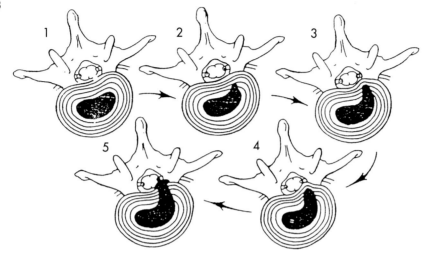

**45.** In protruded (prolapsed) intervertebral discs, the nuclear material is confined by a few of the outermost fibers of the annulus and PLL. Prominence of the annulus is noted at surgery with the demonstration of nuclear material upon incision of the remaining fibers of the annulus and PLL. An extruded intervertebral disc demonstrates nuclear material that has blown out through the annulus and PLL. Sequestrated intervertebral disc herniations consist of free fragments in the spinal canal.

**46.** Degenerative disc disease, a progressive condition, is radiographically characterized by decreased space between the vertebral bodies, osteophytes of the superior and inferior margins of the vertebral bodies, and sclerosis of the superior and inferior surfaces of the vertebral bodies.

**47.** Not necessarily. Many people have dramatic findings of degenerative disc disease on radiographic evaluation and are asymptomatic. A degenerative spine potentially has a decreased threshold to injury. Thus relatively minor trauma may cause LBP in people with this condition.

**48.** Lateral flexion-extension radiographs of the spine can demonstrate abnormal motion, provided the patient is not in so much pain that splinting of the spine occurs. Also indicative of segmental instability is the traction spur seen about 1 to 2 mm above the vertebral body edge, projecting horizontally. The third sign is gas in the disc.

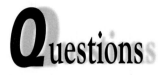

49. What is end-stage degenerative disc disease?

50. How does degenerative disc disease lead to nerve root compression?

51. A midlateral disc herniation at the L4-5 level most frequently compresses which nerve root?

52. A midlateral disc herniation at the L5-S1 level most frequently compresses which nerve root?

53. Under what circumstances would an L5 nerve root be compressed by an L5-S1 disc herniation?

54. Massive central sequestration involving several roots of the cauda equina with bowel and bladder paralysis is most commonly seen with what level of disc herniation?

55. What are the clinical findings associated with an L4-5 herniated disc?

56. What are the physical findings associated with L4 nerve root compression?

57. What is adhesive radiculitis?

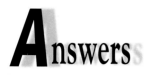 **A**nswers

**49.** Disc space narrowing occurs with overriding and subluxation of the posterior joints. The posterior joints assume a posture of hyperextension. As the facet joints assume a position of extreme extension, there is no cushioning effect at these joints, and pain occurs with minor provocation. The subluxated posterior joints are thereby repeatedly traumatized and develop degenerative osteoarthritis. (See Figure 3-4.)

**Figure** 3-4

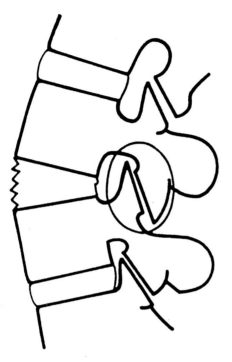

**50.** Through disc protrusion (disc herniation), bony root entrapment (lateral recess stenosis, subarticular stenosis), and redundant ligamentous entrapment (central stenosis from the ligamentum flavum).

**51.** L5.

**52.** S1.

**53.** A lateral disc protrusion could compress the exiting L5 nerve root in the neural foramina.

**54.** L4-5.

**55.** This would produce a deficit most frequently in the L5 nerve root, which would produce weakness in the extensor hallucis longus, and sensory changes in the dorsum of the foot.

**56.** This might be seen with an L3-4 herniated disc. Weakness would be seen in the anterior tibial muscle, and the patellar reflex might be depressed. Sensory changes would be noted along the medial side of the leg.

**57.** The nerve roots are bound down by fibrotic tissue in association with some cases of degeneration. A persistent nagging pain results because the nerve roots are tethered and unable to slide normally, producing this constant pain with activity.

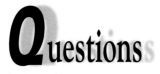

# Questions

58. What is the mechanism that causes the radicular pain characteristic of sciatica in a patient with a herniated disc?

59. What physical examination test is the most sensitive to the presence of a herniated lumbar intervertebral disc which results in sciatica?

60. What are the five categories of low back pain?

61. What is viscerogenic low back pain?

62. What is vascular back pain?

63. What is neurogenic back pain?

64. What is psychogenic back pain?

65. What is spondylogenic back pain?

66. What is an outcome measure?

67. What are appropriate outcome measures for patients with LBP?

68. Do the Waddell signs and symptoms of psychological distress indicate that a patient with LBP is malingering?

# Answers

58. Although pressure on the nerve root from herniated disc material has long been considered the cause of sciatica, this mechanism is probably only in effect if the nerve is hypersensitized by scarring. Recent evidence suggests that the pain of sciatica is associated with inflammatory mediators at the interface of the epineurium of the dorsal root ganglion. The mediators stem from an autoimmune reaction caused by contact with nuclear material.

59. A positive straight leg test has a sensitivity of over 0.90 in the presence of a herniated disc which results in sciatica.

60. (1) Viscerogenic pain; (2) neurogenic pain; (3) vascular pain; (4) psychogenic pain; and (5) spondylogenic pain.

61. This back pain is referred from the kidneys, pelvisacral lesions of the lesser sac, or retroperitoneal tumors. This type of pain is neither aggravated by activity nor relieved by rest. This differentiates it from back pain that is localized to spinal disorders.

62. Vascular back pain results from aneurysms or peripheral vascular disease. Intermittent claudication tends to be associated with these problems. These symptoms are sometimes mimicked by spinal stenosis. Both conditions are aggravated by walking short distances. Pain due to abdominal aneurysms tends not to be associated with activities that would normally worsen spinal pain. This pain tends to be deep-seated and is usually unrelated to activity. Intermittent claudication associated with peripheral vascular disease may mimic spinal stenosis. Both conditions are aggravated by walking short distances. Spinal stenosis-type pain, however, is not relieved by standing still, whereas intermittent claudication is.

63. Neurogenic back pain is most commonly caused by neurofibromas, neurilemmoma, ependymoma, cysts, and tumors arising from nerve roots in the lumbar spine. Symptoms are similar to disc herniation. Unlike disc herniation, these patients will describe night pain, which may cause them to get out of bed to obtain relief.

64. Pain resulting from nonorganic causes. Purely psychogenic back pain is uncommon. You must rule out organic causes prior to making this diagnosis.

65. Spondylogenic back pain is derived from the spinal column, sacroiliac joint, or from changes occurring in the soft tissues. It is aggravated by activities and relieved by rest.

66. An outcome measure is any measure that indicates a change in a patient's status over time.

67. There are numerous outcome measures including range of motion (ROM), strength, and pain. Interestingly, these measures of impairment are often poorly correlated with function and disability. This is especially true for patients with chronic LBP. As a result, many people are advocating the use of self-report measures which ask a patient to rate his or her ability to perform various functional tasks. The Oswestry Low Back Pain Disability Questionnaire and the Roland-Morris Disability Questionnaire have been shown to be valid outcome measures for LBP.

68. No. The Waddell signs and symptoms of psychological distress are designed to identify patients who report symptoms and demonstrate behaviors that are not consistent with the typical clinical picture of a person with LBP. These are described as abnormal illness behaviors that may be linked to psychological disorders and are in no way specific for malingering.

# Questions

69. A 34-year-old truck driver presents with a chief complaint of acute low back pain that refers to his left posterior thigh. His symptoms are worsened when he sits for more than 30 minutes and tend to decrease in intensity when he walks. He has no lower extremity weakness, his lumbar ROM is full, but painful in flexion, and full, but not painful in extension. He can recall no trauma. His symptoms have been present for 6 weeks. His lumbar radiographs are normal. He has no other illnesses. Given this information, what is the most likely diagnosis?

70. How would the patient in question 69 be assigned in the McKenzie Classification?

71. What would be the logical initial management of the patient in question 69?

72. A 74-year-old man presents with a complaint of pain in the sacroiliac region on the left. He can recall no trauma and states that his symptoms began 2 weeks ago. He indicates that his symptoms are worsened when he rotates to the left and right. He states that he has a considerable increase in pain at night, especially if he has played golf the previous day. His left innominate is rotated anteriorly as determined by palpation. What is the appropriate physical therapy management of this patient?

73. When palpating a patient's lumbar spine, you conclude that the L5 spinous process is deviated to the left. Which way is the vertebral body rotated?

74. What is the Patrick test?

75. A 14-year-old boy presents with a complaint of pain along the posterior-lateral portion of both iliac crests. His symptoms are increased with active and passive trunk rotation. He states that these symptoms began 2 weeks ago when he started an intensive exercise program to prepare for preseason football. Given only this information, what is the most likely diagnosis?

76. How should you treat a patient with acute apophysitis of the iliac crest?

77. A 22-year-old man presents with a complaint of intense, midback pain. He states that he slipped on some grease while working in the kitchen of a local restaurant. He states that he landed on his buttocks and developed an immediate onset of symptoms. He had plain film radiographs performed that evening that were interpreted as normal. What is the probable diagnosis?

78. If the patient in question 77 was found to have a fractured vertebral end plate, how should this be treated initially?

79. A 58-year-old man presents with a complaint of burning pain in his midbuttock that is present after he walks 10 minutes. It goes away after he sits or lies down for 5 minutes. What are three primary musculoskeletal sources for this condition?

80. Following a detailed musculoskeletal examination of the patient in question 79, you are unable to identify any abnormalities. His radiographs are normal. What is a probable diagnosis?

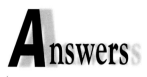
**Answers**

69. In the absence of radiculopathy distal to the knee and in the presence of normal radiographs for this otherwise healthy 34-year-old man, you must consider some form of lumbar joint or sacroiliac dysfunction and/or some form of soft tissue dysfunction in the lumbosacral spine. Because of the lack of examination procedures with acceptable diagnostic accuracy for this condition, the exact diagnosis is rarely agreed upon. This has led to the popularity of clinical classifications for low back pain.

70. Postural syndrome.

71. Because this patient's symptoms are worsened with lumbar flexion and prolonged sitting and are reduced with lumbar extension (as a component of walking), prone press-ups performed q.i.d. for 10 repetitions as well as use of a lumbar roll when sitting would be a logical initial treatment.

72. This patient should be referred immediately to his primary care physician. Although his symptoms may mimic a sacroiliac joint dysfunction, the presence of atraumatic sacral pain that is worsened at night in an elderly man suggests prostate cancer.

73. There is no way to determine that from this information. Anatomic variations and anomalies of the spinous processes are quite common in the lumbar spine. Thus, the finding of a deviated spinous process is not meaningful by itself.

74. A test to detect pathologic conditions in the hip as well as the sacroiliac (SI) joint. With the patient in a supine position, the foot of the involved side is placed on the opposite knee. This places the hip into a flexed, abducted, externally rotated position. Inguinal pain generally indicates a hip disorder. In this position, the SI joints can be stressed by placing one hand on the flexed knee joint and the other on the anterior superior iliac spine of the opposite side of the pelvis and pressing down simultaneously. A complaint of increased pain indicates a SI joint disorder.

75. Apophysitis of the iliac crests. Complete fusion of the apophysis of the iliac crest to the ilium may not occur until age 21 to 25. In skeletally immature individuals, repeated trunk rotation may inflame the apophysis of the iliac crest from the stress created by the oblique abdominal muscles.

76. This is a self-limiting condition with most people returning to full activity in 6 weeks. During the early stages, ice and rest from activities that exacerbate symptoms will hasten healing. Some clinicians recommend the use of crutches for a short period if the symptoms are increased with walking.

77. This is a very difficult case. One major possibility is a fracture of the vertebral end plate. This is a common finding in young adults who sustain compression trauma to the lumbar spine and should be ruled out by a bone scan or MRI before initiating any vigorous physical therapy.

78. The patient should be treated with a lumbar orthosis for a short period of time followed by lumbar stabilization exercises. Activities that involve enhanced compression of the spine such as heavy lifting or running should be avoided for several months.

79. (1) Local sources include a strain of the gluteal muscles, or hip lateral rotators, and inflammation of the gluteal bursa. (2) Sources that typically refer to this area include a sprain of the sacroiliac joint or a strain of various soft tissue structures of the lower lumbar spine. (3) An atypical source of pain referral to this area would be hip joint sprain or arthrosis.

80. This may be vascular insufficiency to the muscles of the midbuttock, perhaps resulting from thrombosis of one of the gluteal arteries.

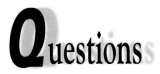

**81.** What is the relationship of the piriformis muscle to the sciatic nerve?

**82.** What clinical findings suggest piriformis syndrome?

**83.** A 22-year-old man injured his back in a work-related lifting accident 2 weeks prior to presenting as an outpatient. He complains of back pain that radiates down his right posterior thigh to the lateral border of the foot. The referring family practice physician has already ordered a computerized tomographic (CT) scan (see Figure 3-5). Physical examination shows that the patient has a positive straight leg raise at 45° and a diminished Achilles reflex. There is no motor weakness. What is your treatment plan?

**Figure** 3-5

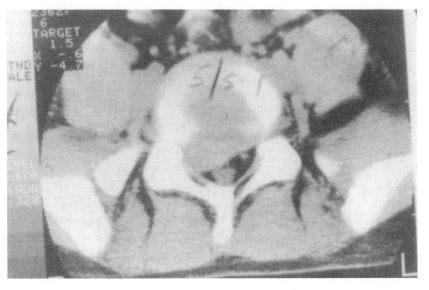

**84.** The patient's pain has increased in intensity and is exacerbated with all conservative treatment at 8 weeks following the injury. What is the recommended treatment plan?

**85.** While awaiting surgery, the patient vigorously sneezes and notes the acute onset of bilateral radiating leg pain and perianal anesthesia. He also has difficulty emptying his bladder. What is now the treatment plan?

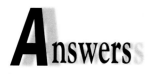
# Answers

81. The piriformis muscle spans the middle of the greater sciatic foramen. The sciatic nerve along with the posterior femoral cutaneous nerve and inferior gluteal artery exits the greater sciatic foramen just inferior to the piriformis muscle. In approximately 10% of cases, the common peroneal division of the sciatic nerve exits the greater sciatic foramen within the piriformis muscle. The clinical significance of this is unknown.

82. This poorly defined condition is presumed to result from irritation of the sciatic and/or posterior femoral cutaneous nerves caused by swelling or spasm of the piriformis muscle. Patients will often complain of midbuttock pain that refers posteriorly into the ipsilateral thigh and perhaps calf. Often there is a history of blunt trauma or sustained compression to the buttock. The motion of hip internal rotation is often limited and reproduces the symptoms.

83. The CT scan shows a right-sided L5-S1 disc herniation. The right S1 nerve root is posteriorly displaced. However, the patient has had symptoms for only 2 weeks. Initial treatment to reduce the acute painful symptoms should involve low back modalities such as moist heat and traction, reduction of activities, and nonsteroidal antiinflammatory drugs (NSAIDs). Physical therapy and back rehabilitation exercises are instituted when the patient can tolerate increased activity levels.

84. The patient is a surgical candidate; he has failed a 6-week trial of conservative therapy. The large extruded disc fragment precludes the use of chymopapain or percutaneous nuclectomy. A standard unilateral discectomy or microdiscectomy are the surgical treatment options.

85. The patient has developed the clinical symptoms of cauda equina syndrome. The patient should be treated with an open discectomy as soon as possible.

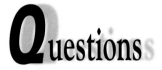

86. A 68-year-old woman has a 3-month history of low back pain and bilateral radiating leg pain. Her leg pain is worse than her back pain. The leg pain radiates down her posterior thigh and involves her feet and calves. The patient reports that her leg pain is exacerbated by walking and relieved by sitting and bending forward. The patient has already tried a course of physical therapy and a course of epidural and oral steroids. A myelogram of the patient's lumbar spine is shown (Figure 3-6). What is the recommended treatment plan?

**Figure** 3-6

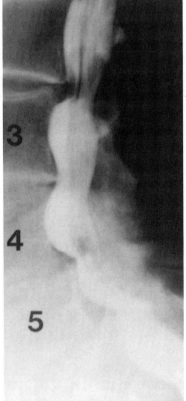

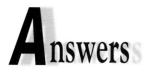

# Answers

86. The lateral myelogram shows multiple levels of narrowing of the spinal canal. At the L2-3 level, there is retrolisthesis of L2 on L3, disc space narrowing, and decreased sagittal diameter of the spinal canal. At L3-4, there is diffuse spondylosis but no significant narrowing of the spinal canal. At L4-5, there is a grade 1 degenerative spondylolisthesis associated with a severe narrowing of the spinal canal and a high-grade block of the myelographic dye. At L5-S1, there is some narrowing of the spinal canal consistent with spinal stenosis. The patient has failed the conservative treatment regimen. She now requires surgery. Treatment would involve multilevel posterior decompression laminectomies and posterolateral fusion between L4 and L5. The fusion must be performed because of the degenerative spondylolisthesis.

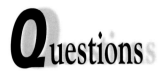

# Questions

87. A 35-year-old man presents with a 2-week history of neck pain radiating into his left arm. He states that his left arm pain is worse than his neck pain. There is no history of trauma. His primary care physician evaluated this patient with an MRI and then referred him to an orthopedist. His physical examination reveals weakness in his triceps and a decreased triceps reflex on the left. He has decreased sensitivity to light touch in his long finger. His MRI is shown in Figure 3-7, A and B. What is your diagnosis?

**Figure** 3-7

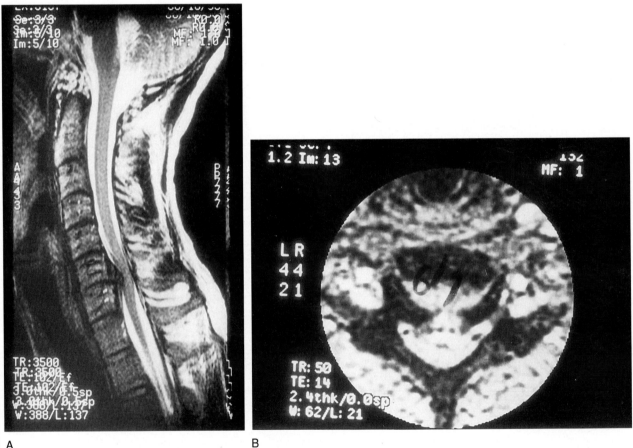

A                                                      B

88. What is the appropriate initial management of this patient?

89. A 15-year-old teenager sustains a bony flexion distraction injury (Chance fracture) through the body, pedicles, and posterior bony elements of L2. He complains of back pain but is neurologically normal. What type of treatment do you recommend?

90. A 25-year-old woman sustains an L1 burst fracture in a motor vehicle accident. She has substantial weakness in her gastrosoleus and anterior tibial muscles on the right, absent extensor hallucis longus (EHL) muscle function on the left, and patchy sensory deficits in her lower extremities below the knees. Rectal tone, perianal sensation, and the bulbocavernosus reflex are normal. A CT scan of her injured vertebra reveals 50% canal occlusion with no laminar fracture. Describe the anatomic location of her deficits (i.e., cord versus conus versus roots).

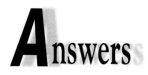

# Answers

87. This patient has an acute C7 radiculopathy secondary to a C6-C7 herniated nucleus pulposus.

88. This patient is best managed initially with nonoperative treatment, consisting of short-term immobilization in a cervical orthosis and cervical traction, combined with NSAIDs and analgesics. Most patients respond to this type of treatment regimen with significant improvement over 6 to 12 weeks.

89. In this young patient with a pure bony flexion distraction injury, you can anticipate excellent bone healing after adequate immobilization. Such an injury has minimal soft-tissue disruption, and stability will be obtained once bony union has occurred. This patient should be treated in a hyperextension cast. You can anticipate and strive for normal spinal alignment in the cast. If the patient had evidence of significant ligamentous disruption or a nonreducible kyphotic deformity, a single-level posterior compression arthrodesis would be preferred.

90. This patient has a significant nerve root injury. Her spinal cord appears to be functioning adequately because she has maintained conus medullaris function, has no spasticity, and has no discrete functional level. Her patchy sensory deficits, asymmetric weakness, and sacral sparing are suggestive of nerve root compression as opposed to spinal cord compression. This significantly affects the prognosis because root recovery is better than cord recovery after such an injury.

# Questions

91. A 46-year-old man injures his lower back while lifting a bag of groceries. He is otherwise healthy and has no history of back injury and no prior complaint of back pain. His neurologic examination is unremarkable. What is the role of routine radiographic evaluation in this patient?

92. What is the role of MRI in the patient with acute low back pain in question 91?

93. What is the incidence of asymptomatic lumbar HNP in an adult population?

94. A 55-year-old man presents with gradually increasing midback discomfort. This began several days ago after drainage of a dental abscess. The patient complains of persistent midback pain despite activity modification or rest. He has no complaint of leg symptoms. Figure 3-8, A, B, and C are from this patient's initial workup. What is this patient's working diagnosis at this time?

**Figure** 3-8

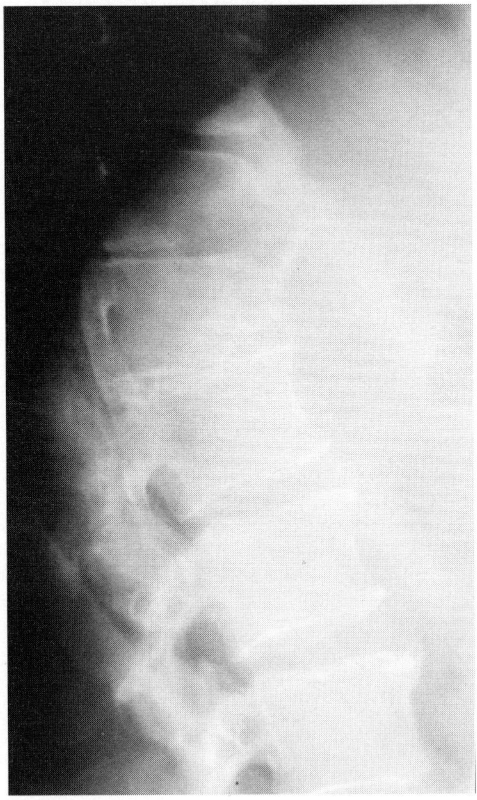

A

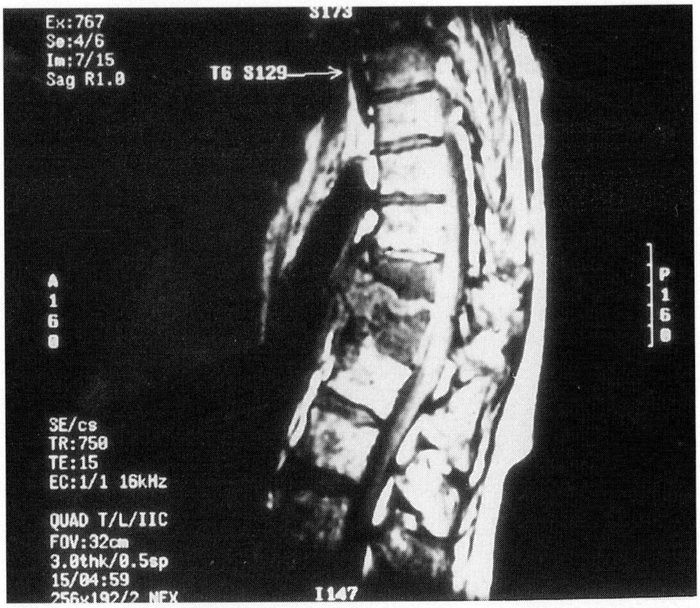

B

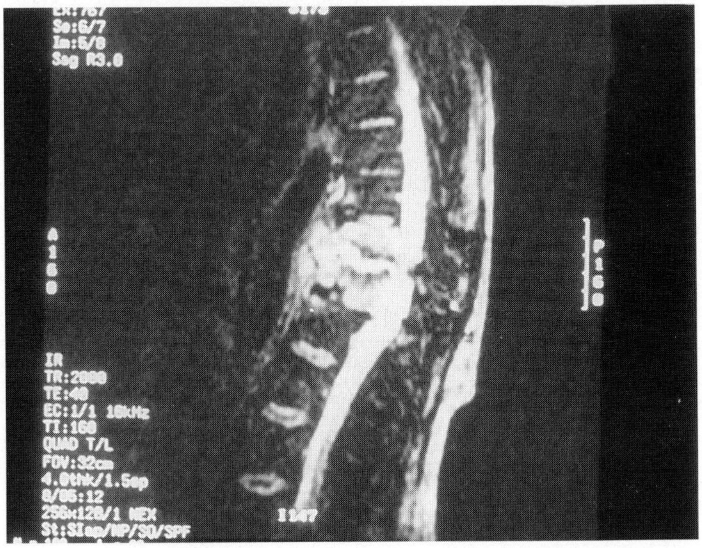

C

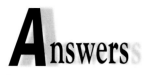

# Answers

91. Plain radiographic films of the lumbar spine are frequently nondiagnostic and not helpful in the evaluation of acute low back pain without trauma. Routine radiographic examination at this patient's initial encounter is not indicated.

92. MRI is also not indicated in this patient on his initial examination. He has no history of previous back pain and no history of significant trauma. He has a normal neurologic examination and no radicular complaints. Because of its extreme sensitivity, MRI in the lumbar spine is not a good screening tool.

93. Boden and associates (*Journal of Bone Joint Surgery*, 1990) suggest an overall incidence of approximately 33% asymptomatic HNP in the lumbar spine. This incidence increases in the patient older than 55 years of age. Greenberg and Schnell (*Journal of Neuroimaging*, 1991) and Jensen and associates (*New England Journal of Medicine*, 1994) also agree with an approximately one-third incidence of asymptomatic HNP. Use of MRI as a screening tool is thus limited due to its high incidence of significant findings in the asymptomatic patient.

94. This patient's history and radiographic examination are consistent with early pyogenic vertebral osteomyelitis of the thoracolumbar spine.

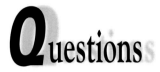

**95.** What radiographic findings are consistent with infection in this patient?

**96.** How could you differentiate between spinal tumors and spinal infections with the use of MRI?

**97.** The patient in Figure 3-9, A and B has had 12 weeks of persistent left lower extremity burning pain and weakness. What physical findings would you expect upon examination of this patient?

**Figure** 3-9

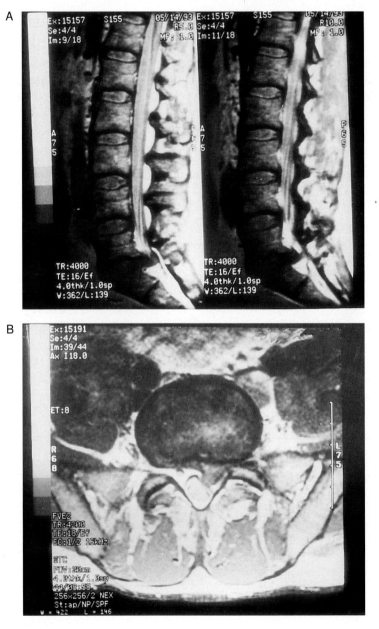

**98.** What is the appropriate initial management of this patient?

**99.** What is the role of lumbar fusion in this patient with an acute S1 radiculopathy refractory to nonoperative therapy?

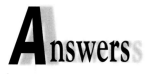
# Answers

95. This patient demonstrates loss of disc space height with gross bony destruction. There appears to be loss of end plate clarity and evidence of a soft-tissue abscess. The MRI shows edema in both vertebral bodies without gross vertebral body destruction. The central focus of the pathologic process appears to be the disc space. These findings are all consistent with a vertebral osteomyelitis.

96. According to An and associates (*Spine*, 1991), the most consistent finding in spinal infection is involvement of the disc space and the adjacent vertebral bodies. These vertebral bodies have decreased signal intensity on T1 weighted images and increased signal intensity on T2 weighted images. The disc space is usually spared in spinal destruction associated with tumor growth. Irregularities in the vertebral end plates are more common with infection than with tumor growth. Soft-tissue changes are more diffuse with infection, and contiguous vertebral involvement is most consistent with infection.

97. The patient in Figure 3-9, A and B has a left-sided paracentral L5-S1 herniated nucleus pulposus. A herniated disc at this location most commonly involves the nerve root for the level below the disc space involved. This would therefore involve the S1 nerve root on the left. A left S1 radiculopathy would produce weakness in the gastrosoleus muscle group and a decreased or diminished ankle jerk on the left side. A positive straight leg raise with pain radiating below the knee and into the foot may also be expected.

98. This patient should be initially managed with limited activity and analgesics. Prolonged bed rest is thought to be detrimental. Deyo and associates (*New England Journal of Medicine*, 1986) demonstrated no additional improvement from bed rest greater than 2 days. Numerous mechanical interventions such as traction, posture modification, and manipulation are controversial and not clearly beneficial. The benefit of exercise is also questioned. A McKenzie exercise program may have a prognostic value. Patients who are able to obtain normal lumbar extension are frequently able to be successfully treated nonoperatively as opposed to patients who cannot obtain normal lumbar extension (Kopp, et al., *Clinical Orthopedics and Related Research*, 1986). Your attention should be directed toward prevention of back disability with appropriate activity modification and an early return to work with appropriate work restrictions (Dillin, *Seminars in Spine Surgery*, 1989).

99. A lumbar fusion is not indicated in the initial treatment of the patient with leg pain secondary to a herniated nucleus pulposus. White and associates (*Spine*, 1987) showed no improvement in their prospective series of excision versus excision and fusion. The fusion group had an overall less satisfactory rate and higher complication rate. First-time lumbar herniated nucleus pulposus is best treated with disc excision without fusion.

100. Two weeks after an uncomplicated lumbar disc excision, a patient develops increasing back pain, including pain at rest and increased pain with activity. He has no radicular symptoms. Upon physical examination, he has a well-healed wound and limited motion with flexion and extension of his lumbar spine. He has tenderness to deep palpation in the area near his incision and has a negative straight leg raise. The erythrocyte sedimentation rate (ESR) is 42. What is this patient's diagnosis?

101. A 28-year-old man has an 18-month history of midback and buttocks pain with activity. He has difficulty running because of pain, which radiates down his lower extremity. He has noticed a certain "jumpiness" in his lower extremity over the last 6 months. He has no difficulty with bowel or bladder control. Physical examination reveals hyperreflexia in his lower extremity and no motor weakness. Sensory examination is within normal limits. The patient's studies are shown in Figure 3-10, A and B. What is the diagnosis?

**Figure** 3-10

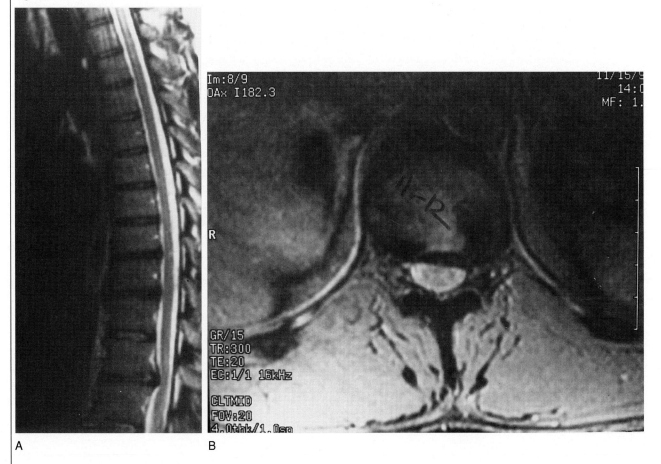

A                              B

102. What is the best form of treatment for this patient?

103. A 77-year-old woman complains of bilateral calf pain that is present after she walks for 15 minutes. This pain goes away when she sits down. What are the two most likely causes of this condition?

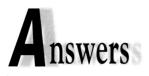# **A**nswers

**100.** This patient most likely has a postoperative deep wound infection versus a disc space infection. Postlaminectomy disc space infections typically develop in a slightly delayed fashion. They can occur without wound drainage, and the most significant finding is frequently persistent back pain. The ESR rate is extremely sensitive in diagnosing a deep infection after lumbar spine surgery (Jonsson, et al., *Spine*, 1991). After 2 weeks, the ESR values have typically returned to normal in the majority of normally healing postoperative patients.

**101.** This patient has a T11-T12 herniated nucleus pulposus with resultant myelopathy.

**102.** This patient has a history of prolonged back and buttocks pain with activity. He has failed previous nonoperative therapy for his back pain. His condition has continued to worsen, and he has demonstrated spinal cord involvement by his increased spasticity and hyperreflexia. This patient should be treated surgically at this time. Not all patients require surgical treatment for thoracic disc herniations (Brown, et al., *Spine*, 1992). However, the patient with persistent pain refractory to nonoperative treatment and any significant neurologic deficits should be treated surgically.

**103.** Vascular impairment to the distal lower limb (intermittent claudication) and spinal stenosis causing intermittent claudication of the spinal cord or cauda equina.

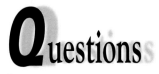
# Questions

104. What are simple clinical tests that differentiate between vascular impairment to the distal lower limb and spinal stenosis?

105. Describe efficacious nonoperative treatment for patients with spinal stenosis causing intermittent claudication of the spinal cord or cauda equina.

106. What symptoms associated with spinal stenosis would require immediate consultation with an orthopedist or neurosurgeon?

107. An 18-year-old woman who is a competitive springboard diver presents with a complaint of acute central low back pain. Her pain is worsened during the combined movements of extension, ipsilateral rotation, and side bending of her lumbar spine. She denies lower extremity pain, dysesthesia, or motor weakness. Her symptoms began following an acceleration in the intensity of her training 3 weeks ago. Given only this information, what is the most likely diagnosis?

108. How is the diagnosis of spondylolysis confirmed?

109. How should an acute fracture of the pars intraarticularis be treated?

110. What are the five types of spondylolisthesis?

111. How should children with symptomatic and asymptomatic type I spondylolisthesis be treated?

112. What are the indications for surgery in spondylolisthesis?

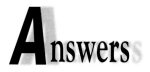**A**nswers

**104.** When a patient is walking uphill on a treadmill or riding a stationary bicycle, the lumbar spine is somewhat flexed, relatively increasing the diameter of the vertebral foramen, so resulting calf pain is probably due to vascular impairment of the lower limbs. If the patient's symptoms of calf pain are brought on during sustained lumbar extension when standing or lying prone, the cause is probably spinal stenosis causing intermittent claudication of the spinal cord or cauda equina.

**105.** Flexion-based exercises such as William's flexion may help relieve symptoms.

**106.** Any indication of compression of the spinal cord or cauda equina leading to neuropathy is of great significance. Clinicians should always be concerned with reports of abnormal bowel or bladder function, lower extremity motor loss, or the presence of true anesthesia in the lower extremities. Severe night pain or unexplained weight loss, although not typically associated with spinal stenosis, may indicate a neoplastic disorder and thus should be carefully investigated.

**107.** An acute fracture of the pars intraarticularis (spondylolysis). This condition is extremely common in divers because of the forceful hyperextension of the spine during diving and entry into the water. The presence of this condition is reinforced by the absence of radiculopathy/neuropathy and by the reproduction of symptoms with the posterior quadrant test (extension, with ipsilateral rotation and side bending of her lumbar spine).

**108.** Oblique view radiographs of the lumbar spine will often demonstrate this fracture (the "scotty dog sign"). However, when there is strong clinical evidence despite normal films, MRI or bone scan is a more sensitive test.

**109.** During the early stages, rest from the offending activity is very important. Many clinicians recommend the use of a lumbar orthosis to dramatically reduce lumbar spine motion for 3 to 6 weeks. Following this, a flexion-oriented exercise program may be very helpful.

**110.** Dysplastic spondylolisthesis (type I) is secondary to congenital malformation of the sacrum or neural arch of L5, which allows forward slippage of L5 on the sacrum. Isthmic spondylolisthesis (type II) is the most common form; it involves a lysis or elongation of the pars. Separation or dissolution of the pars allows forward slippage; elongation of the pars may be secondary to healing of repeated microfractures. Degenerative spondylolisthesis (type III) results from the loss of the ligamentous integrity of the annulus fibrosus and the facet joints. This is associated with the normal aging process of lumbar spinal segments. Traumatic spondylolisthesis (type IV) results from an acute fracture of the pars and requires casting. Pathologic spondylolisthesis (type V) results from bone tumors involving the pars.

**111.** If they are asymptomatic, do not treat but perhaps follow-up with lateral spine films every 6 months until age 15, then every 1 to 2 years until age 20. If they are symptomatic (mild to moderate symptoms), treat conservatively with decreased activities, antiinflammatory drugs, analgesics, bed rest, hamstring stretching, and occasionally a cast for 6 weeks to 3 months. No surgery is performed unless conservative treatment is not helpful for 6 months to 1 year. A patient with a recent fracture of the pars requires a cast for 3 to 6 months, which often leads to healing.

**112.** Greater than 50% slippage, persistent symptoms after an adequate trial of conservative treatment, neurologic findings, documented progression, postural deformity, and abnormal gait secondary to hamstring tightness.

**113.** A 33-year-old man complains of low back pain that radiates into his buttocks and down into the posterior thighs. He states that the pain in his legs occurs mostly with vigorous activity, such as running or heavy lifting. He complains of a relatively constant ache in his lower back that has been significantly worsened by some recent heavy lifting. The physical examination reveals some midline lumbosacral tenderness with a slight, palpable step-off between the spinous processes of L4 and L5. He has normal reflexes and no appreciable motor weakness. His radiographic films are shown in Figure 3-11, A and B. What is the radiographic diagnosis?

**Figure** 3-11    A

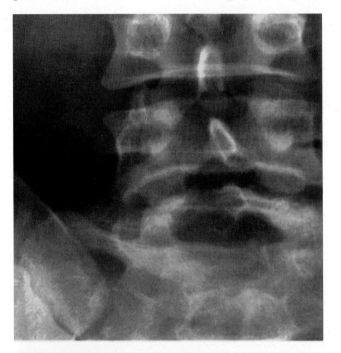

B

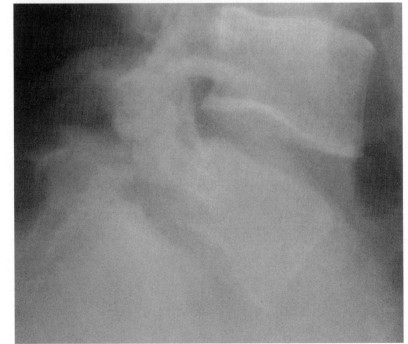

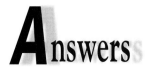

# Answers

**113.** This patient has a grade I, L5 on S1 spondylolisthesis. This appears to be the isthmic type.

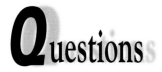

**114.** What is the approximate incidence of spondylolisthesis in the U.S. population?

**115.** What is the most common nerve root that is irritated with an L5 on S1 spondylolisthesis?

**116.** A 15-year-old soccer player has an acute onset of low back pain that radiates into his posterior thighs but not below his knees. Upon physical examination, he has tight hamstrings but no objective neurologic deficits. Radiographs demonstrate a grade 1 isthmic lytic spondylolisthesis. How should this patient be treated?

**117.** A 9-year-old girl with a 1-year history of intermittent low back pain is referred. She is a member of a gymnastic team. She has no objective neurologic deficits and no limitation in motion of her lumbosacral spine. Radiographs demonstrated a 55% spondylolisthesis of L5 on the sacrum. What is the treatment plan?

**118.** Is the radiographic finding of spondylolisthesis usually associated with LBP?

**119.** Are prone press-ups a useful exercise for patients with symptomatic spondylolisthesis?

**120.** A 54-year-old active woman complains of back and leg pain. She states that her back pain is almost constant and that her legs bother her after standing 10 minutes or walking farther than one block. This pain is relieved by sitting. Her symptoms have been getting gradually worse over the last 6 months despite bracing, physical therapy, and NSAIDs. Her studies are shown in Figure 3-12, A and B. What is the diagnosis?

**Figure** 3-12

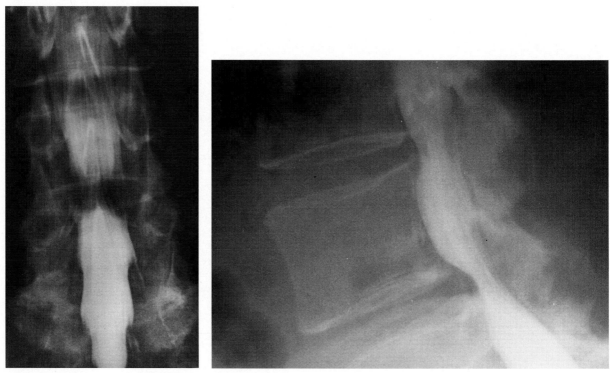

A                                    B

**121.** What is the etiology of this skeletal deformity?

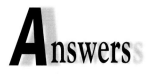**A**nswers

**114.** The best natural history study was performed by Frederickson and associates (*Journal of Bone and Joint Surgery*, 1984), which reported the overall incidence of spondylolisthesis to be approximately 6%. This percentage is the approximate incidence found at the end of adolescence. There does not appear to be a significant number of new cases of isthmic spondylolisthesis that develop after adolescence.

**115.** The L5 nerve root is the most commonly irritated nerve root in an L5 on S1 spondylolisthesis. The L5 root is impinged by the hypertrophic nonunion at the pars associated with residual foraminal and lateral recess stenosis. In addition, there is some pressure applied by the L5 pedicle as the L5 vertebral body descends into the pelvis with the higher grade spondylolisthesis slips.

**116.** With a lumbosacral orthosis and restriction of vigorous physical activities for 3 months. Once he is pain-free, he may resume all physical activities.

**117.** The patient is a surgical candidate. Slips of greater than 50% are at risk for progression of the deformity.

**118.** Not necessarily. Symptoms are more common in those people with an anterior translation of more than 50% of one vertebral body relative to the adjacent vertebral body. It is important to note that it is the instability associated with the spondylolisthesis rather than the actual degree of slippage that is the probable cause of symptoms.

**119.** Typically not. Lumbar extension may create forces that accentuate the anterior displacement of the vertebral body. Most practitioners recommend lumbar flexion exercises and a stabilization program.

**120.** This patient has a high-grade spinal stenosis associated with a degenerative spondylolisthesis of L4 and L5.

**121.** Degenerative spondylolisthesis is a result of segmental spine degeneration. The studies show no mechanical malformation (i.e., abnormal facets) as in type I dysplastic spondylolisthesis or bone defect as in type II isthmic spondylolisthesis. In this condition, the posterior elements are found to be intact, and there is believed to be gradual remodeling of the facet joints and increased motion caused by disc degeneration (Taillard, *Clinical Orthopedics and Related Research*, 1976). The associated disc space collapse and forward subluxation of L4 on L5 result in narrowing of the spinal canal thus leading to spinal stenosis.

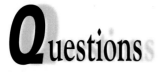

# Questions

122. What is the best treatment for this patient?

123. What are some possible observations and findings in the initial evaluation of a cervical spinal cord injury?

124. Describe the neurologic examination for sensation in cervical spinal cord injuries.

125. What are the sensory areas associated with C2, C3, C4, C5, C6, C7, C8, and T1?

126. What muscles are associated with C4, C5, C6, C7, C8, and T1?

127. Describe the two classifications of neurological injuries in the cervical spine.

128. What are the four types of incomplete spinal cord lesions?

129. Describe the clinical features and prognosis for each type of incomplete lesion.

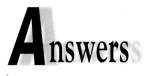
# Answers

122. This patient should be treated by a lumbar decompression at the involved level with a single segment posterior fusion. Herkowitz's prospective study (*Journal of Bone and Joint Surgery*, 1991) has suggested that patients treated with decompression and a posterior arthrodesis have less limiting back and leg pain, and a better functional result than patients treated with decompression without fusion.

123. Observe voluntary movements of the extremities. Palpate the neck. Hypotension in the range of 90/50 mm Hg is not uncommon in quadriplegic patients secondary to temporary generalized sympathectomy. This should not be confused with hemorrhagic shock since treatment is much different. Excessive fluids do not raise the blood pressure in neurogenic shock and may cause a serious overload of fluid. Pulse rate is usually normal (70 to 90 bpm). Look for associated injuries.

124. Pin prick and light touch are used to evaluate sensation transmitted in the anterior column. Deep pressure, vibration, and position sense are used in examination of the posterior column.

125. C2, the back of the scalp; C3, the anterior neck; C4, the anterior clavicles to the second rib interspace; C5, the deltoid area; C6, the radial forearm, thumb, and index and long fingers; C7, the ring and small fingers; C8, the ulnar border of the hand and forearm; T1, the medial arm.

126. C4, diaphragmatic muscle, trapezius, sternocleidomastoid; C5, deltoid and biceps; C6, extensor carpi radialis brevis and longus; C7, pronator teres, flexor carpi radialis, triceps, finger extensors; C8, flexor digitorum superficialis and profundus; T1, intrinsic muscles of the hand.

127. (1) Root injury; these are peripheral nerve injuries, which can recover somewhat; and (2) spinal cord injury; any sparing distal to the injury constitutes an incomplete lesion, and recovery varying from minimal to full is possible. Complete spinal cord injury demonstrates no function below the level of the injury.

128. (1) Brown-Sequard; (2) central cord; (3) anterior cord; and (4) posterior cord syndromes.

129. (1) Brown-Sequard syndrome (injury to the lateral half of the spinal cord) causes ipsilateral muscle paralysis and loss of proprioception, vibratory sense, and two-point discrimination. It causes contralateral loss of pain and temperature sensation. The prognosis for partial recovery is good. Most patients are able to ambulate and control their bowels and bladders once recovery is complete. (2) The central cord lesion is the most common incomplete syndrome. It is usually caused by an extension injury to an osteoarthritic spine. On radiograph, there is no fracture or dislocation. However, there is almost complete flaccid quadriplegia. The cause is cord compression by anterior osteophytes and the posterior ligamentum flavum, resulting in severe flaccid lower motor neuron paralysis of the fingers, hands, and arms. Damage to the central portion of the corticospinal and spinothalamic tracts in the white matter causes upper motor neuron spastic paralysis of the trunk and lower extremities. Sacral sparing is present when careful examination is performed. Sacral tracts, positioned on the periphery of the cord, are usually spared from injury. The prognosis is fair. Progressive return of motor and sensory function to the lower extremities and trunk can occur. However, there is poor recovery of hand function. Patients ambulate with a spastic gait. (3) The anterior cord syndrome is characterized by complete motor paralysis and sensory anesthesia, with the exception of dorsal column sparing, providing deep pressure and proprioception. The prognosis is good if recovery progresses during the first 24 hours. After 24 hours, if sacral motor function or sensation has not returned, prognosis is poor— less than 10% of patients make a functional recovery. (4) In the posterior cord syndrome, there is loss of deep pressure, deep pain, and proprioception, but with intact motor function, pain, and temperature sensation. Patients walk with a slapping gait similar to tabes dorsalis. This is a rare syndrome.

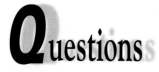

130. What complications are associated with early care of quadriplegia?

131. When is a urethral catheter placed in a spinal-cord-injured patient?

132. How often should you turn a spinal-cord-injured patient?

133. What steps can be taken to prevent pulmonary complications in the spinal-cord-injured patient?

134. How is the bladder managed in quadriplegia?

135. What is the bowel program in quadriplegia?

136. A patient sustained an L3 fracture-dislocation with loss of sensory and motor function below the L3 level. What type of neurologic injury did the patient sustain?

137. An 8-year-old boy sustained a complete spinal cord lesion at the T2 level. What are his chances of developing scoliosis?

138. What is spinal shock?

139. What is the significance of spinal shock?

140. What is sacral sparing?

141. What is the significance of sacral sparing in patients with spinal cord injuries?

142. What is the bulbocavernosus reflex?

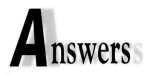

# Answers

130. Respiratory insufficiency and pneumonia, pressure ulceration, gastrointestinal bleeding, urinary retention with bladder distension and calculus formation, joint contracture, skeletal osteoporosis, and psychologic withdrawal.

131. A urethral catheter is placed for the first 24 to 48 hours. These patients have low blood pressure and demonstrate a sympathectomy-type picture. Urine output is usually low and therefore intravenous (IV) and oral fluids should be restricted during the first 24 to 48 hours. When urinary diuresis occurs at 36 to 48 hours, oral and IV fluids can be administered accordingly. The paralyzed bladder should be treated with intermittent catheterization.

132. Every 2 hours for skin care or use a side-to-side rotating bed.

133. Intermittent positive pressure breathing several times daily to maintain full expansion of the lungs with proper humidification is essential. Tracheostomy must be used if secretions cannot be cleared by nasal or oral suctioning. Pulmonary edema and right congestive heart failure may occur during the first week secondary to excessive fluid overload.

134. Catheterization for 24 to 40 hours followed by an intermittent catheterization program to develop automatic reflex emptying of the bladder. Consult a urologist.

135. Reflex emptying of the bowels with a suppository is the goal of bowel training. Every 2 to 3 days, a glycerine or bisacodyl Dulcolax suppository is introduced, occasionally with digital stimulation. Stool softeners are given p.r.n.

136. The patient sustained an injury to his cauda equina. Below the L1 level, lumbar and sacral nerve roots are injured; the spinal cord ends above this level in the conus medullaris. A spinal cord injury produces an upper motor neuron spastic paralysis; a cauda equina lesion produces a lower motor neuron flaccid paralysis. The lumbar and sacral root injuries may demonstrate progressive recovery whereas complete cord injuries do not.

137. All patients who are skeletally immature at the time of injury will develop a neuromuscular scoliosis.

138. Spinal shock is a transient phenomenon that occurs immediately following spinal cord injury when the reflex activity of the entire spinal cord is depressed. During spinal shock, the reflex arcs below the level of the spinal cord injury are absent. An example of this is the bulbocavernosus reflex, a sacral nerve root reflex mediated distal to the level of the cervical cord injury, that is often absent immediately following a cervical cord injury. Spinal shock usually begins to resolve within 24 hours. Return of reflex activity below the level of injury indicates the end of spinal shock.

139. The diagnosis of a complete or incomplete spinal cord injury cannot be made until the patient is out of spinal shock.

140. Sacral sparing is the presence of any voluntary control of the anal sphincter or toe flexor muscles or the presence of any perianal (saddle) sensation.

141. The presence of sacral sparing indicates the transmission of neural signals across the proximal level of the spinal cord injury. Preservation of this distal spinal cord functioning indicates that the patient has a partial spinal cord injury and may demonstrate some neurologic recovery.

142. The bulbocavernosus reflex is a spinal reflex in which there is anal sphincter contraction following glans penis or clitoris compression.

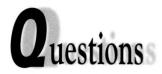

**143.** What is the significance of the bulbocavernosus reflex?

**144.** If a patient with a T8 spinal cord lesion has return of distal spinal reflexes (i.e., the bulbocavernosus reflex) and has no return of any distal voluntary motor or sensory function, what are his or her chances of having any significant functional recovery?

**145.** Which partial spinal cord injury has the best prognosis for functional recovery?

**146.** A 70-year-old man fell at home and struck his forehead on a night stand. He was brought directly to the emergency room. Upon physical examination, the patient demonstrated flaccid paralysis of the upper extremities, spastic involvement of the lower extremities, and intact sacral sensation and motor function. No fractures were seen on radiographs. The radiographs did demonstrate degenerative changes in the midcervical spine. What type of spinal cord injury pattern does the patient have?

**147.** If no fractures are present, what is the mechanism of injury to the spinal cord?

**148.** Why are the upper extremities involved more than the lower extremities?

**149.** What is the prognosis for recovery of the patient in question 146?

**150.** A 30-year-old woman is stabbed in the back at the midthoracic level with an ice pick. In the emergency room, she is noted to have no motor strength but preservation of sensation in her left leg and motor preservation without sensation in her right leg. What type of spinal cord injury did the patient sustain and which portion of the cord was injured?

**151.** A patient with a C5-C6 fracture-dislocation who demonstrates significant root recovery will need what rehabilitative appliances?

**152.** A patient sustained a C3-4 injury and has a C3 functional level. What rehabilitative appliance and apparatus is the patient a candidate for?

**153.** A patient with C5-level quadriplegia will have what functioning muscle groups and will need what type of upper extremity orthoses?

**154.** What type of ambulatory patterns are expected in thoracic-level paraplegia?

**155.** What type of ambulatory status and orthotics would be expected for a patient with L3-level paraplegia?

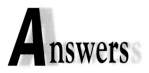

# Answers

143. Its absence indicates spinal shock. Its return indicates the end of spinal shock. With return of the bulbocavernosus reflex and the end of spinal shock, if the patient has no motor or sensory function below the level of injury or no sacral sparing, the spinal cord lesion is complete.

144. Patients with complete spinal cord injuries heralded by the return of distal spinal reflexes show no significant functional recovery.

145. Ninety percent of patients with Brown-Sequard syndrome make functional recoveries.

146. Central cord syndrome.

147. When the cervical spine is acutely hyperextended, the cervical cord is pinched between anterior bony spurs and the posterior infolded ligamentum flavum. This causes an ischemic insult to the central matter of the spinal cord.

148. Within the corticospinal and spinothalamic tracts, the upper extremity neural elements are positioned centrally and the lower extremity neural elements are positioned more peripherally. The hemorrhage and necrosis do not progress to the periphery, so these fiber tracts are left intact.

149. Fifty percent of patients recover some function. Flaccid paralysis in the upper extremities has a poor prognosis secondary to central gray matter necrosis.

150. The patient has a Brown-Sequard syndrome (spinal cord hemitransection). This unilateral injury to the spinal cord results in loss of ipsilateral motor function and contralateral sensation. The left half of the cord was injured.

151. A C6 quadriplegic patient will have voluntary wrist extension. He can be independent with sliding board transfers from bed to chair and able to propel a manual wheelchair with quadriplegic pegs on the wheel rim. He will require a wrist-driven flexor-hinge splint for prehension and may develop independent living skills, including feeding and personal hygiene.

152. A patient with a C3-level quadriplegia will have head and neck control but will require a ventilator at least at night. She will have loss of phrenic nerve function and is a candidate for an internal phrenic pacemaker. The patient may be able to propel an electric wheelchair with a chin-controlled device.

153. A patient with C5 quadriplegia will demonstrate voluntary shoulder abduction and elbow flexion. The patient will be unable to move his wrists or hands and will be dependent for transfers, feeding, and hygiene. An arm-control electric wheelchair may be necessary along with mobile arm supports and externally powered hand splints for prehension.

154. Patients with thoracic-level paraplegia may stand in parallel bars and are independent wheelchair ambulators.

155. Patients with L3 paraplegia have voluntary knee extension and can be expected to become community ambulators with knee–ankle–foot orthoses (KAFOs) or ankle–foot orthoses (AFOs).

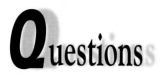

**156.** What is autonomic dysreflexia?

**157.** A 21-year-old rugby player is brought into the emergency room with an inability to move his arms and legs. This began 1 hour ago after injury during a contest. The patient's physical examination reveals flaccid paralysis of his lower extremities, complete absence of motor function in his left upper extremity, and trace firing of his right deltoid muscle. The patient has patchy sensation over the superior lateral aspects of both arms with the absence of sensation below the elbows bilaterally; there is no sensation to light touch or pin prick below the nipple lines bilaterally. The bulbocavernosus reflex is intact. His radiographs are shown in Figure 3-13, A through D. What is the clinical diagnosis?

**Figure** 3-13

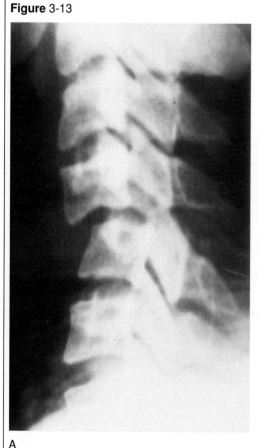

A

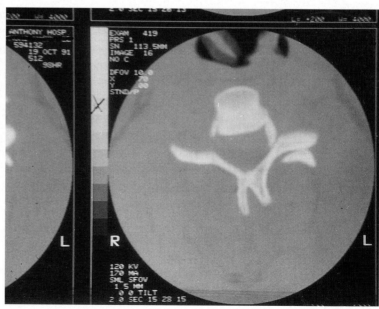

B

# Answers

**156.** Autonomic dysreflexia is associated with cervical cord lesions. Stimulation of the sympathetic nervous system in the thoracic region may result from bladder irritation or distension. Stimulation of the thoracic sympathetics causes peripheral arterial constriction and elevated systemic blood pressure. The rise in blood pressure stimulates the carotid sinus to slow the heart rate. The parasympathetics cannot modulate the sympathetic response because of the cervical cord injury. As a result, the blood pressure can continue to rise and the heart rate to fall. The patient complains of headache and presents with systolic pressures of 200 to 300 mm Hg and bradycardia. Treatment is through removal of the thoracic sympathetic stimulus and usually responds to simple bladder drainage.

**157.** The clinical diagnosis for this patient is C5 quadriplegia secondary to a C5-C6 facet dislocation-subluxation. You can say that this patient has a complete spinal cord injury because of his physical examination and the presence of a bulbocavernosus reflex. If this patient were in spinal shock (i.e., absence of the bulbocavernosus reflex within the first 24 hours after the injury), it would be impossible to make the diagnosis of a complete spinal cord injury at this time.

**Figure** 3-13 continued

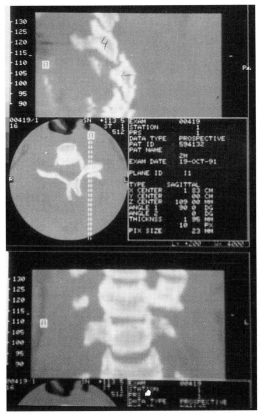

C

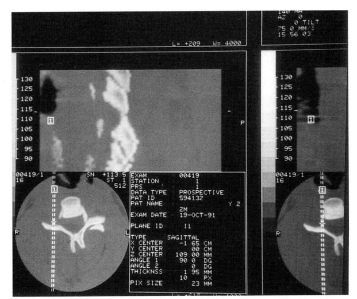

D

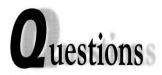

**158.** What is the role of steroids in the treatment of this patient?

**159.** What further treatment should be immediately instituted for the patient in question 157?

**160.** A 13-year-old boy sustained an abdominal injury from blunt trauma after being struck by a car. The patient developed midthoracic level paraplegia 2 hours after the accident while being prepared for abdominal surgery in which a ruptured spleen was removed. He had a normal spine series taken on admission. What is the cause of this neural deficit?

**161.** What caused injury to this artery?

**162.** How can this diagnosis be confirmed?

**163.** What is the prognosis for improvement through immediate decompression of the spinal cord in the patient described in question 160?

**164.** Four hours after admission, a previously intact 10-year-old girl with an unstable L2 fracture-dislocation notices loss of feeling in her legs and weakness in attempts to move her legs. Your examination confirms these findings. Further evaluation fails to demonstrate any thoracic or abdominal trauma, or hypotensive episodes. What should be done?

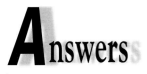 **nswers**

158. Treatment with high-dose methylprednisolone is recommended based upon the study by Bracken and associates (*New England Journal of Medicine*, 1990) that suggested there was improved neurologic recovery in patients with complete spinal cord injuries who are treated with high-dose methylprednisolone within the first 8 hours after their injuries. Though the neurologic recovery was small and not always functionally significant, there was a statistically significant improvement in these patients' motor and sensory scores if treated with methylprednisolone as compared with a placebo.

159. In this awake, alert, cooperative patient with an acute complete spinal cord injury, early spinal alignment should be achieved. Numerous studies by Rizzolo (*Spine*, 1994) and others have reported a significant benefit and safety from early cervical traction for reduction of such an injury. There is little to lose and much to gain in terms of potential early neurologic recovery through spinal reduction in the patient with complete quadriplegia by instituting early cervical traction. The functional return of even one root level is significant in this situation.

160. In contrast to cervical paraplegia associated with spinal cord injury without radiographic abnormality (SCIWORA) noted in infants and newborns, delayed midthoracic paraplegia in a teenager with normal spine films is suggestive of a vascular insult to the cord in the watershed area served by the artery of Adamkiewicz.

161. Vascular injury is usually associated with blunt chest or abdominal trauma, severe hypotension from a ruptured spleen, or retroperitoneal hematoma.

162. MRI is the best imaging option.

163. The prognosis for neurologic improvement is poor. In this patient, paraplegia from a vascular injury to the cord is usually permanent and complete. Surgical decompression is not indicated.

164. The problem is a deterioration in neurologic status in a previously neurologically intact patient. In the absence of findings suggestive of an isolated vascular injury to the cord, the patient should be taken to the operating room to align the spine and decompress the cord. Immediate intravenous administration of steroids has advocates as a preoperative measure to decrease edema about the cord.

**165.** Identify the structures shown in Figure 3-14.

**Figure** 3-14

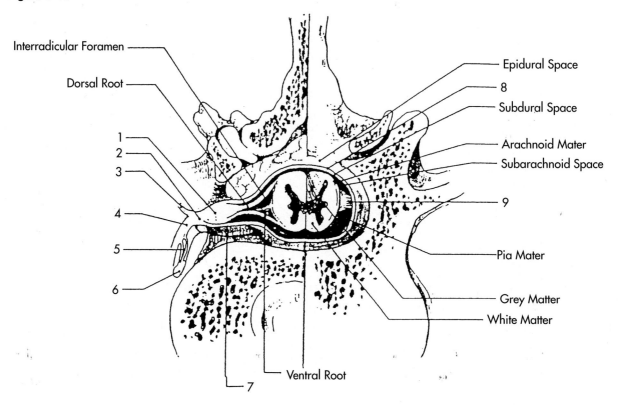

Interradicular Foramen

Dorsal Root

Epidural Space

8

Subdural Space

Arachnoid Mater

Subarachnoid Space

1
2
3

9

4

5

6

Pia Mater

Grey Matter

White Matter

Ventral Root

7

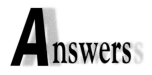

**165.** (1) Dorsal root ganglion; (2) spinal n.; (3) dorsal primary ramus; (4) ventral primary ramus; (5) rami communicans; (6) sympathetic ganglion; (7) sinuvertebral n.; (8) dura mater; and (9) denticulate lig.

# Chapter 4

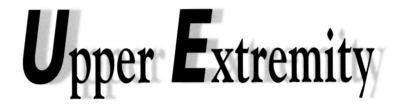

# Upper Extremity

CASEY JONES, MD

DAVE STREGE, MD

CAROLYN T. WADSWORTH, MS, PT, OCS, CHT

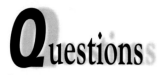

# Questions

1. A 42-year-old man sustains a closed fracture of the distal third of the humeral shaft after a fall from a ladder. Immediate evaluation reveals an ipsilateral wrist drop. Closed reduction of the fracture results in satisfactory fracture alignment without bayonet opposition, but there is no immediate change in his neurologic status. How should this patient be managed?

2. Injury of the axillary nerve results in what functional deficits?

3. The rotator cuff of the shoulder is composed of which muscles?

4. Which muscles insert on the greater and lesser tuberosities of the proximal humerus?

5. Describe the ligaments that stabilize the acromioclavicular joint.

6. Horizontal stability of the acromioclavicular joint is controlled by which ligaments?

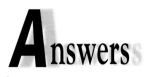**nswers**

1. Because of the close proximity of the radial nerve to the humeral shaft in distal third humeral fractures, radial nerve injuries are probably the most common complication of these fractures. Holstein and Lewis are credited with describing this relationship in these fractures. As the majority of these radial nerve palsies (approximately 90%) are neurapraxias, resolution would be expected with time. Appropriate management would be to wait for at least 3 to 4 months until clinical or electromyographic (EMG) evidence of muscle reinnervation should have occurred before considering nerve exploration.

2. (1) Weakness of shoulder flexion, abduction, and extension due to paralysis of the anterior, middle, and posterior deltoid muscle; (2) weakness of shoulder external rotation due to paralysis of the teres minor muscle; and (3) decreased sensation in a variable region over the lower half of the deltoid area due to loss of the cutaneous sensory branch of the axillary nerve—the superolateral brachial cutaneous nerve.

3. Subscapularis, supraspinatus, infraspinatus, and teres minor muscles.

4. The greater and lesser tuberosities of the proximal humerus are separated by the bicipital groove through which passes the tendon of the long head of the biceps. The supraspinatus, infraspinatus, and teres minor insert into the greater tuberosity. The subscapularis inserts into the lesser tuberosity.

5. The acromioclavicular joint is a diarthrodial joint with a fibrocartilaginous intraarticular disc. It is stabilized by two sets of ligaments. The acromioclavicular joint capsular ligaments are the superior, inferior, anterior, and posterior ligaments, of which the superior is the strongest. Additionally, the coracoclavicular ligament provides support to the acromioclavicular joint. The coracoclavicular ligament is a strong ligament composed of two components: the conoid and trapezoid (see Figure 4-1).

**Figure** 4-1

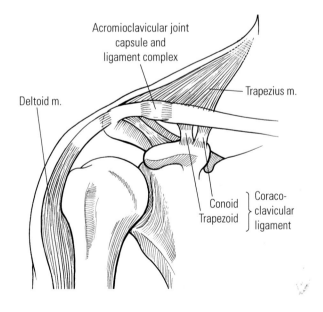

6. The acromioclavicular ligaments control horizontal stability. Vertical stability is controlled by the coracoclavicular ligaments.

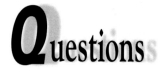

7. Rockwood classifies acromioclavicular joint injuries into six types. What are they?

8. What is the treatment of choice for each type of acromioclavicular joint injury?

9. How should a sternoclavicular injury be treated?

10. The site for safe aspiration of the elbow joint is defined by what anatomic landmarks?

11. The mobile wad of Henry is composed of which muscles?

12. What is the normal carrying angle of the elbow?

13. Bifurcation of the brachial artery occurs at what level?

14. Describe the relationship of the median nerve to the brachial artery in the arm.

15. What functional arc of motion at the elbow is considered necessary for most daily activities?

16. A 20-year-old woman falls while playing volleyball, landing on her left elbow. She complains of poorly localized elbow pain. Radiographs demonstrate no evidence of fracture or dislocation, but anterior and posterior fat pads are noted (see Figure 4-2). What is the significance of this finding?

**Figure** 4-2

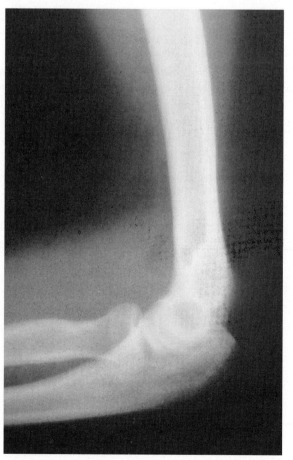

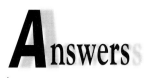

# Answers

7. Type I: sprain of the acromioclavicular ligament with no disruption of the acromioclavicular or coracoclavicular ligaments (no instability); type II: acromioclavicular ligament disruption leading to horizontal acromioclavicular instability (subluxation); type III: " classic" acromioclavicular dislocation with disruption of the acromioclavicular and coracoclavicular ligaments; type IV: posterior dislocation of the acromioclavicular joint (into or through the trapezius); type V: superior dislocation of the acromioclavicular joint with severe displacement; and type VI: inferior dislocation of the acromioclavicular joint.

8. Types I and II: symptomatic treatment with sling and early range-of-motion (ROM) exercises; type III: for patients older than 25 and nonlaborers, only symptomatic treatment is required. For the heavy laborer or those less than 25 years of age, operative repair with some type of internal fixation (commonly a coracoclavicular screw); and types IV, V, and VI: attempted closed reduction. If reduced, treat as type III. If unreduced, proceed to open reduction and internal fixation.

9. A type I injury (mild sprain) is treated with ice, a sling for 3 to 5 days, and then a return to daily activities. A type II injury (subluxation) is reduced and placed in a figure-eight clavicle strap, or the arm is supported in a sling for 1 to 2 weeks followed by gradual use of the arm. In a type III injury (dislocation), closed reduction can be performed for anterior or posterior dislocation and a figure-eight clavicle strap worn by the patient for 4 to 6 weeks. If an anterior dislocation recurs after reduction and application of figure-eight dressing, the deformity is accepted, since this is less risky than the potential problems of operative repair and internal fixation. A sling is worn for 2 weeks and then ROM exercises are begun when the patient is comfortable. A posterior stenoclavicular dislocation is usually stable after reduction and can be maintained in a figure-eight dressing.

10. Elbow joint aspirations are safely performed laterally within the triangle formed by the lateral epicondyle of the humerus, radial head, and the tip of the olecranon.

11. Brachioradialis, extensor carpi radialis longus, and extensor carpi radialis brevis muscles.

12. The angle formed by the intersection of the long axis of the humerus and the axis of the ulna with the elbow in full extension is a measure of the carrying angle of the elbow. Normally, the carrying angle measures 10° valgus in males and 13° valgus in females.

13. The brachial artery bifurcates into the ulnar and radial arteries within the proximal forearm at the level of the radial head.

14. In the upper arm, the median nerve lies lateral to the brachial artery. In the midarm at the intramuscular septum, the nerve crosses anterior to the artery so that in the distal arm, the nerve lies medial to the brachial artery.

15. The normal ROM at the elbow is from 0° to 145° of flexion. However, most daily activities can be carried out within a functional arc of 30° to 130°. Additionally, normal pronation of 75° and supination of 85° is well beyond the functional arc of 50° of pronation and  50° of supination necessary to carry out most daily activities.

16. A fat pad sign is a radiolucent stripe found within the soft tissue shadow of extremity radiographs and is due to the low radiodensity of adipose tissue. At the elbow, anterior and posterior fat pads are most easily seen on the lateral projection. These fat pads are intracapsular but extrasynovial. The anterior fat pad is normally visible anterior to the coronoid fossa of the humerus. The posterior fat pad is normally obscured on the lateral view owing to its position within the olecranon fossa. If the posterior fat pad is viewed or the anterior fat pad is enlarged, intraarticular pathology is suspected due to increased intraarticular fluid collections from inflammation or hemarthrosis after trauma. (If no posterior fat pad is viewed, the presence of an anterior fat pad is probably a normal finding.)

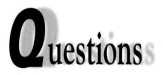

17. What role does the elbow play in upper extremity function, and what is the significance of elbow injury?

18. How is a nondisplaced transcondylar distal humeral fracture treated?

19. A 72-year-old woman slips and falls in an icy parking lot, landing on her elbow. Radiographs of the swollen elbow reveal an extensively comminuted T intercondylar humeral fracture. How should this fracture be managed?

20. After initiating postinjury elbow rehabilitation, why are passive manipulation and stretching generally not recommended?

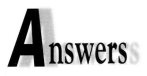

# Answers

17. The importance of the elbow in upper extremity function is often overshadowed by the versatility of the shoulder or the intricacy of the hand, but it serves as a vital link in a mechanical chain of levers. The elbow is an effective accelerator and is critical to positioning and manipulating the hand.

    The elbow is the most commonly injured joint in children, and is frequently affected by overuse disorders in adolescents and adults. Painful dysfunction and restricted motion in the elbow can impose severe restrictions on use of the upper extremity and the accessibility of the hand to other body areas, as well as to the environment.

18. A nondisplaced transcondylar distal humerus fracture is immobilized for 1 to 2 weeks in a long-arm posterior splint with the elbow at 90° to 110° of flexion. This is followed by early active ROM exercises and frequent radiographic evaluations for signs of displacement.

19. Owing to poor results with open reduction and internal fixation of extensively comminuted fractures and the osteopenic bone of the elderly, closed treatment with either olecranon traction or the "bag of bones" technique is recommended. In the latter, the elbow is placed in maximum flexion within the limits dictated by swelling and circulatory compromise. The arm is placed in a collar and cuff with the elbow hanging free so that gravity can be used to obtain ligamentotaxis and possible fracture reduction. At 2 weeks, motion is begun in flexion at the elbow. The sling is gradually loosened in order to increase extension motion and the sling is discarded at 6 weeks. In the younger population with better-quality bone, these fractures are treated with open reduction internal fixation.

20. There is a high risk of heterotopic bone formation and subsequent ankylosis.

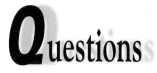

21. A 12-year-old boy is brought to your office by his mother. She relates a history of an elbow fracture when the boy was 9 years old, which required manipulation and casting in an operating room. The injury was then treated in a cast for several weeks after which her son began ROM exercises. He did not regain full motion for a number of months. When he did, he was noted to have an elbow deformity. The parents were told by the treating physician that the deformity would correct with time, but after 3 years, they can detect no improvement. Clinically, he appears as shown in Figure 4-3, A and B. His current radiographic films are seen in Figure 4-3, C and D. The elbow fracture is likely what specific type of fracture?

**Figure** 4-3

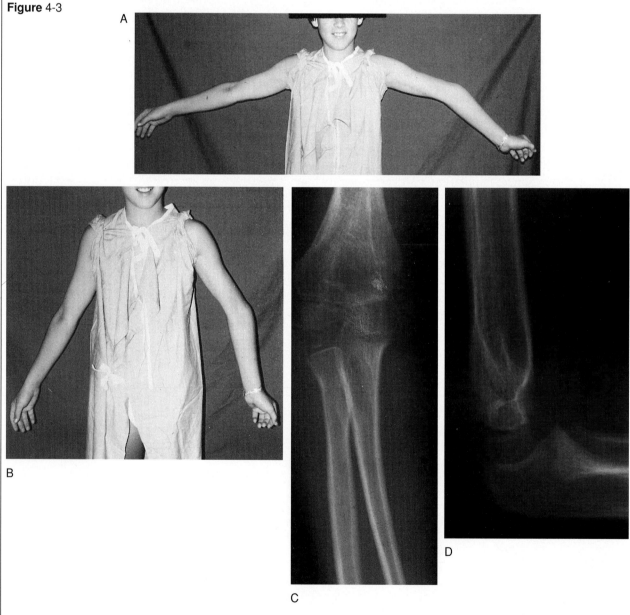

22. How likely is it that this 12-year-old boy with open physes will yet remodel his distal humerus and correct his deformity?

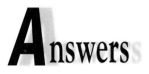**nswers**

21. The most common type of fracture around the elbow in skeletally immature individuals is the supracondylar fracture. A well-recognized complication of this fracture is cubitus varus (gunstock deformity). Men and boys predominate in this type of fracture. The ratio of males to females is 2 to 1. The supracondylar fracture occurs most frequently in children in the 3- to 10-year-old age group, and this is most likely the diagnosis in this case.

22. Several studies have confirmed that after a supracondylar humeral fracture, even in skeletally immature patients, the varus–valgus configuration of the elbow does not change or remodel.

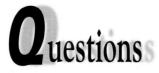

23. In children, what other fractures of the distal humerus, if any, can produce cubitus varus?

24. How are childhood supracondylar fractures classified?

25. What nerve is most commonly injured with childhood supracondylar fracture?

26. How are supracondylar fractures of the elbow in children treated?

27. A worried couple brings their 3-year-old daughter to the emergency room for severe pain and decreased function of her left elbow. An hour earlier, the child's older brother was playfully swinging her by the arms, when suddenly she experienced discomfort and refused to use her left arm. Her parents are concerned that she has a fracture. Is this likely?

28. How are radial head fractures classified?

29. A 24-year-old man undergoes radial head excision at the time of injury for a comminuted radial head fracture involving the entire radial head. The patient regains excellent ROM of the right elbow, but his postoperative course is complicated by increasing ipsilateral wrist pain. What is the likely cause of this wrist pain?

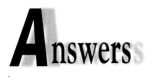

**23.** Cubitus varus is the most common osseous deformity produced by both medial and lateral humeral condylar fractures in children. Although both medial and lateral condylar fractures can produce valgus, they both more commonly result in varus. In medial and lateral condylar fractures of the immature distal humerus, the varus which may be produced is usually mild and rarely requires treatment.

**24.** A number of classifications have been proposed, but the most commonly used classification separates these fractures into flexion type (5% of supracondylar fractures) and extension type (95% of supracondylar fractures).

  The flexion type results from direct trauma against the posterior aspect of the flexed elbow. The distal fragment lies anterior to the humerus and is flexed at the elbow.

  The extension type occurs as a result of a fall on the outstretched arm. The distal humeral fragment is displaced posteriorly and proximally secondary to the pull of the triceps. Extension-type fractures are further classified as type I, nondisplaced; type II, angulated but with an intact cortical hinge; and type III, completely displaced. Type III extension fractures are then usually subclassified as posteromedial or posterolateral. Of these, posteromedially displaced fractures account for 75% of cases.

**25.** The radial nerve is injured with the greatest frequency. This is reasonable when you consider that posteromedial, type III extension injuries are the most common type III injuries and are the type to most likely put the radial nerve at risk.

**26.** If possible, obtain accurate anatomic alignment with closed manual reduction or traction, and splint the elbow in 120° of flexion for 3 weeks in a posterior shell; then change the splint to 90° for an additional 3 weeks. Displaced, unstable fractures may require Kirschner wire (K-wire) fixation, with splinting at 90°. Open fractures, articular fractures, and fractures with significant neurovascular compromise require open reduction and internal fixation (ORIF) and splinting.

**27.** It is unlikely that this child sustained a fracture from relatively mild trauma. Rather, she has "nursemaid's elbow," a distally displaced radial head. This is manually reduced by supinating the forearm, then flexing the elbow. The patient should be able to resume normal function and requires no further treatment.

**28.** Radial head fractures are classified into four types: type I: nondisplaced; type II: marginal fracture with displacement; type III: comminuted fracture involving the entire radial head; and type IV: any radial head fracture with simultaneous elbow dislocation.

**29.** The association of a radial head fracture with disruption of the distal radioulnar joint is called an Essex-Lopresti injury. Disruption of the interosseous membrane of the forearm as well as the ligamentous support of the distal radioulnar joint is believed to occur concurrently with the radial head fracture. This ligamentous disruption after radial head excision allows greater than normal proximal radial migration. With time, this results in an increasing ulnar positive variance with subsequent subluxation of the distal radioulnar joint and increasingly painful ulnar abutment at the wrist. Various treatment alternatives have been advised for this problem, including Silastic radial head replacement, radiocapitellar joint replacement, tightening of the interosseous membrane, ulnar shortening, ulnar head excision, and radioulnar synostosis. At this time, there is no ideal solution.

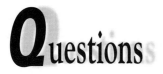

30. A patient with an elbow injury demonstrates radiographic evidence of a comminuted radial head fracture and a fracture of the coronoid process. What is the significance of this injury and how is it treated?

31. A patient is seen in the emergency room and found to have an acute posterior dislocation of the elbow. How should this be treated?

32. After successful closed reduction of a posterior dislocation of the elbow, how should postreduction care and rehabilitation proceed?

33. What is the most common nerve injury seen after an elbow dislocation?

34. What are the most common sites of involvement of heterotopic ossification after elbow dislocation?

35. Four months after elbow dislocation, a patient is noted to have a 60° flexion contracture with radiographic evidence of mild heterotopic ossification in the anterior capsule. How should treatment proceed?

36. A patient is noted to have a 30° flexion contracture at the elbow 12 months after elbow dislocation. The patient has undergone extensive physical therapy including dynamic splinting prior to this time. How should management proceed?

37. A 3% to 5% incidence of ectopic bone formation is noted to occur after fractures or dislocations about the elbow. What are the risk factors that increase the likelihood of ectopic bone formation?

38. What is the functional loss resulting from distal biceps tendon rupture and how should this problem be managed acutely?

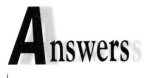
# Answers

30. Combined fractures of the radial head and coronoid process tend to be very unstable and may be associated with medial or lateral collateral ligament disruption. This requires ORIF of the coronoid process fracture or reattachment of the brachialis muscle to the proximal ulna as well as repair of torn medial or lateral collateral ligaments. If salvage of the radial head is not possible due to comminution, prosthetic radial head replacement is usually necessary to maintain stability at the elbow.

31. After initial examination and assessment of neurovascular function of the involved upper extremity and after administration of appropriate sedation or general anesthetic, closed reduction should be attempted. Most reduction maneuvers involve application of countertraction to the arm as traction is applied to the wrist and forearm. Medial or lateral displacement is corrected first. As distal traction is continued, anterior pressure is directed on the olecranon and the elbow is gradually flexed. This unlocks the coronoid out of the olecranon fossa. Most practitioners recommend avoiding hyperextension maneuvers owing to the potential for injury to the brachialis muscle and for heterotopic ossification. If after several attempts, closed reduction cannot be accomplished, proceed with open reduction. After reduction is accomplished, the elbow should be brought through a full ROM and neurovascular status again assessed.

32. The elbow should be splinted at 90° of flexion. The splint is removed within a few days and early active ROM exercises are begun. A removable elbow splint may be used for comfort between exercise periods during the first 1 to 2 weeks. Passive motion and stretching are avoided during the early rehabilitation period.

33. Injuries to the median, radial, and ulnar nerves at the time of elbow dislocation are relatively common. Therefore, careful neurovascular assessment of the involved extremities is important before and after attempted reduction maneuvers. Most commonly, the ulnar nerve is injured, resulting from valgus stress at the time of dislocation. Injury to the radial nerve is least commonly reported.

34. The medial and lateral collateral ligaments, the anterior capsule, and the brachialis muscle.

35. Surgical intervention should be delayed until the osseous elements are completely mature. While this is believed to occur at 9 to 12 months after time of injury, there is no reliable means of predicting tissue maturation. Radioactive isotope scanning has not been shown to be completely reliable as an indicator for tissue maturation. This patient would most likely benefit from physical therapy including heat, ultrasound, dynamic splinting, and gentle active assisted stretching exercises.

36. Since the results of surgical release in obtaining extension beyond 30° are unpredictable, the general recommendation is to refrain from surgery for flexion contractures of less than 45°. Additionally, as the functional ROM is 30° to 130°, a lack of the last 30° of full extension does not tend to be an overwhelming functional deficit. In this case, no further treatment need be offered.

37. Head injury increases the likelihood of ectopic bone formation to 89%. Dislocation combined with fracture about the elbow, frequent manipulation in reduction attempts, delayed reduction, and delayed motion at the elbow all increase the likelihood of ectopic bone formation. Ectopic ossification also occurs in 1% to 3% of patients with burns. Injuries in the younger patient population decrease the likelihood of ectopic bone formation.

38. If left untreated, distal biceps tendon ruptures result in approximately 40% loss of strength of both flexion and supination at the elbow. Therefore the treatment of choice is surgical repair of the complete distal biceps tendon rupture within 7 to 10 days of injury. However, as other muscles surrounding the elbow are available to assume the function of the biceps muscle, surgical repair in the elderly patient, in whom demands on the upper extremity are minimal, may not be warranted.

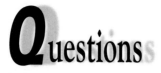

39. Lateral epicondylitis is the most common cause of lateral elbow pain. What other entities should be considered before making this diagnosis?

40. What is the pathologic process and the specific anatomic site of involvement of lateral epicondylitis?

41. What provocative tests are used to support the diagnosis of lateral epicondylitis?

42. How is lateral epicondylitis treated?

43. Would the presence of calcification in the extensor origin seen on a radiograph affect your recommended treatment?

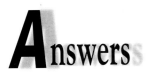

**Answers**

39. Injury or fracture of the radial head or capitellum, lateral elbow instability, and radial tunnel syndrome.

40. Lateral epicondylitis (or "tennis elbow") is the term frequently used to describe an overuse syndrome resulting in lateral elbow pain. This results in a tendinitis occurring at the origin of the extensor carpi radialis brevis (ERCB) muscle. The pathologic findings consist of replacement of normal tendon collagen fibers with tissue composed of fibroblasts and vascular granulation-like tissue described by Nirschl as "angiofibroblastic proliferation."

41. Pain over the lateral epicondyle is produced by resisted wrist extension or passive wrist flexion with the elbow extended. It can also be provoked by resisted middle finger extension with the forearm supinated and the elbow extended. Another maneuver is Mill's test, which involves flexing the wrist and pronating the forearm, **then** extending the elbow.

42. Symptoms usually respond to nonsurgical treatment. Initial management should consist of rest and refraining from activities that aggravate the condition and use of aspirin or nonsteroidal antiinflammatory drugs (NSAIDs). Then use physical therapy modalities (heat, ultrasound, cortisone phonophoresis) followed by aggressive stretching and strengthening exercises. This may be supplemented with wrist cock-up or lateral elbow counterforce bracing. Long-term management includes activity and tool modification and continued exercise to maintain flexibility, strength, and endurance. If there is no response to this treatment, consideration should be given to local corticosteroid injection. In the rare case where symptoms continue to persist after nonsurgical management, surgical intervention should be considered. This involves excision of the abnormal angiofibroblastic tissue at the origin of the extensor carpi radialis brevis muscle.

43. Such calcifications are seen in approximately a quarter of the cases of lateral epicondylitis. They have no prognostic significance and should not alter your planned treatment.

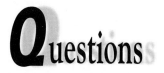

**44.** A 34-year-old woman, employed as a seamstress in a factory, complains of pain in her left forearm. She has no history of trauma, but feels that her work aggravates her symptoms. Upon examination, you note localized dorsal tenderness 5 cm distal to her lateral epicondyle. There is no apparent swelling or structural change. Sensation is intact. What is her probable diagnosis, and what provocative tests would help confirm it?

# nswers

**44.** This patient likely has radial tunnel syndrome, i.e., posterior interosseous nerve compressive neuropathy. The nerve may be compressed by fibrous bands anterior to the radial head, a vascular arcade (leash of Henry), the tendinous margin of the ECRB muscle, beneath the Arcade of Frohse (proximal edge of the supinator muscle), or between the two heads of the supinator muscle (see Figure 4-4).

Provocative tests include: fully pronating the forearm with the wrist flexed, resisting elbow flexion with the forearm supinated, resisting supination with the elbow extended, and resisting middle finger extension with the elbow extended. Infrequently, patients with this syndrome demonstrate weakness in the extensor digitorum communis (EDC), extensor carpi ulnaris (ECU), abductor pollicis longus (APL), extensor digitiminimi (EDM), extensor pollicis brevis (EPB), extensor pollicis longus (EPL), and/or extensor indicis proprius (EIP) muscles.

**Figure** 4-4

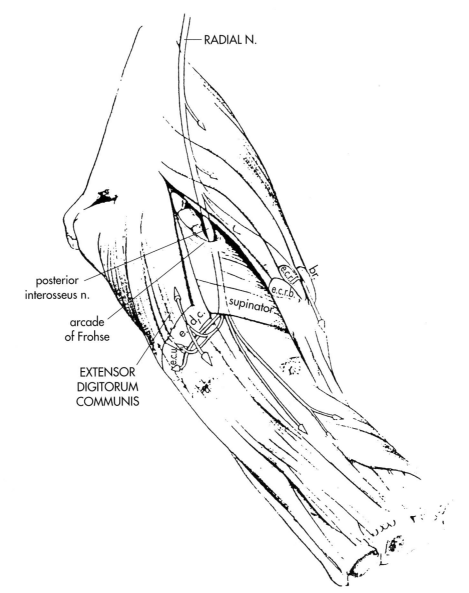

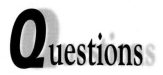

45. What structures at the elbow are most susceptible to injury in the throwing athlete?

46. What are the radiographic and physical findings associated with "Little Leaguer's elbow"?

47. How is "Little Leaguer's elbow" treated?

48. A 10-year-old boy complains of a dull, aching pain in his right, dominant elbow. He has no history of acute trauma, but is completing his second season of baseball where he usually plays first base. Examination reveals localized tenderness and swelling over the lateral joint line. He lacks 14° of elbow extension. Radiographs show the capitellar epiphysis is slightly irregular and smaller than the opposite normal epiphysis. What are your recommendations for management of this patient?

49. A 15-year-old girl has developed right dominant elbow discomfort over the last month. She is a member of her high school girl's golf team and plays daily. Her pain is over the medial side of the joint and is increased by valgus stress and resisted pronation and wrist flexion. What conditions must be considered in a differential diagnosis?

50. Before attempting elbow arthrodesis, what other upper extremity functions should be taken into consideration?

# Answers

**45.** Repetitive valgus stress occurs at the elbow of the throwing athlete. The primary stabilizer to valgus stress is the relatively strong anterior oblique medial collateral ligament, and the secondary restraint to valgus stress is the radiocapitellar articulation at the elbow. With repetitive valgus stress, there is attenuation or incompetence of the medial collateral ligament and secondary injury to the radiocapitellar joint (see Figure 4-5).

**Figure** 4-5

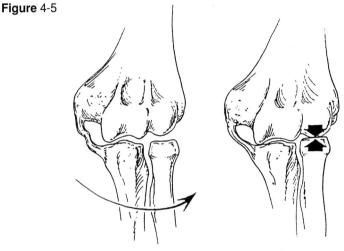

**46.** "Little Leaguer's elbow," a condition found in young, throwing athletes, is manifested by progressive medial elbow pain, especially with throwing. Owing to the repetitive valgus stress of throwing as well as the strong pull of the flexor muscles off the medial epicondyle, this condition is thought to be due to a subtle stress fracture through the physis of the medial epicondyle. Upon physical examination, there is point tenderness over the medial epicondyle as well as an elbow flexion contracture, frequently greater than 15°. Radiographic findings, if present, consist of subtle widening or even fragmentation of the epiphyseal line of the medial epicondyle when compared with the opposite normal elbow.

**47.** Treatment is always nonoperative. Most patients respond to a period of rest and refraining from the aggravating activity for a period of 2 to 3 weeks. This should be followed by supervised physical therapy with progressive strengthening and reconditioning before returning to throwing activities.

**48.** This patient has osteochondrosis of the capitellum, or Panner's disease. It is the most common source of elbow pain in 7- to 12-year-old children. The process begins as a degeneration or necrosis of the capitellar ossification center, followed by recalcification. It is usually self-limiting, but activity modification is required. The patient must refrain from throwing that increases valgus loading of the elbow and radiocapitellar compression. He should be placed on an exercise program to restore full ROM and strength of the upper extremities. When he is asymptomatic, he may begin a controlled return to activity, with instruction in throwing mechanics.

**49.** This patient could have medial epicondylitis (involving the origin of the pronator teres and flexor carpi radialis [FCR] muscles), avulsion of the medial epicondyle, or attenuation of the ulnar collateral ligament.

**50.** The function of the shoulder and elbow is to position the hand in space. When considering elbow arthrodesis, satisfactory motion of the shoulder is absolutely essential, or the patient will lose his or her ability to position the hand. Bilateral elbow arthrodesis should not be considered because the functional limitation is too great.

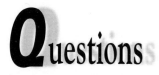
# Questions

**51.** What is the optimal position for elbow arthrodesis?

**52.** What anatomic structures are responsible for impingement tendinitis of the shoulder?

**53.** Why is the supraspinatus tendon most commonly involved in impingement tendinitis and rotator cuff tears?

**54.** In addition to supraspinatus tendinitis and rotator cuff tears, impingement can predispose the patient to what other conditions?

**55.** What is the function of the rotator cuff?

**56.** Neer has classified impingement tendinitis into three stages. What are these stages?

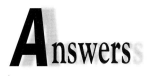

# Answers

51. In the patient with satisfactory motion at the elbow and wrist, arthrodesis at 90° of flexion will optimize functioning. With adaptive motion at the neck, shoulder, and wrist, the hand can reach the mouth and writing can also be done comfortably.

52. Structures which cause narrowing of the subacromial space. Bony changes and osteophyte formation tend to occur on the anteroinferior surface of the acromion, along the coracoacromial ligament, especially as it inserts into the anteromedial portion of the acromion (see Figure 4-1). Osteophytes also occur at the acromioclavicular joint.

53. Involvement of the supraspinatus tendon in impingement tendinitis and rotator cuff tears is probably related to the vascularity of this tendon. The area of the tendon just proximal to the site of insertion tends to be hypovascular, a "watershed zone." Vascular filling within this area is dependent upon shoulder positioning. With the arm in an adducted position, the tendon is compressed over the humeral head and vascular filling is prevented. With the arm in abduction, compression of the tendon across the humeral head is decreased and vascular filling occurs. Hypovascularity, in addition to mechanical impingement of the supraspinatus tendon at this site, can then result in inflammation as well as the impaired ability to heal and repair small tears within the rotator cuff. The tendon's location directly between the greater tuberosity and the anterior acromion place it at risk for impingement during arm elevation.

54. Impingement can produce subacromial bursitis with acute painful limitation of shoulder movement. Also, degenerative changes within the rotator cuff, often secondary to impingement, can irritate the overlying bursa.

    Impingement can contribute to degenerative changes of the long head of the biceps tendon, eventually leading to rupture. Tendon rupture then becomes part of the cycle involving additional impingement secondary to the loss of humeral head restraint.

55. The rotator cuff serves multiple functions. It assists with shoulder abduction, internal rotation (produced by the subscapularis muscle), and external rotation (provided by the infraspinatus and teres minor muscles). The rotator cuff additionally serves to stabilize the glenohumeral joint by depressing the humeral head in the glenoid fossa. When portions of the rotator cuff are selectively contracted, these muscles can serve to resist displacing forces, thereby preventing shoulder subluxation and dislocation.

56. Stage I is edema and hemorrhage, stage II is fibrosis and tendinitis, and stage III is tendon degeneration and rupture.

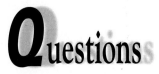
# Questions

57. How do the Neer stages of impingement tendinitis differ by history and physical examination?

58. What is an impingement sign?

59. What is an impingement test?

60. What radiographic findings are consistent with impingement tendinitis and rotator cuff tear of the shoulder?

61. What is the diagnostic study of choice to demonstrate rotator cuff tears?

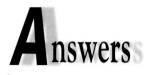
nswers

57. Stage I can occur at any age, but most frequently under age 25. An aching shoulder pain is brought on by activities involving the upper extremity. Positive physical findings include tenderness over the greater tuberosity and anterior acromion; painful motion of the shoulder, especially in abduction, which is increased with resistance at 90° of abduction; and a positive impingement sign. The biceps tendon is also frequently involved, demonstrated by tenderness over the biceps tendon and pain elicited with resisted forward flexion of the humerus with the forearm in supination and extension at the elbow (straight arm raising test). Stage I is a reversible lesion.

Stage II usually occurs between the ages of 25 and 40. Shoulder discomfort occurs not only with strenuous activities but also with activities of daily living and at night. Pain has occurred over a prolonged period of time. Signs are similar to those noted in stage I, but increased shoulder stiffness and tenderness over the acromioclavicular joint are more commonly found in stage II. Because of repeated insults, the supraspinatus tendon, the biceps tendon, and subacromial bursa become thickened and fibrotic making this lesion irreversible.

Stage III usually occurs after the age of 40. The usual history is prolonged, recurrent shoulder problems with pain occurring at night and with work-related activities. Signs are similar to stages I and II, but shoulder weakness is significant (especially with shoulder abduction and external rotation). Infraspinatus and supraspinatus muscle wasting and bone spurs may also be noted.

58. An impingement sign is demonstrated by having the patient place the affected arm in neutral rotation, while the examiner forcibly forward flexes the humerus. This causes the greater tuberosity of the humerus to be jammed against the undersurface of the acromion. Eliciting pain with this maneuver is a positive impingement sign. A less reliable, but commonly used, maneuver to demonstrate impingement is performed with the patient's humerus at 90° of forward flexion and forcibly internally rotating the shoulder. Once again, this causes the greater tuberosity to be driven further underneath the acromion and produces pain in cases of impingement tendinitis.

59. After a positive impingement sign has been elicited, 10 ml of 1-percent lidocaine is injected into the subacromial bursa of the shoulder. If local anesthetic relieves the pain of the repeated impingement sign, this further confirms the diagnosis of impingement tendinitis.

60. The findings on plain radiographs of the shoulder are subtle. Frequently the glenohumeral joint appears normal. Osteophyte formation will be noted over the anteroinferior surface of the acromion and at the acromioclavicular joint with cystic degeneration at the greater tuberosity of the humerus. The space between the humeral head and the acromion is also frequently narrowed in large rotator cuff tears, because the rotator cuff has lost its ability to function as a humeral head depressor. Less than 7 mm of space between the humeral head and the acromion is suggestive of a rotator cuff tear.

61. Although ultrasonography and magnetic resonance imaging (MRI) are used in some centers, these methods require considerable experience, which leads to variability in diagnosis. The "gold standard" for diagnosis of a full-thickness rotator cuff tear is the shoulder arthrogram. The escape of dye into the subacromial or subdeltoid space after injection of the glenohumeral joint demonstrates a full-thickness rotator cuff tear. The accuracy of this study is 95% to 100%. Although the size of the rotator cuff tear cannot be demonstrated by routine shoulder arthrography, supplementation with a double contrast arthrogram or arthrotomogram may assist in defining the size.

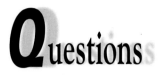

# Questions

62. An 18-year-old high school shortstop has a 3-week history of considerable discomfort in his dominant right shoulder after baseball games or prolonged practice. There has been no history of trauma and no night pain. Upon examination, the patient has full active motion of the shoulder with tenderness over the greater tuberosity of the humerus and a positive impingement sign. Radiographs of the right shoulder are negative. How should this patient be managed?

63. A 62-year-old woman presents with a 6-month history of increasing shoulder discomfort. Pain occurs with any activity involving use of the affected extremity as well as at night. There has been no history of trauma. Upon examination, there is tenderness over the lateral acromion and anteriorly over the biceps tendon. Active ROM is full, but there is significant weakness, especially with abduction and external rotation. The impingement sign is positive. Radiographs demonstrate a normal glenohumeral joint with small subacromial osteophyte formation. How should management of this patient proceed?

64. Describe the rehabilitation protocol following subacromial decompression and rotator cuff repair.

65. A 38-year-old woman has a 9-month history of persistent shoulder pain. The pain limits her work-related activities. There has been no specific trauma. She maintains full active ROM of the shoulder with a positive impingement sign. The patient has undergone 4 months of conservative treatment measures for impingement tendinitis without significant improvement. Radiographs of the right shoulder demonstrate minimal osteophyte formation in the subacromial region. A shoulder arthrogram is negative. How should this patient be managed?

66. A 42-year-old man falls down several steps injuring his shoulder. He is unable to abduct his shoulder beyond 30° actively, but maintains full passive ROM. Plain radiographs of the shoulder are negative for a fracture or dislocation. How should this patient be managed?

67. When acromioplasty is selected for treatment of impingement tendinitis, what part and how much of the acromion is resected?

68. A 47-year-old physical education teacher noticed a snapping sensation in her dominant shoulder while playing racquetball approximately 1 month ago. During the past 2 weeks, she has developed increasing tenderness over her anterior shoulder. Your examination reveals crepitus in the bicipital groove during shoulder flexion. Her pain is reproduced by resisting supination and elbow flexion with the elbow at 90°, as she internally rotates her shoulder. What is causing her symptoms, and how would you treat her?

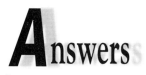# Answers

62. This patient's symptoms and signs are consistent with impingement tendinitis and would be classified as stage I in Neer's classification. These are reversible lesions and generally respond to nonoperative treatment. This would include a period of rest, refraining from aggravating activities (i.e., baseball) antiinflammatory medications, and physical therapy modalities followed by progressive shoulder rehabilitation after the pain has subsided. Rehabilitation should emphasize cuff strengthening in internal and external rotation.

63. This patient demonstrates stage III of Neer's classification for impingement tendinitis with possible chronic rotator cuff tear. A trial of conservative treatment measures should be initiated including rest, antiinflammatory medications, and physical therapy. If these measures fail and pain persists, an arthrogram should be performed to demonstrate suspected rotator cuff tear. Treatment should proceed with surgical subacromial decompression (acromioplasty and resection of the coracoacromial ligament) with repair of a rotator cuff tear, if present.

64. The patient is immobilized for 3 weeks in 45° abduction to relax the tension on the repair. She is assisted with PROM of her shoulder beginning on the fourth postoperative day. Four weeks postoperatively, she is instructed in active assistive exercises, but is to avoid active abduction. Eight weeks postoperatively, she progresses to full AROM, then begins progressive resistive exercise (PRE) on week 12. She progresses to full function and resistance from month 8 to month 12.

65. This patient demonstrates impingement tendinitis of the shoulder without a rotator cuff tear that is resistant to conservative treatment. Since pain is interfering with her activities, surgical intervention with subacromial decompression (acromioplasty and coracoacromial ligament resection) is warranted. Simple coracoacromial ligament resection alone may relieve pain but tends to be short-lived, so this procedure along with acromioplasty is generally recommended.

66. Suspicion of an acute rotator cuff tear should be confirmed with a shoulder arthrogram to demonstrate that weakness of abduction is not due to other causes of abduction weakness (e.g., suprascapular nerve palsy). In a very active person with an acute rotator cuff tear, the treatment of choice is surgical repair.

67. Since the anterior portion of the undersurface of the acromion is the actual site of impingement, the anteroinferior portion of the acromion should be resected. This is accomplished by resecting a wedge-shaped piece of bone measuring approximately 9mm anteriorly and approximately 2cm in length from the undersurface of the acromion. At the time of acromioplasty, the coracoacromial ligament should always be resected. Additionally, the acromioclavicular joint should be resected if it is noted to be arthritic and symptomatic, or if this joint is enlarged by periarticular osteophytes and is causing further impingement on the supraspinatus tendon.

68. This patient presents with long head of the biceps tendinitis, a degenerative condition that may result from either acute trauma or repetitive stress. Inflammation within the tendon or its sheath produces swelling and pain in the anterior shoulder. Treatment involves rest in a sling, ice, and NSAIDs. After the acute symptoms subside in 5 to 7 days, heat modalities and a progressive exercise program emphasizing rotator cuff strengthening should be started.

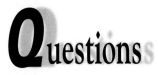

# Questions

69. A 53-year-old farmer felt a "pop" in his shoulder while attempting to lift a bag of seed. He is noted to have a bulge ("Popeye arm") in the anterior aspect of his right arm. How should this patient be managed?

70. A 58-year-old man comes into your office Monday morning with severe right shoulder pain. He spent most of the weekend painting his house. He has tenderness with palpation over the anterolateral aspect of his shoulder. Abduction produces pain beginning at 60° and is limited to 100° by pain. Internal and external rotation are full and pain-free when his arm is at his side. Isometric resisted movement is strong and only slightly uncomfortable with his arm at his side, but pain increases as he elevates his arm. The patient has no previous history of shoulder problems, and his health is good. What is your diagnosis and how would you treat him?

71. Is glenohumeral joint stability dependent on surrounding musculature?

72. What is the most common type of anterior dislocation of the shoulder?

73. What is the most common mechanism of action causing anterior dislocation of the shoulder?

74. What is the most common mechanism of action causing posterior dislocation of the shoulder?

75. Why are electric shock and convulsive seizures more likely to be associated with posterior dislocations of the shoulder?

76. In examination of the shoulder, what is the significance of an apprehension sign and how is it elicited?

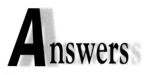

# **A**nswers

**69.** This patient has a rupture of the proximal long head of the biceps tendon. Because of the high association of proximal biceps tendon rupture with impingement tendinitis and rotator cuff tears, a shoulder examination for signs of impingement as well as a shoulder arthrogram should be performed. In an active patient, the biceps tendon should be repaired by suturing it to the intertubercular groove of the humerus. The intraarticular portion of the biceps tendon should be excised and acromioplasty and repair of a rotator cuff tear, if present, should be performed. Although disability related to biceps tendon rupture is minimal, attention to shoulder impingement and rotator cuff tear is of importance with this tendon rupture.

**70.** This patient has symptoms of acute subacromial bursitis. He should initially be treated with rest, NSAIDs, cold application, and support in a sling. Within 2 to 3 days, he should be instructed in pendulum exercises and progressed to A and PROM within a relatively pain-free range. In 2 weeks, he can begin resisted internal and external shoulder rotation with his arm at his side, then progress to resisted rotation and abduction throughout a full ROM. He should remain on a rotator cuff strengthening program and be instructed in measures to prevent recurrence.

**71.** In the resting state and with minimal loads across the joint, glenohumeral joint stability does not depend upon surrounding musculature. Passive joint stability is provided by ligamentous and capsular restraints, the concavity of the glenoid surface and its labrum, negative intraarticular pressure produced by a finite joint volume, and by the adhesive and cohesive properties of the joint fluid. The stability provided by these passive restraints is noted in the anesthetized and paralyzed patient where shoulder stability is maintained, as well as in the fresh cadaveric specimen in which the glenohumeral articulation is also maintained. When larger loads are placed across the glenohumeral joint, dynamic stability is provided by the surrounding musculature.

**72.** Subcoracoid dislocation. Subglenoid, subclavicular, and intrathoracic anterior dislocations are less common.

**73.** Anterior dislocations of the shoulder are most commonly the result of an indirect force with the arm axially loaded in an abducted, extended, and externally rotated position.

**74.** A posterior dislocation of the shoulder is most commonly the result of axial loading of the arm in an adducted, flexed, and internally rotated position.

**75.** Electric shock and convulsive seizures result in violent contracture of all of the muscle groups surrounding the shoulder. When this occurs, the stronger internal rotators (pectoralis major, latissimus dorsi, and subscapularis muscles) simply overwhelm the weaker external rotators (teres minor and infraspinatus muscles), resulting in posterior dislocation of the shoulder.

**76.** A positive apprehension sign is one in which manipulation of the shoulder elicits apprehension or a sensation that the shoulder is about to dislocate. This suggests shoulder instability. In the most common apprehension test, or crank test, to demonstrate anterior shoulder instability, the examiner holds the patient's arm in 90° of abduction and applies progressive external rotation to the arm while stabilizing the posterior shoulder with the opposite hand. Similarly, posterior instability can be tested with the jerk test, in which the examiner axially loads the humerus while grasping the elbow and placing the arm in 90° of forward flexion and internal rotation. With continued axial loading, the arm is moved horizontally across the body into an adducted position. This may produce a jerk as the humeral head subluxates posteriorly over the posterior glenoid rim. Additionally, this frequently elicits apprehension on the part of the patient. Although pain may be elicited with these maneuvers, the presence of pain alone without signs of apprehension does not demonstrate instability, and other conditions should be considered.

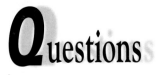
# Questions

77. A 72-year-old obese woman complains of shoulder pain after a fall. She holds the affected extremity in the "sling position" with the forearm across the abdomen. She resists attempts to abduct the shoulder because it causes pain. The neurovascular status of the upper extremity and the remainder of the physical examination are otherwise normal. An AP radiograph of the shoulder is read as negative. How should this patient be managed?

78. AP radiographs of the shoulder in the case of subacromial posterior dislocation may appear quite normal. What subtle radiographic signs suggest posterior dislocation in an AP radiograph?

79. What is a Hill-Sachs lesion, and how is it best demonstrated radiographically?

80. What is a Bankart lesion and what is its significance?

81. What is the West Point view and what is its significance?

82. How frequently are rotator cuff tears associated with anterior dislocations of the shoulder?

83. A patient has sustained an anterior dislocation of the shoulder which is easily reduced. After reduction, the patient is noted to have significant weakness in shoulder abduction. Sensation over the lateral aspect of the shoulder and arm is normal. The remainder of the neurovascular examination is negative and postreduction radiographs of the shoulder are negative. What is the likely cause of abduction weakness and how should this be managed?

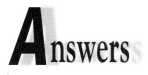

# Answers

77. The physical findings of posterior dislocation are minimal, especially in the obese patient. Additionally, a single AP radiograph is inadequate for examination of the shoulder after trauma. Subacromial posterior dislocation may appear deceptively normal on the AP radiograph. Additional views (axillary or transcapular) are necessary in diagnosing shoulder dislocations.

78. Posterior dislocation places the humerus in an internally rotated position. Thus the normal profile of the neck of humerus is not seen on the AP view. In the normal shoulder, overlap between the glenoid and the humeral head creates an elliptic shadow and the humeral head fills the majority of the glenoid cavity. With posterior dislocation, this shadow is lost and the humeral head no longer fills the majority of the glenoid cavity. A "trough line" or longitudinal radiodense line formed within the humeral head, representing an impaction fracture of the anterior humeral head, may be demonstrated with posterior dislocation. Additionally, posterior dislocation is suggested if there is greater than 6mm of space between the anterior rim of the glenoid and the humeral head.

79. The Hill-Sachs lesion is a compression fracture of the posterolateral aspect of the humeral head resulting from anterior dislocation of the shoulder. Radiographic views used to demonstrate the Hill-Sachs lesion are the Stryker Notch view or the Hill-Sachs view. In the Stryker Notch view, the X-ray cassette is placed under the shoulder of the supine patient. The palm of the hand of the affected extremity is placed behind the head, the elbow is placed straight upward, and the X-ray beam is centered over the coracoid process tilting 10° cephalad. In the Hill-Sachs view, an AP radiograph of the shoulder is made with the humerus in extreme internal rotation.

80. A Bankart lesion is an avulsion of the capsule and glenoid labrum off of the anterior rim of the glenoid resulting from traumatic anterior dislocations of the shoulder. The importance of this lesion is that it may contribute to shoulder instability resulting in recurrent dislocation. Although the Bankart lesion is probably not the only "essential" lesion leading to recurrent anterior dislocation, this lesion, combined with a posterolateral defect in the humeral head (Hill-Sachs lesion) and erosion or fracture of the anterior rim of the glenoid, is a good predictor of instability.

81. The West Point axillary view of the shoulder is most commonly used to detect fractures or defects of the anteroinferior rim of the glenoid resulting in anterior dislocations of the shoulder. This view is obtained by placing the patient prone, with the X-ray cassette placed under the involved shoulder, and the involved extremity placed on a 7.5-cm pad. After the head and neck are turned away from the involved shoulder, the X-ray beam is directed toward the axilla, raised 25° off the horizontal, and aimed 25° toward the patient's midline.

82. Rotator cuff tears are thought to occur relatively frequently after anterior dislocations of the shoulder. The incidence increases with increasing age of the patient, exceeding 30% after age 40 and 80% after age 60.

83. Injury of the axillary nerve is the most common nerve injury after anterior dislocation of the shoulder. This is thought to occur with an overall incidence of approximately 30% and occurs more often in the elderly population. With axillary nerve injury, cutaneous sensation over the lateral shoulder is frequently normal and therefore sensory examination is an unreliable indicator of injury. After anterior dislocation of the shoulder, these nerve injuries are most often traction neuropraxias and should simply be treated by observation. Most will recover within 10 weeks from the time of injury. However, the prognosis is poor for axillary nerve palsies persisting beyond 10 weeks.

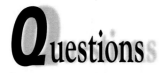

# Questions

84. After anterior shoulder dislocation, what factors place the patient at risk for recurrence?

85. How should postreduction management proceed in a patient with an uncomplicated traumatic anterior shoulder dislocation?

86. A 22-year-old college football lineman has had three episodes of traumatic anterior dislocation of the shoulder. The first occurred after trying to make an arm tackle 4 years ago. Upon physical examination, he has evidence of anterior instability of the shoulder. Radiographs of the shoulder are negative. How should this patient be managed?

87. Limiting external rotation is the goal of most surgical procedures to treat anterior instability of the shoulder. What are the risks of this method of treatment and for which patients should this procedure generally not be recommended?

88. A 20-year-old man demonstrates the ability to cause a "clunk" sensation in his shoulder with certain maneuvers which result in a bony prominence posteriorly in the shoulder. The patient has noted the ability to do this since a young age. This does cause intermittent pain in the shoulder and some difficulty with his job as a construction worker. How should this problem be managed?

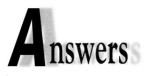
**A**nswers

84. Recurrence is the most common complication following traumatic anterior dislocation of the shoulder. Age at the time of the initial dislocation is probably the most important factor. Patients under the age of 20 are thought to have a recurrence rate in the range of 80%. Athletes are at a greater risk for recurrence than nonathletes. After the age of 40, the recurrence rate falls to approximately 10%. Males have a higher recurrence rate than females and the majority of the recurrences occur within 2 years of the initial traumatic dislocation. Extremity dominance is unrelated to recurrence. Recurrence varies inversely with the severity of the initial trauma, such that if a minor traumatic event caused the initial dislocation, the likelihood of recurrence is relatively high.

85. Postreduction management after traumatic anterior dislocation of the shoulder is controversial, especially in the younger patient in whom risk of recurrence is relatively high. However in the younger patient (less than 30 years old), sling immobilization in a position of comfort of adduction and internal rotation for a period of 3 to 5 weeks is recommended. In the older patient (more than 30 years) in whom the risk of developing stiffness is greater and the risk of recurrence is decreased, sling immobilization for 1 to 2 weeks is recommended. During the period of immobilization, progressive isometric exercises, especially for internal and external rotation, are initiated. More vigorous strengthening exercises are initiated after the period of immobilization. ROM of the glenohumeral joint is rarely a problem after dislocation, but more vigorous ROM exercises may be initiated 6 weeks after the time of injury if this is a problem. Return to overhead labor activities or athletic activities is not allowed until normal rotator strength and full forward elevation of the shoulder have been demonstrated.

86. Initial treatment of any anterior dislocation of the shoulder should begin with strengthening of the internal and external rotators to improve dynamic stability. If instability persists, surgical intervention is recommended. Although  many procedures have been described, current recommendations favor repair of the Bankart lesion (if present) with anterior capsulorrhaphy or a subscapularis muscle tightening procedure, or both. It is important to ensure that instability is solely anterior with these procedures. Anterior glenoid osteotomies have, for the most part, fallen out of favor.

87. For patients who require normal or supranormal ROM of the shoulder (swimmers, baseball pitchers) a surgical procedure resulting in limitation of external rotation is likely to cause significant limitation, so that they would not be able to return to their presurgical level of activity. Not only is limitation of motion a problem with these procedures, but if the anterior repair produces excessive tightness (e.g., inability to externally rotate beyond 0°), these patients are at greater risk to develop osteoarthritis of the glenohumeral joint due to a change in joint mechanics. Aggressive strengthening of the rotator muscles is preferred over surgery for such patients.

88. The patient who is able to voluntarily dislocate the shoulder frequently has multidirectional instability and a history where minimal trauma has resulted in the initial dislocation. Frequently, these patients have other emotional or psychiatric problems, and they should be referred for psychiatric evaluation. Surgery for these patients is rarely recommended. Those patients without psychiatric problems who are voluntary dislocators usually respond to a rehabilitation program involving strengthening of the rotator muscles of the shoulder increasing dynamic stabilization. Only after 6 to 12 months of intensive physical therapy and after the patient has demonstrated the desire to discontinue voluntary dislocation should surgical stabilization be considered.

# Questions

89. An 18-year-old swimmer complains of increasing bilateral shoulder pain with swimming activities. There has been no history of shoulder dislocation. Physical examination is remarkable because of the patient's ability to hyperextend at the knees and elbows bilaterally. Multidirectional instability of both shoulders can be demonstrated. Radiographs of the shoulders are negative. How should this patient be treated?

90. Modifications of the Bristow procedure have been previously used for treatment of anterior shoulder instability, in which the tip of the coracoid process is transferred to the anterior glenoid. What muscles are attached to the coracoid process, what nerve is at risk for injury, and why is this procedure generally no longer recommended for the treatment of anterior shoulder instability?

91. A 51-year-old woman complains of left nondominant shoulder pain of 3 weeks duration. She has no history of trauma or unaccustomed use of her shoulder. She is quite protective of her arm and uses a "shoulder hunching" maneuver to elevate her arm. What characteristic clinical and arthrographic findings are necessary to make a diagnosis of frozen shoulder?

92. What is the recommended treatment for the patient in question 91?

93. Does frozen shoulder ever spontaneously resolve?

94. The C5 nerve root emerges superior or inferior to the C5 cervical vertebral body?

95. After emerging from the vertebral foramina, nerve roots of the brachial plexus descend between what anatomic structures?

96. What is the function of the dorsal rami of C5-T1?

97. The phrenic nerve arises from which nerve root(s)?

98. The phrenic nerve lies in what position relative to the scalene muscles?

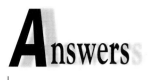

# Answers

89. In patients with atraumatic shoulder instability, this tends to occur bilaterally, with multidirectional instability and generalized ligamentous laxity as demonstrated in this case. These patients frequently respond to rehabilitation. Aggressive physical therapy with strengthening of the rotators of the shoulder frequently provides sufficient dynamic stability. If the patient does not respond to conservative treatment, an inferior capsular shift should be included as part of the surgical procedure.

90. Three muscles attach to the coracoid process. The pectoralis minor muscle inserts proximally and the origin of the conjoined tendon (i.e., the short head of the biceps muscle and the coracobrachialis muscle) arises distally from the tip. The musculocutaneous nerve runs medial to the coracoid process and obliquely through the coracobrachialis muscle at variable distances from the coracoid process and is at risk for injury. Because of the multiple complications of this procedure, including recurrent subluxation, coracoid nonunion, screw-related problems, injury to the musculocutaneous nerve, and shoulder weakness, this procedure is no longer the treatment of choice.

91. Frozen shoulder (adhesive capsulitis) involves chronic capsular inflammation with fibrosis, adhesions, and obliteration of the joint cavity. It typically affects persons between 40 and 60 years of age and is more common in women. A patient usually presents with spontaneous onset of gradually progressive shoulder pain and severe limitation of movement. Motion is limited in a capsular pattern, with the greatest limitation in external rotation, followed by abduction, then internal rotation. Arthrography reveals joint volume to be reduced by at least 50%; the volume may be 5 to 10 ml, as compared with a normal volume of 20 to 30 ml.

92. Modalities and medication should be administered for pain relief. She should be placed on an exercise program that includes active, passive, and resistive exercises and joint mobilization. If she fails to respond to conservative treatment, infiltration brisement or manipulation under anesthesia may assist in expanding the capsule. She will require an ongoing exercise program to assure that she regains full function.

93. Yes, many authorities describe frozen shoulder as a self-limiting condition. It may progress through stages as follows: a "freezing stage," lasting 2½ to 9 months; a "frozen stage," lasting 4 to 12 months; and a "thawing stage" lasting 1 to 3 years. However, due to the lengthy nature of this condition, and the possibility of residual dysfunction, most patients prefer medical intervention rather than letting it run its course.

94. The brachial plexus is normally composed of the C5-T1 nerve roots. The C5-7 nerve roots emerge superior to their respective cervical vertebral bodies. C8 emerges below C7 and T1 below the T1 vertebral body.

95. The anterior primary rami of the nerve roots forming the brachial plexus descend between the anterior and middle scalene muscles.

96. The dorsal rami of C5-T1 supply innervation to the muscles and skin of the dorsal neck.

97. The phrenic nerve arises primarily from the C4 nerve root. However, there may be additional contributions from C3 or C5. Determination of the functioning of the C4 neurologic level is especially important when determining if the tetraplegic patient will be respirator-dependent.

98. The phrenic nerve lies anterior to the anterior scalene muscles. This differs from the remainder of the nerves to the brachial plexus which descend **between** the anterior and middle scalene muscles.

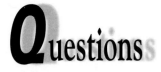

# Questions

99. The lateral cord of the brachial plexus is composed of which nerve divisions?

100. The cords of the brachial plexus are named relative to the position of what anatomic structure?

101. What are the terminal branches of the lateral cord of the brachial plexus?

102. What are the terminal branches of the medial cord of the brachial plexus?

103. What are the terminal branches of the posterior cord of the brachial plexus?

104. What is the innervation of the pectoralis minor muscle?

105. What is the innervation of the teres major muscle?

106. What is a Horner's syndrome?

107. Horner's syndrome results from injury to or interruption of which nerve fibers?

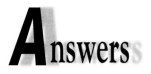

# Answers

99. The lateral cord is composed of the anterior divisions of the upper and middle brachial plexus trunks. The anterior division of the lower trunk becomes the medial cord and the posterior divisions of the upper, middle, and lower trunks become the posterior cord.

100. The lateral, medial, and posterior cords of the brachial plexus are named with respect to their positions surrounding the axillary artery.

101. The lateral cord of the brachial plexus arises from the C5-7 nerve roots. The terminal branches of the lateral cord include the lateral pectoral nerve, the lateral root of the median nerve, and the musculocutaneous nerve.

102. The medial cord of the brachial plexus arises from the C8 and T1 nerve roots. The terminal branches of the medial cord include the medial pectoral nerve, the medial brachial cutaneous nerve, the medial antebrachial cutaneous nerve, the medial root of the median nerve, and the ulnar nerve.

103. The posterior cord of the brachial plexus arises from the C5-T1 nerve roots. The terminal branches of the posterior cord include the upper and lower subscapular nerves, the thoracodorsal nerve, the axillary nerve, and the radial nerve.

104. The medial pectoral nerve innervates the pectoralis minor muscle. The pectoralis major muscle is innervated by both the medial and lateral pectoral nerves.

105. The lower subscapular nerve innervates the teres major muscle. The upper and lower subscapular nerves innervate the subscapularis muscle.

106. Horner's syndrome results from loss of sympathetic innervation and produces the characteristic physical findings of ptosis, enophthalmus, and miosis as well as anhydrosis to the ipsilateral side of the face.

107. The sympathetic nerve fibers arise from the cervicothoracic ganglia and the C8-T1 nerve roots that accompany the trigeminal nerve to the orbit, where they become the ciliary nerves. These fibers control the tarsal muscles, the orbital muscles of Muller, and the dilator muscles of the pupil. Interruption of these sympathetic nerve tracts due to injury or local anesthetic instilled at the C8-T1 nerve root level or cervicothoracic ganglia will produce Horner's syndrome.

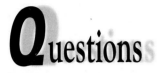

108. After a motorcycle accident, a patient is found to have a flail and anesthetic upper extremity. Three weeks after the injury, the patient's physical condition is unchanged. Nerve conduction velocity studies obtained at this time reveal absent motor conduction but intact sensory conduction. What is the significance of this finding?

109. When should baseline EMG studies be obtained after a brachial plexus injury? In the presence of denervated muscles, what kind of electromyographic findings can be demonstrated?

110. Cervical myelography is frequently used to demonstrate the presence of nerve root avulsions after brachial plexus injury. What radiographic findings suggest nerve root avulsion?

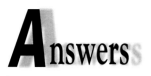

# Answers

108. After brachial plexus injury, the finding of absent motor conduction with intact sensory conduction on nerve conduction velocity studies suggest a preganglionic injury to the involved nerve roots. Since the cell bodies of the afferent sensory fibers reside in the dorsal root ganglion, a lesion proximal to this site (i.e., nerve roots) will not result in wallerian degeneration of these sensory nerve axons and nerve conduction velocity of these fibers will remain normal. As there is interruption of the sensory pathways to the central nervous system, sensation cannot be perceived and the corresponding area remains anesthetic. If nerve conduction velocity studies demonstrate absence of both sensory and motor conduction, this suggests a postganglionic level or a combination of preganglionic and postganglionic injury levels (see Figure 4-6).

**Figure** 4-6

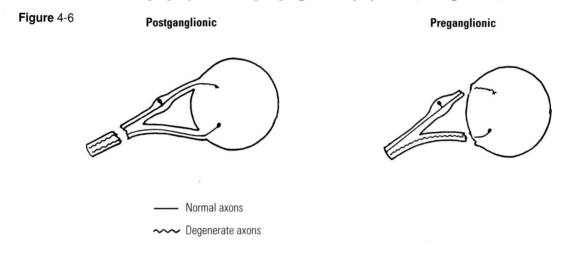

Postganglionic                                        Preganglionic

—— Normal axons

〜〜 Degenerate axons

109. EMG is used to detect muscle denervation. After axonal interruption, wallerian degeneration of the axon occurs over a 3-week period. Muscle denervation potentials are not likely to be demonstrated until wallerian degeneration of the affected axons has occurred. Therefore, baseline EMG studies should probably be postponed until approximately 3 weeks after the time of injury. Under normal conditions, muscle at rest is electromyographically silent. After denervation, small electrical potentials are generated spontaneously by the denervated muscles. Therefore, the positive finding by the EMG study of denervated muscle is one of spontaneous fibrillation potentials.

110. Avulsion injury to the nerve roots of the brachial plexus commonly damages both the nerve root and the surrounding meninges. The characteristic findings with cervical myelography in the presence of an avulsion injury include inability to visualize the nerve root as well as the presence of meningeal diverticula, referred to as a traumatic meningocele at the level of the avulsed nerve root. However, these findings are not pathognomonic of a preganglionic lesion, because cases have demonstrated the presence of traumatic meningocele without nerve root avulsion (false positive) as well as nerve root avulsions existing in the presence of a normal myelogram (false negative). With cervical myelography, positive findings are only suggestive and not conclusive for the presence of a preganglionic nerve root avulsion.

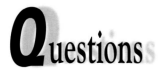

111. After brachial plexus injury, what findings suggest a preganglionic lesion?

112. A 38-year-old mail carrier experienced severe weakness of his nondominant shoulder with abduction and external rotation. He exhibits moderate tenderness over the site where his mailbag strap passes over the scapula. Impingement sign of the shoulder is negative. What diagnostic study should be done to confirm the diagnosis?

113. How should this patient be managed?

114. What anatomic structure(s) pass(es) beneath the superior transverse scapular ligament?

115. Injury to what nerve results in winging of the scapula?

116. An 18-year-old man fell out of a tree and landed on his shoulder. Radiographs obtained at the time of injury were found to be negative. Three weeks after injury, his right shoulder pain resolved, but he noted the onset of winging of the scapula. What is the likely cause of this scapular winging and why was this finding not apparent immediately after the injury?

117. How should traumatic winging of the scapula be treated?

118. Thoracic outlet syndrome (TOS) is most frequently confused with compression neuropathy of which peripheral nerve?

119. What structures are commonly compressed in TOS?

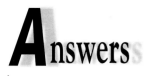

# Answers

**111.** In patients with complete brachial plexus involvement, findings consistent with a preganglionic lesion on physical examination will demonstrate, in addition to a flail arm, Horner's syndrome due to involvement of the sympathetic cervicothoracic ganglia, winged scapula due to interruption of the long thoracic nerve, paralysis of the rhomboid muscles secondary to injury proximal to the dorsal scapular nerve, and diaphragmatic paralysis if there is C4 nerve root involvement. A cervical myelogram may demonstrate traumatic meningoceles. Nerve conduction studies should demonstrate intact sensory conduction with absent motor conduction and EMG will demonstrate denervation of both cervical paraspinal as well as peripheral musculature of the affected extremity.

**112.** Weakness of shoulder abduction and external rotation is not always due to a rotator cuff tendinitis or tear. With a negative impingement sign and evidence of local irritation over the suprascapular notch, suprascapular nerve compressive neuropathy should be suspected. The diagnostic studies of choice are nerve conduction velocity and electromyography.

**113.** Begin with elimination of the activity that precipitated the neuropathy (i.e., removal or change of position of the mailbag). Most suprascapular nerve palsies respond to conservative measures including activity modification, local anesthetic, and cortisone injection into the region of the scapular notch as well as physical therapy to maintain shoulder ROM. If conservative treatment measures fail or fibrillation potentials are noted on EMG studies of the spinatus muscles, then surgical decompression of the suprascapular nerve is indicated.

**114.** The suprascapular nerve. The suprascapular artery passes over this ligament.

**115.** Dynamic winging of the scapula is caused by injury to the long thoracic nerve resulting in paralysis of the serratus anterior muscle.

**116.** Winging of the scapula in this case is likely due to a traction injury to the long thoracic nerve. This results in paralysis of the serratus anterior muscle. Although paralysis of the serratus anterior muscle probably occurred at the time of injury, winging of the scapula will not be clinically evident until stretching of the overlying trapezius muscle has occurred.

**117.** Traumatic winging of the scapula is usually due to a traction neuropraxia of the long thoracic nerve. Therefore, in most cases, these should be treated symptomatically. A short period of rest with sling immobilization of the involved upper extremity should be followed by ROM exercises. Most winging injuries resolve with time and benign neglect. If there is no resolution after approximately 2 years, appropriate stabilization procedures may be undertaken.

**118.** Signs and symptoms consistent with thoracic outlet syndrome are closely related to those associated with ulnar neuropathy. Features which distinguish TOS from ulnar neuropathy are sensory deficit along the ulnar aspect of the forearm or upper arm and motor involvement of the thenar muscles found in thoracic outlet syndrome and not in ulnar neuropathy.

**119.** Neurologic symptoms, which are present in a vast majority of patients, result from compression of the lower trunk of the brachial plexus. Less commonly, there is involvement of the middle trunk of the brachial plexus. Therefore, most neurologic symptoms in TOS are related to C8-T1 motor and sensory symptoms. Less common vascular symptoms are due to compression of the subclavian artery and subclavian vein (distal to the scalene triangle).

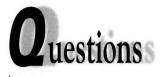

**120.** Describe the four areas associated with the thoracic outlet where compression of neurovascular structures may occur.

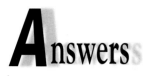

# Answers

**120.** The **sternocostovertebral space** is bounded by the spine dorsally, the first rib laterally, and the sternum anteriorly. The neurovascular bundle can be compressed by lesions in the apices and pleurae of the lungs (Pancoast's tumors). (See Figure 4-7.)

The **scalene triangle** is defined by a triangle formed by the anterior scalene muscle, middle scalene muscle, and the clavicle. It may be narrowed by the presence of fibromuscular bands, a cervical rib, or scalene muscle hypertrophy.

The **costoclavicular space** is located between the clavicle and first rib. It may be compromised by weighting the shoulder girdle (e.g., carrying heavy loads, a backpack, etc.) or descent of the shoulder girdle related to poor posture or aging.

The **coracopectoral space** occurs between the pectoralis minor muscle and the rib cage. Neurovascular structures may be compressed here as they are forced to angulate sharply around the pectoralis minor muscle during overhead activities.

**Figure** 4-7

**A. Sternocostovertebral space**

Sternum  Spine

First rib

**B. Scalene triangle**

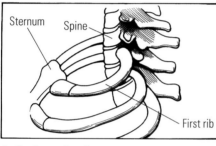

Anterior and middle scalene muscles

Subclavian artery

First rib

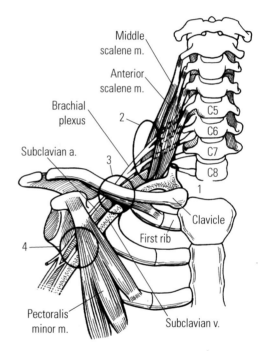

Middle scalene m.

Anterior scalene m.

Brachial plexus

Subclavian a.

2

3

C5

C6

C7

C8

1

Clavicle

First rib

4

Pectoralis minor m.

Subclavian v.

**C. Costoclavicular space**

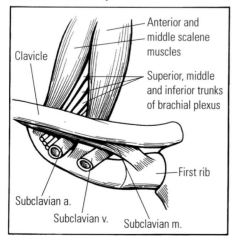

Anterior and middle scalene muscles

Clavicle

Superior, middle and inferior trunks of brachial plexus

Subclavian a.

Subclavian v.  Subclavian m.

First rib

**D. Coracopectoral space**

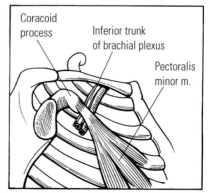

Coracoid process

Inferior trunk of brachial plexus

Pectoralis minor m.

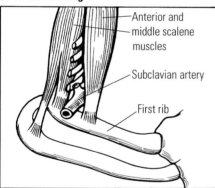

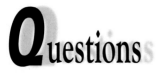

# Questions

121. What is the differential diagnosis of TOS?

122. What are the provocative tests used on physical examination to diagnosis TOS?

123. What diagnostic study confirms diagnosis of TOS?

124. What are the most common complaints and physical findings in a patient with suspected TOS?

125. How should the patient with suspected TOS be treated?

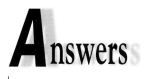

# Answers

121. Cervical radiculopathy; tumors of the apical portion of the lung (Pancoast); and peripheral nerve compression, most notably that of the ulnar nerve.

122. In the classic Adson Test, the patient is seated with the neck extended and rotated toward the ipsilateral side while the breath is held in full inspiration. The disappearance of the radial pulse along with reproduction of the patient's symptoms signifies a positive result.

    In Wright's hyperabduction test, the patient's arm is abducted 90° with the arm in full external rotation. Again, diminution of the radial pulse concurrent with reproduction of symptoms signifies a positive test.

    In the overhead exercise test, the fingers are rapidly and repeatedly flexed and extended, with the arms abducted. Forearm and hand pain, fatigue, and paresthesias occurring in less than a minute of this activity constitute a positive test.

    Finally, the costoclavicular maneuver places the patient's shoulders in a military brace position, with the arms drawn downward and posterior. Diminution of the radial pulse and reproduction of the symptoms constitute a positive test. False-positive results may be obtained in these tests.

123. No specific diagnostic study can be relied upon to confirm the diagnosis of TOS. This diagnosis is strictly made on a clinical basis. Special studies may, however, be beneficial. Radiographs of the cervical spine may demonstrate the presence of cervical ribs, supporting the diagnosis of TOS, or may demonstrate cervical spondylosis suggesting nerve root compression at the level of the intervertebral foramen. Electrophysiological studies may demonstrate slowing of nerve conduction velocities in the region of the supraclavicular fossa, supporting TOS, or may demonstrate compression of other peripheral nerves mimicking TOS. In the event that there is a vascular component to the thoracic outlet syndrome, transfemoral subclavian angiography would be warranted.

124. Symptoms are variable. However, most patients complain of paresthesias radiating from the cervical region of the neck to the shoulder and down along the medial aspect of the limb to the ulnar two to three fingers. Pain frequently accompanies these paresthesias and is described as gnawing or burning. Nocturnal pain and paresthesias are common. Weakness of the hand as well as decreased dexterity are also frequent complaints. Symptoms are usually aggravated by placing the involved extremity in an elevated or overhead position. If there is vascular involvement, intermittent or constant swelling, cyanosis, and cold intolerance may be present. Upon physical examination, sensory changes usually involve the ulnar aspect of the hand as well as the medial aspect of the forearm and arm. Muscle wasting and weakness may be demonstrated in the intrinsic muscles of the hand including the thenar muscles. Vascular changes may include diminished distal pulses, decreased blood pressure compared to the opposite side, color and temperature changes (with the extremity pale, blue, or cold), as well as the presence of a thrill or bruit over the subclavian artery.

125. The treatment of choice for TOS is conservative, if possible. Initially, a period of rest from activities that provoke symptoms is indicated. A physical therapist should instruct the patient in proper posture; strengthening the trapezius, rhomboid, and levator scapulae muscles; and stretching the pectoralis minor and scalene muscles. Activity modification must also be undertaken in order to reduce provocative motions or postures. In the obese patient, weight reduction may be of benefit and proper breast support may be beneficial in women. If after 4 months of conservative treatment, significant symptoms persist or if there is significant vascular component to this disorder, surgical intervention is indicated. In order to provide adequate decompression of the thoracic outlet, most recommend first rib resection with removal of any congenital fibromuscular bands as the procedure of choice.

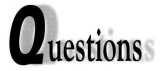

# Questions

126. Name the three types of prostheses used after upper extremity amputations.

127. The aesthetic hand prosthesis is made most commonly of what material?

128. Which prehensile terminal device for body-powered upper extremity protheses is most commonly used—the voluntary-opening or voluntary-closing split hook?

129. What are the advantages of a split hook for the terminal prehensile device of a body-powered prosthesis?

130. With the wrist-powered prosthesis, which wrist motions are commonly used to produce which hand functions?

131. What are the advantages of the myoelectric prosthesis?

132. What are the disadvantages of the myoelectric prosthesis?

133. What is the biggest deterrent to efficient functioning of upper extremity prostheses?

134. For the above-elbow amputee with a body-powered prosthesis, what motion produces elbow flexion?

135. In the above-elbow body-powered prosthesis, motion of the terminal device is dependent on elbow locking. How is this accomplished?

136. For the C4 quadriplegic patient, what is the appropriate upper extremity orthosis?

137. For the C5 quadriplegic patient, what is the appropriate upper extremity orthosis?

138. For the C6 or C7 quadriplegic patient, what is the appropriate upper extremity orthosis?

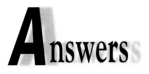

# Answers

126. The three types include: (1) passive prosthesis, which is primarily for cosmesis with minimal functional capacity; (2) body-powered prosthesis, in which motion of the prosthesis is controlled by movements of the remaining, naturally articulated body segments; and (3) externally powered prosthesis, in which motion is provided by some portable external energy source. In reality, most prostheses are "hybrid" prostheses, being a combination of these three types.

127. Silicone polymers are most commonly used for the aesthetic hand prosthesis rather than the previously used polyvinylchlorides. The use of silicone produces more realistic hand detail, natural hand colors, and texture. Its tear strength is relatively high and mechanical properties are not appreciably changed by temperatures within the normal climatic range (it does not become brittle in cold weather). Its chemical inertness allows for easy cleaning with soap and water.

128. The voluntary-opening split hook. The advantage of voluntary opening is that grasp can be maintained without requiring the user's continuous attention and constant tension on the motivating cable.

129. It is strong, lightweight, simple, reliable, and very functional. It resists wear and tear, its cost is relatively low, and maintenance and repairs are relatively simple. Its major disadvantage is that it is less cosmetically appealing.

130. Wrist extension results in hand opening and wrist flexion results in hand closing. This is opposite of the normal tenodesis effect of the natural hand. This motion is, however, better adapted to table surface pick-up.

131. It is much more cosmetically appealing; there is no body harness necessary for its operation; it tends to be more comfortable; it also works more effectively close to the body and with overhead activities than does the body-powered prosthesis.

132. It is not designed for heavy work. It is heavy, which limits its use in short residual limbs; it is prone to breakdown and requires more servicing, and repair and maintenance facilities are not readily available in most locations; its cost is usually 3 to 4 times greater than the body-powered prosthesis; and a battery source must be maintained and recharged for use of this prosthesis.

133. The inability to replicate or reproduce sensory and proprioceptive feedback mechanisms. Visual monitoring or sound cues must be relied upon to control specific motions. This greatly impairs the efficiency of motion and limits the ability to produce finely controlled movements.

134. Motion of the prosthesis is produced by increasing tension on the motivating cable, which passes obliquely from the harness on the contralateral shoulder across the posterior aspect of the thorax. Tension is increased with biscapular abduction and glenohumeral flexion of the amputated extremity. This results in cable shortening and subsequent elbow flexion.

135. Downward rotation of the scapula through shoulder depression, humeral abduction, and slight humeral extension lock as well as unlock the elbow mechanism.

136. The long opponens hand splint. This does not improve function but prevents hand contractures.

137. A flexor-hinged ratchet. Since some shoulder and elbow function should be intact, the wrist and hand can be positioned for functional use with this orthosis.

138. The wrist-driven flexor-hinged orthosis. The tenodesis effect of wrist motion can be used to produce and control grasp-and-pinch motions with this orthosis.

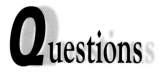

**139.** At what age should prosthetic fitting be considered for congenital upper extremity deficiency?

**140.** What are the advantages of early fitting of prostheses for congenital upper limb deficiency?

**141.** Identify the structures in this cross section of the arm at the midhumeral shaft level. (See Figure 4-8.)

**Figure** 4-8

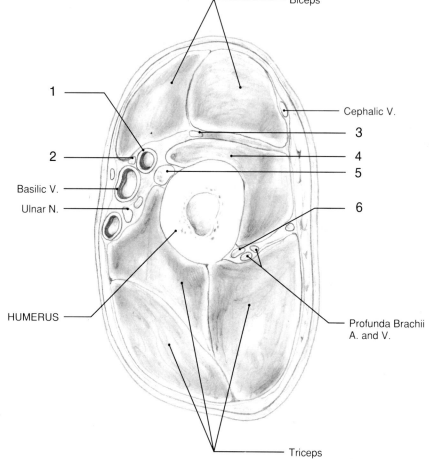

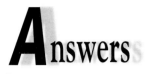
# nswers

139. The timing of prosthetic fitting should coincide with normal development. Since the infant begins to execute useful gross grasping motions at the age of 3 months, most recommend placement of at least a primitive passive prosthetic fitting at this time. This encourages bilateral activities.

140. Early prosthetic tolerance, equalization of limb lengths (for crawling), bimanual pattern of activity, and acceptance of the prosthesis as an integral part of the body (it becomes a part of the infant's self-image).

141. (1) Brachial artery; (2) median nerve; (3) musculocutaneous nerve; (4) brachialis muscle; (5) coracobrachialis tendon; and (6) radial nerve.

142. Identify items 1 through 7 in Figure 4-9.

**Figure** 4-9

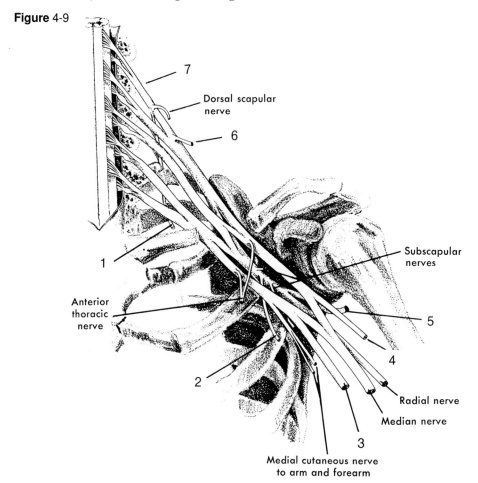

143. An 81-year-old woman has chronic, unremitting shoulder pain, but is otherwise in good health. Her condition has not responded to a course of NSAIDs, or intraarticular corticosteroid injection, and it interferes with both function and sleep. Examination reveals abduction to 100°, flexion to 100°, internal rotation of 45°, external rotation of 30°, and extension of 15°. There are no clinical signs of subacromial impingement nor clinically significant pathology at the acromioclavicular joint. Crepitation is felt with any glenohumeral motion. Is shoulder implant arthroplasty indicated; and if so, is the primary indication loss of motion, relief of pain, or improvement in strength and function?

144. In considering shoulder implant arthroplasty, of what importance is the status of the rotator cuff— its presence, its clinical function, and its repairability if torn?

145. What long-term results can you tell your patient he or she may expect? How do these results compare with the results of total joint arthroplasty (TJA) in weight-bearing joints such as the hip and knee?

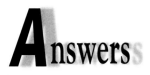
# Answers

**142.** (1) Long thoracic nerve; (2) thoracodorsal nerve; (3) ulnar nerve; (4) musculocutaneous nerve; (5) axillary nerve; (6) suprascapular nerve; and (7) C5 nerve root.

**143.** The limiting parameter is the health of the patient and her ability to tolerate surgery. The primary indication for shoulder implant arthroplasty is pain relief. Motion improvement is unreliable and is dependent on multiple factors that include the condition of the rotator cuff, the condition prompting the surgery, the general condition of the patient, the surgical technique, and postoperative rehabilitation. Improvement in motion can generally be expected; however, this improvement is secondary to pain relief and osteophyte removal. Improvement in postoperative strength is similarly dependent on multiple factors and is, as a result, unreliable. However, the subjective patient assessment of strength may increase if pain relief is good.

**144.** The condition of the rotator cuff may be the **single** greatest determinant of postoperative motion, stability, and strength. An intact rotator cuff is ideal, a repairable rotator cuff is desirable, and an unrepairable rotator cuff is a relative contraindication to shoulder implant arthroplasty. In the face of a marginally repairable or un-repairable rotator cuff, the patient must be counseled regarding the more limited expectations of surgery.

**145.** Significant pain relief after shoulder implant arthroplasty reaches 90%. Long-term results compare favorably with lower extremity TJA revision rates. At 10 years, shoulder arthroplasty revision rates are reported in various studies as being between 10% and 25%. Motion and strength results are less predictable. Motion and strength are dependent on multiple factors as noted, but can be excellent. The best **general** predictor of postoperative strength and motion is preoperative strength and motion.

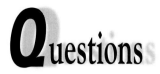

146. A 68-year-old man is referred for loss of motion and chronic pain in his right shoulder. He is a retired truck driver who remains active with low demand hobbies. His referring physician has had him on NSAIDs for several years, but his pain and motion loss have progressed despite the medication. He is now unable to engage in his avocations and awakens several times each night as a result of shoulder pain. His examination demonstrates active abduction to only 40°, active flexion to 65°, weak and deficient active internal and external rotation, and pain on virtually all motion. His initial radiographs are shown (Figure 4-10, A and B). There are several contraindications and relative contraindications to total shoulder arthroplasty (TSA). Are any of these evidenced by the radiographic films? Would shoulder fusion be a more reasonable alternative for function and pain relief?

**Figure** 4-10   A

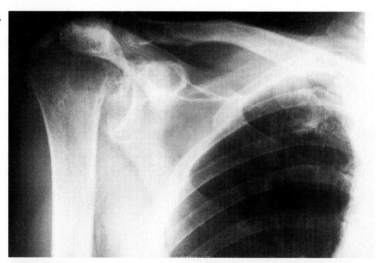

B

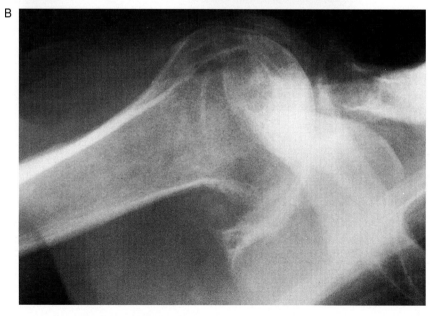

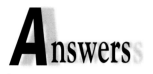

# Answers

**146.** Contraindications or relative contraindications to TSA include a history of sepsis, a neuropathic joint, and paralysis or loss of effective deltoid and rotator cuff function. Because these radiographic films give evidence of rotator cuff pathology, a fusion would be a reasonable consideration. Another option might be TSA or tendon transfer to close the cuff defect and then treat with "limited goals" rehabilitation.

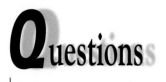

**147.** What is the likely condition of the rotator cuff? Is it repairable? Would this shoulder require a constrained prosthesis?

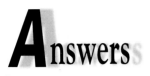

# Answers

147. Because the humeral head is articulating with the acromion, there is obviously a massive rotator cuff defect that may not be amenable to repair or effective reconstruction. This patient might be best served by glenohumeral arthrodesis. More marginal considerations include shoulder implant arthroplasty with a superiorly constrained glenoid prosthesis or humeral replacement with an oversized or bipolar prosthesis. As indicated earlier, constrained prostheses have very limited indications, and are usually for salvage revision.

   After detailed discussion with the patient, the shoulder in Figure 4-10, A and B, was treated by shoulder implant arthroplasty using an oversized humeral head and no glenoid component. The rotator cuff was judged to be unrepairable at surgery. The patient has some, though not complete, relief of pain. He is now able to perform most desired activities and is not awakened by shoulder pain. He requires only occasional, nonnarcotic pain medication for discomfort caused by heavy use of his arm. His only complaint is an inability to fully abduct actively, although he can hold his arm in an overhead position once it has been assisted there by the other arm. Other active motion is nearly equal to the contralateral unaffected shoulder. His current radiographic films are shown (Figure 4-11, A and B).

**Figure** 4-11    A

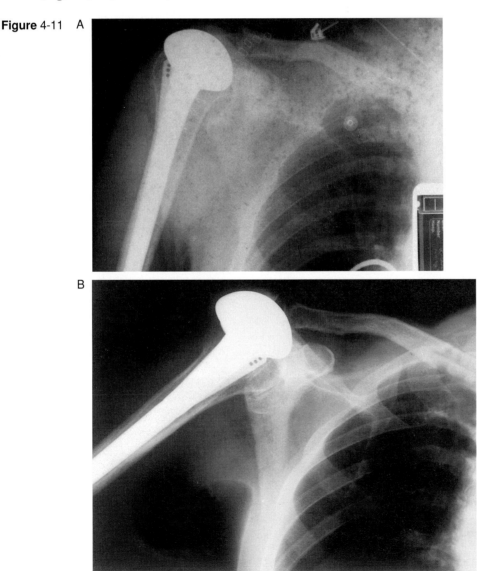

B

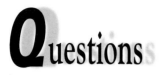

**148.** A patient with a 17-year history of renal cell carcinoma has, of late, experienced steadily increasing bone pain. A bone scan has demonstrated multiple areas of increased uptake. A plain-film survey of these areas reveals the radiographic lesion shown (Figure 4-12, A and B). The oncologist informs you that the patient's current life expectancy is 6 to 12 months. The patient is frail but still ambulatory, living at home with his wife and remains capable of managing his own activities of daily living. His shoulder and elbow motion are full, but motion causes pain in the midbrachium area. What role should radiation therapy play in the treatment of metastatic bone lesions?

**Figure** 4-12

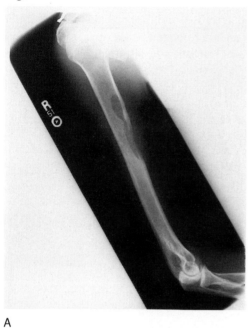

A

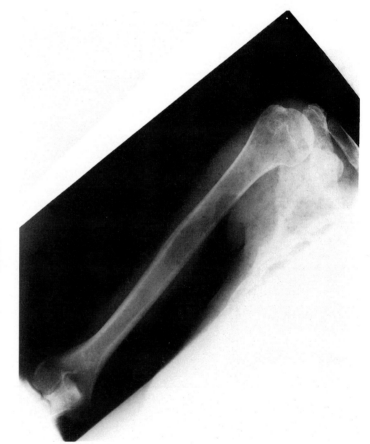

B

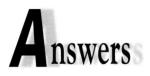

# Answers

148. Radiation therapy can be used before or after prophylactic surgical stabilization in lesions likely to respond. For smaller lesions with a low likelihood of fracture, radiation therapy may prevent further cortical destruction, relieve pain, and avoid the necessity for future surgery. Lesions with a high likelihood of pathological fracture should be stabilized. The choice of preoperative versus postoperative irradiation should be made in conjunction with the patient's oncologist, bearing in mind that radiation therapy initially weakens the bone and may increase the possibility of fracture. Consideration should also be given to the fact that irradiation can compromise options for surgery or impair wound healing. It is therefore desirable, when possible, to plan incision sites away from sites of irradiation. In this case, although irradiation might be of some benefit, renal cell carcinoma is typically not highly sensitive to radiation therapy.

149. A 57-year-old school teacher fell from a chair while changing a ceiling light and injured her arm. The radiographic films ordered by the emergency room physician reveal the fracture shown (Figure 4-13, A and B). Your examination reveals no obvious deficits of either sensory or motor function in the median, ulnar, or radial nerve distributions. The biceps, triceps, and deltoid muscles fire, but the patient resists moving the shoulder or elbow because of pain. Distal pulses are strong, and capillary refill is less than 3 seconds. There is crepitation and pain on movement around the shoulder, and you note a prominent indented area anterolaterally, proximal to the insertion of the anterior deltoid muscle. You assess that the distal fracture spike has impaled the overlying soft tissue. Measurement of the radiographic films shows the apical anterior angulation to be 47°. Is the degree of angulation of this fracture acceptable? Would healing in this position result in significant motion deficits? Cosmetic deformity?

**Figure** 4-13

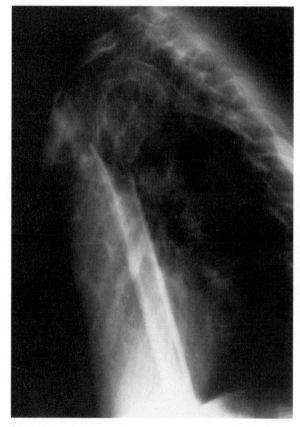

A

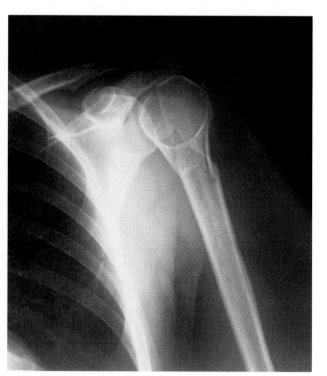

B

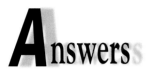

**A**nswers

149. Because of the generous soft tissue coverage of the humerus, even this degree of angulation would likely be cosmetically unnoticeable. The tremendous ROM of the glenohumeral joint coupled with the contributions of the scapulo-thoracic joint is also rather forgiving of residual angulatory deformity. The generally accepted parameter for residual angulation is 45° or less. Healing in the degree of apical anterior angulation would not result in significant flexion deficit or impingement.

# Questions

150. An active, healthy, 67-year-old man sustains the fracture shown (Figure 4-14, A and B) in a low-speed motor vehicle accident. He has no injuries other than this closed fracture. He is vascularly intact but has a complete motor and sensory radial nerve palsy. Does the nerve injury necessitate exploration and rigid stabilization of the fracture?

**Figure** 4-14

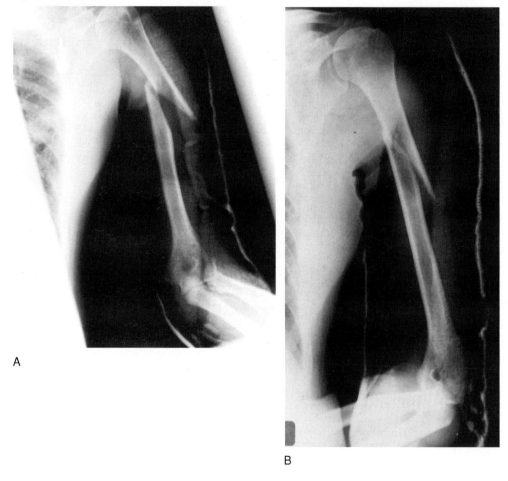

A

B

151. If this were a type II open fracture being debrided in the operating room, should the radial nerve be explored as part of the surgery?

152. At 4 months from the time of injury, the patient has painless, gross motion at the fracture site, and no significant callus formation is seen on radiographic films. The patient has been treated in a well-fitting fracture brace. His radial nerve palsy has resolved completely. At what point in treatment can this be classified as a nonunion?

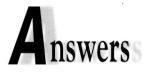
# Answers

150. Various sources report that from 5% to 18% of patients with humeral shaft fractures have some radial nerve injury. Traditionally, some types of humeral fractures (Holstein), when associated with complete radial nerve palsy, were believed to require exploration. Secondary radial nerve palsies were also believed to be an indication for immediate exploration. More recent study has shown that the vast majority of radial nerve injuries associated with humeral fractures are injuries in continuity and will resolve without exploration. Those that do not, will, in most cases, do as well with late nerve repair as with immediate nerve repair. There are some data which indicate that some nerve injuries in continuity actually yield worse long-term clinical results if immediately explored. Injuries in continuity do not require rigid fracture stabilization to resolve.

151. Exploring the radial nerve for palsy in conjunction with humeral fracture surgery performed for other reasons is the one instance in which there is general agreement that such exploration is indicated.

152. Four months is usually the least amount of time required to establish a diagnosis of humeral nonunion.

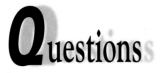

**153.** At this point, should the patient be advised to undergo internal fixation, internal fixation with grafting, or continued nonsurgical treatment?

**154.** While standing next to a ski lift stanchion, a 28-year-old skier was run into by an out-of-control snowboarder. He was struck from the side and pinned between the stanchion and the snowboarder, compressing his shoulders transversely. In the emergency room, he is complaining of pain at the base of his neck anteriorly and difficulty swallowing. A chest radiographic films shows no pneumothorax. His physician's examination reveals asymmetry of the medial ends of the clavicles and marked tenderness at the left sternoclavicular joint. There seems to be less fullness at the left sternoclavicular joint, and the superomedial corner of the manubrium is possibly palpable on the left. His anteroposterior radiographic film is shown (Figure 4-15). Is there sufficient information to make a diagnosis and to initiate treatment?

**Figure** 4-15

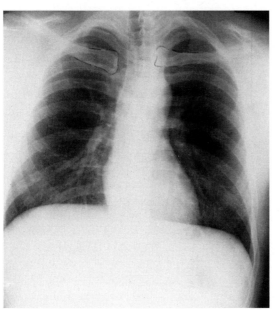

**155.** Should the diagnosis be made with special plain radiographic films, tomograms, computerized axial tomography (CT), or MRI?

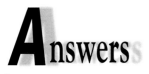

# Answers

**153.** At least two series have reported fracture bracing for humeral shaft fractures to yield a high rate of union. Average time to union for closed fractures treated in a fracture brace is less than 12 weeks. Assuming good compliance and no treatment difficulties and given the findings noted, this case could be classified as a nonunion. Some practitioners recommend continued nonsurgical treatment; however, it is reasonable at this point to discuss with the patient options for treatment of nonunion. Electrical stimulation has not enjoyed great success or popularity in the treatment of humeral nonunion. Reamed and unreamed, locking and nonlocking intramedullary devices have been used in the treatment of this problem. The best and most consistent results to date have been obtained using meticulous AO/Association for the Study of Internal Fixation (ASIF) technique for compression plating with concurrent, **cancellous** bone grafting. Locking intramedullary devices have been reported to yield good results, but experience with these devices is less extensive than with compression plating and cancellous grafting.

**154.** There is an obvious asymmetry of the medial ends of the clavicles on the anteroposterior radiographic film. This, along with the history and examination, strongly suggests a sternoclavicular dislocation. Though earlier wisdom stated that this diagnosis could be made clinically, imaging tools now available allow the diagnosis to be made definitively and should be used. Because the consequences of anterior and posterior dislocations differ significantly, his physician is obligated to clarify the diagnosis and cannot do so with just clinical evaluation.

**155.** The sternoclavicular joints are notoriously difficult to visualize with plain radiographic films. Numerous special views have been recommended by different practitioners but are not well-known and can be difficult to interpret. Perhaps the best known is the serendipity view, but this too can be confusing. Tomograms can be helpful. The imaging modality of choice is CT. MRI can also clarify the diagnosis.

**156.** The patient described in question 154 was sent for CT imaging. Representative cuts are shown (Figure 4-16, A, B, and C). What is your diagnosis?

**Figure** 4-16

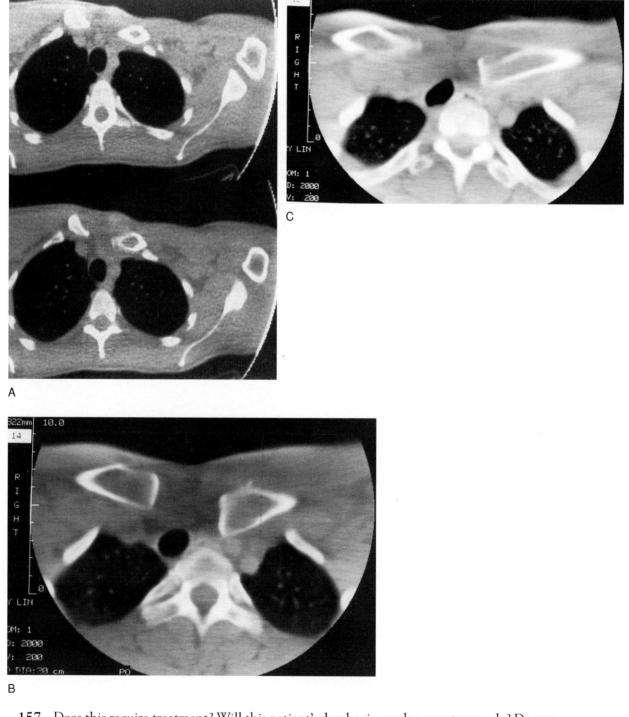

**157.** Does this require treatment? Will this patient's dysphagia resolve spontaneously? Do any consequences attend a chronically unreduced posterior sternoclavicular dislocation?

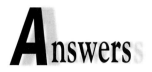

# Answers

156. The correct diagnosis is posterior sternoclavicular joint dislocation. Although the ratio of posterior to anterior dislocations of the sternoclavicular joint has not been clarified, posterior dislocations are far less common than anterior dislocations.

157. Unreduced, posterior dislocations of the sternoclavicular joint can compress vessels to the head or to the ipsilateral arm causing vascular compromise. They can also cause dysphagia and breathing problems or can compress the thoracic outlet. Posterior sternoclavicular dislocations should be reduced.

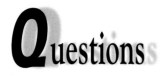

# Questions

**158.** Should this dislocation be reduced closed? Should the procedure be performed in the emergency room, clinic, or operating room?

**159.** What treatment is recommended for an unstable sternoclavicular dislocation?

**160.** A 37-year-old police officer injured his right shoulder when he fell off a rope slide during training. He landed with his proximal anterior brachium impacting against the corner of a low brick wall. A shoulder trauma series that is ordered when he is seen in the emergency room does not show any fracture or dislocation. However, examination reveals that he is unable to abduct the shoulder more than minimally, and external rotation is markedly weak. You can detect no muscle tone in any part of the deltoid muscle on attempted abduction, but the supraspinatus muscle fires. What is your clinical diagnosis?

**161.** At this point should his surgeon explore the axillary nerve, consider tendon transfers for the deltoid muscle paralysis, order electrodiagnostic tests, or treat expectantly?

**162.** At 1 month, electrodiagnostic tests on the patient in question 160 show fibrillation potentials in the teres minor muscle and all three parts of the deltoid muscle. What implication does this have?

**163.** Although you continue physical therapy, 3 months later the patient in question 160 is still unable to abduct more than minimally, and external rotation remains weak and questionably functional. Flexion is present actively, but beyond 60°, the patient has difficulty preventing the brachium from going into internal rotation. Electrodiagnostic testing continues to show fibrillation potentials. Can return of active abduction ever be expected if the deltoid muscle remains paralyzed?

**164.** Should the shoulder now be fused or the axillary nerve explored?

**165.** A 55-year-old man, who was unaware that the suitcase he was removing from a high shelf was full, sustained a sudden pronounced load on his flexed, abducted shoulder. He had immediate shoulder pain that has not resolved in the intervening month. He complains of inability to elevate his arm and persistent pain that disturbs his sleep. Upon examination, he has a positive impingement sign and a positive drop arm test. His shoulder outlet view, demonstrating a type III acromion, is shown (Figure 4-17). Diagnosed as a rotator cuff tear, this patient's symptoms have not improved over a period of 1 month. What kind of treatment is recommended: surgical, pharmacological, or physical therapy?

**Figure** 4-17

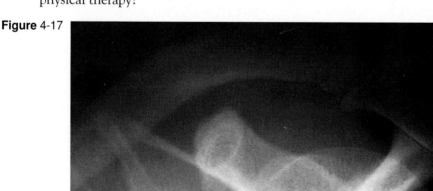

**166.** After a 3-month trial of physical therapy, the patient in question 165 is still unacceptably symptomatic. Is an acromioplasty, rotator cuff repair, or both indicated?

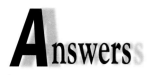

# Answers

158. Although some practitioners advocate reduction maneuvers in a clinic or emergency room, most recommend closed reduction under general anesthesia. Before reduction, a careful assessment should be carried out to determine the status of major vessels and pulmonary structures. It is probably wise to have a surgeon available who can deal with injury to these structures should any become apparent during closed or open reduction.

159. **Anterior dislocations** of the sternoclavicular joint are often unstable and difficult to hold using a figure-eight sling or a shoulder harness. They often do not cause clinical symptoms if left unreduced. Given the potential complications of stabilization procedures, anterior dislocations should probably be allowed to heal in the unreduced position if they cannot be held using closed means. Anterior dislocations can be treated late if they cause unacceptable, chronic symptoms. **Posterior dislocations** are usually stable following reduction. If surgical stabilization is desirable for an anterior or posterior sternoclavicular dislocation, either biological or synthetic materials can be used to stabilize the joint. The use of metal implants at the sternoclavicular joint has resulted in horrendous complications, including death, and is to be condemned.

160. Traumatic axillary nerve palsy.

161. The injury to the axillary nerve may be any magnitude, from a traction neurapraxia to an avulsion of the nerve from the muscle. **Immediate** exploration would be difficult to justify. Tendon transfer for a deltoid muscle palsy is a legitimate treatment for this condition, but not before the nature or the permanency of the injury is determined. Electrodiagnostic tests are unlikely to yield useful information until 3 to 4 weeks following injury. Support or immobilization for comfort followed by physical therapy are probably the best early treatment.

162. Fibrillation potentials are indicative of denervation. The posterior branch of the axillary nerve supplies the teres minor muscle and the posterior portion of deltoid muscle. The anterior branch supplies the middle and anterior portions of deltoid muscle.

163. In some cases, intact rotator cuff muscles will abduct the glenohumeral joint. Failure to achieve active abduction after 4 months of physical therapy makes it unlikely that this patient will achieve active abduction without deltoid muscle recovery.

164. It is desirable to maintain mobility of the glenohumeral joint if possible. Fusion for a paralytically unstable shoulder is an option, but an attempt to return motion by repairing or reconstructing the nerve or by tendon transfers is probably a better consideration at this point.

165. Depalma found that approximately 90% of patients diagnosed as having a rotator cuff tear will have adequate resolution of their symptoms without surgery. NSAIDs can be of benefit as can subacromial steroid injections using local anesthetics or steroids. Physical therapy and activity limitation, or a combination of these, will often resolve symptoms and deserve a trial prior to considering surgery.

166. With a type III acromion, most authorities would recommend an acromioplasty for this patient, whether or not a rotator cuff repair is performed. Controversy exists regarding the necessity of rotator cuff repair. Some prominent shoulder surgeons believe that the pain associated with cuff tear responds well to acromioplasty alone and that cuff repair adds little to the result. Neer has described "cuff arthropathy" which may lead to destruction of the glenohumeral joint and is an argument in favor of rotator cuff repair.

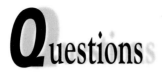

167. In counseling this patient regarding rotator cuff surgery, what likely outcomes can you predict regarding pain relief and strength and motion?

168. Following repair, what is the likelihood of a recurrent defect in the rotator cuff?

169. Does failure of a rotator cuff repair generally cause a recurrence of pain symptoms?

170. A 20-year-old college student fell while snowboarding and landed on her right elbow, suffering immediate pain. Her radiographic films are shown (Figure 4-18, A and B). Her examination reveals a swollen and ecchymotic elbow with no skin breaks. Any motion at the elbow is painful and not tolerated. Wrist and digital motion seem unimpaired and nonpainful. There are no apparent vascular or neurologic deficits. She is otherwise healthy. Describe and classify this fracture.

**Figure 4-18**

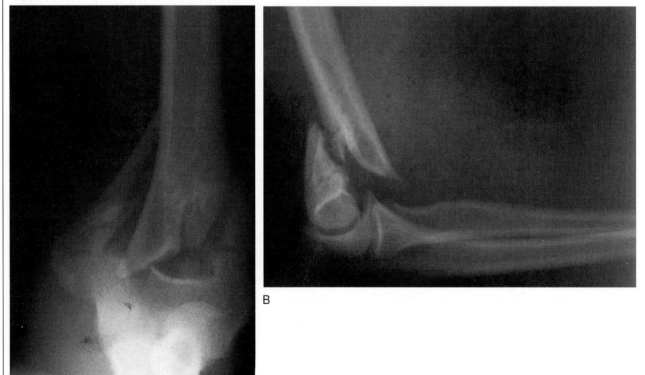

A

B

171. Would the treatment of choice for this injury be closed reduction and immobilization, the "bag of bones technique" of Eastwood, traction, or ORIF?

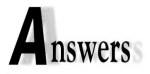
# Answers

**167.** Acceptable levels of pain relief are reported to be achieved up to 95% of the time. Various practitioners have indicated strength recovery of 75% to 90% after rotator cuff repair. Some have related success to the length of time between injury and surgery, indicating that a delay in repair compromises the results. Other practitioners find no such correlation. Several practitioners have related success regarding motion and strength to the size of the rotator cuff lesion. Motion is generally less in virtually all planes than in a normal shoulder. Recovery of motion and strength is significantly dependent on patient motivation and the postoperative rehabilitation program and may require as long as 6 to 12 months for maximal improvement.

**168.** Harryman, et al. found that 65% of 105 rotator cuff repairs remained intact at an average 5-year follow-up. The probability of remaining intact was inversely proportional to both age of the patient and size of the tear.

**169.** If there is sufficient subacromial decompression, most patients continue to have satisfactory pain relief despite recurrence of a cuff defect. Some have used this as an argument in favor of decompression without repair. Function, however, seems to be better with an intact cuff repair.

**170.** This is a displaced and comminuted intercondylar fracture of the distal humerus in a skeletally mature individual. There are several accepted systems by which this fracture could be classified. Muller's system for classification of distal humeral fractures is reasonably comprehensive and would label this a C3 distal humerus fracture (bicondylar, comminuted); however, the more accepted system for classification of humeral intercondylar fractures is that proposed by E. J. Riseborough and Radin. In their system this fracture would be a type III (T-intercondylar with displacement and rotation).

**171.** Before the advent of modern implants and surgical techniques, fractures such as this did poorly with open treatment; consequently, many practitioners recommended closed management for all distal humeral fractures. Currently, the principle of early motion in the treatment of elbow fractures is widely espoused and should be the primary goal in management. Most closed means of treating this fracture would require an unacceptable length of immobilization.

An exception to this would be the "bag of bones technique" of Eastwood. This technique involves a collar and cuff (initially keeping the elbow in marked flexion) and a rapidly advanced program of elbow motion. This method is generally recommended for elderly patients with types III and IV fractures, a group in whom the results of open treatment have been less than satisfying. It is also recommended for patients in whom, for other reasons, surgery is not an option.

Traction is an acceptable alternative, allowing initiation of early motion and reportedly yielding reasonable results, but requiring prolonged hospitalization and bed rest. Results are probably inferior to optimal internal fixation and early motion, although no comparative studies have been done.

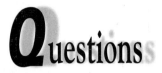

172. After ORIF to restore the articular surface and secure the intercondylar portion of the fracture with screws and the medial and lateral columns with plates (see Figure 4-19), what functional outcome can this patient expect to achieve?

**Figure** 4-19

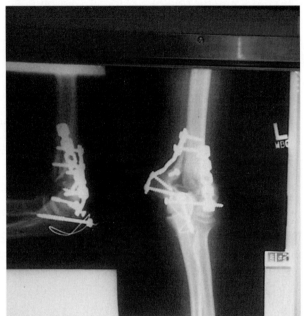

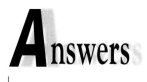

nswers

172. Ideally, she can expect to regain functional elbow motion, close to full forearm pronation and supination, and a relatively painless joint. These results require strong motivation to complete an extended rehabilitation program. This patient began progressive stretching and strengthening exercises after several weeks of immobilization. She also worked to develop endurance. She experienced a temporary setback after surgery at 8 months to remove the hardware. Approximately 1 year postinjury, she demonstrated active elbow ROM of 14° to 112°, forearm supination of 75° and pronation of 85° (see Figure 4-20, A through D). A music major training to become a professional flutist, the patient could play her flute up to 2 hours per session, twice a day, and was also playing the organ for an hour a day.

**Figure** 4-20

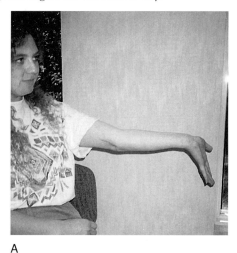

A

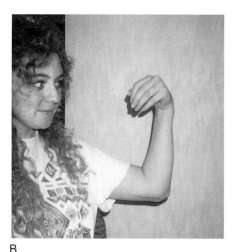

B

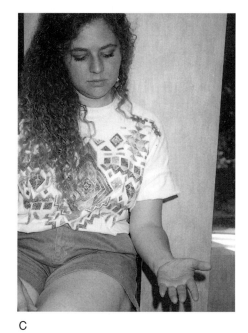

C

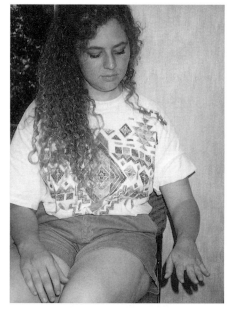

D

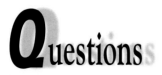

**173.** A 36-year-old athletic woman complains of elbow "dislocation" every time she fully extends her elbow. This condition was the result of an injury sustained 4 years earlier while she was engaged in a karate practice session. During this session, there was a collision of the ulnar border of her forearm with her opponent's foot, causing a severe valgus stress at her elbow. At the time, she was not noted to have a fracture or dislocation and was treated in a sling for comfort. Recovery took several weeks. Since that injury, she has had a feeling of elbow instability, which has prevented vigorous activity involving the affected arm. Your examination does not demonstrate dislocation on extension but does show gross valgus instability. Radiographic films are remarkable for an old radial head injury that healed with mild deformity. Of the structures seen in Figure 4-21, which is the primary valgus stabilizer of the elbow?

**Figure** 4-21

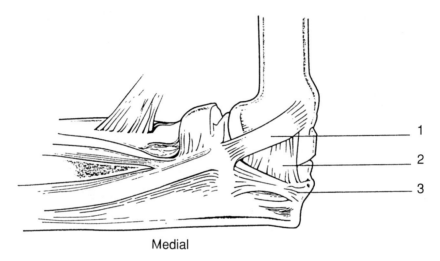

Medial

**174.** What is the most important secondary valgus stabilizer of the elbow?

**175.** What are the relative contributions of soft tissue and bony valgus stabilizers at this joint?

**176.** What long-term problem may result from valgus instability of the elbow?

**177.** Would radial head replacement afford relief from this patient's valgus instability?

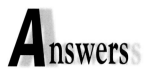
**173.** Structures (1), (2), and (3) constitute the medial collateral ligament of the elbow. Of these, the transverse portion (3) contributes little to stability. The anterior oblique bundle (1) is the most active in the functional ROM at this joint and is considered to be the primary valgus stabilizer of the elbow.

**174.** The radial head is the predominant secondary valgus stabilizer of the elbow.

**175.** According to Morrey et al., the medial collateral ligament (MCL) complex accounts for 54% of stability against an applied valgus stress in flexion. The osseous articulation, predominantly the radial head, accounts for 33%. The majority of the balance of stability is from the joint capsule.

**176.** The most notable long-term sequela from chronic valgus instability at the elbow is ulnar neuropathy.

**177.** Although there is a clear relationship between MCL and radial head injury in creating valgus instability at the elbow, radial head replacement has been used for valgus stabilization in acute elbow trauma and is now recommended only when no other options are available. Jobe has described both MCL repair and MCL reconstruction as yielding good results in chronic valgus instability at the elbow.

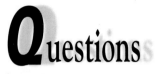

178. A 38-year-old man complains of numbness and weakness in his right hand. He does not relate the problem to a traumatic event and notes its onset to have been gradual over a period of several months. He says his symptoms are more pronounced when he has his elbow flexed, such as when he is holding a newspaper. He is sometimes awakened at night with marked numbness in his small finger. Upon questioning, he indicates that during childhood, he had a fracture about the right elbow that was "set" and then treated in a cast. Upon examination, you find he has full and symmetrical flexion and extension of the elbow and wrist. There is a mild but definite increase in cubitus valgus at the right elbow. Distally, there is 6-mm static two-point discrimination (2PD) in the ulnar 1½ digits of the right hand compared to 4-mm static 2PD in the remainder of the right hand and all of the left. There seems to be some weakness of finger abduction and adduction in the right hand compared with the left hand. There is some decrease of first dorsal interosseous mass on the right, despite it being the dominant hand. There is a positive Tinel's sign just posterior to the medial epicondyle and also just distal and radial to the pisiform, though this is much less prominent. You diagnose an ulnar neuropathy. At what level is ulnar nerve compression most likely?

179. With your clinical diagnosis and examination findings, should you proceed with further diagnostic testing or treat the patient on the basis on your current evaluation?

180. What diagnostic test(s) will most likely confirm your diagnosis?

181. If you choose to treat this problem nonsurgically for a time, what treatment would you recommend?

182. What is the recommended surgical treatment for cubital tunnel syndrome?

183. What theoretical advantage do decompression and epicondylectomy have over transposition of the ulnar nerve?

184. What are the disadvantages of decompression and epicondylectomy when compared with anterior transposition?

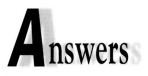
# Answers

178. The most common site of compression of the ulnar nerve is the cubital tunnel. This patient's history of childhood elbow fracture with a presumably resultant cubitus valgus also suggests that the elbow is the likely site of compression, because chronic cubitus valgus has been associated with an increased likelihood of tardy ulnar nerve palsy (ulnar neuropathy).

179. Although the history and examination strongly suggest a cubital tunnel syndrome, Guyon's canal is another potential area of compression. Other unusual causes of peripheral nerve compression (tumor, vascular anomaly) can exist virtually anywhere along the course of the nerve. Because of the existence of atrophy, expectant treatment is not prudent, and further diagnostic evaluation is indicated.

180. The accepted method to confirm a compressive ulnar neuropathy at the elbow is electrodiagnostic testing. Eversmann has stated that slowing of nerve conduction velocity greater than 33% across the elbow is always significant. Electromyographic testing of ulnar innervated muscles helps to confirm the diagnosis. In cases where a mass is suspected to be causing compression, CT or MRI imaging may be helpful. An X-ray film of the right elbow permits objective measurement of cubitus valgus and identification of bony elements impinging at the cubital tunnel.

181. Specific options for the nonsurgical treatment of cubital tunnel syndrome include elbow pads, avoidance of prolonged elbow flexion, and elbow extension night splints. The rationale for these treatments is the relative superficial course of the ulnar nerve as it traverses behind the medial epicondyle and the decrease in the cross-sectional area of the cubital tunnel as the elbow flexes. Considering the presence of intrinsic atrophy in this case, prolonged nonoperative treatment is probably not indicated, and surgery is the treatment most likely to either halt or reverse the clinical deficits.

182. Several surgical options have been described for the treatment of this problem. Although different practitioners advocate different operative procedures, simple decompression, medial epicondylectomy, and anterior transposition (subcutaneous, submuscular, or partially submuscular) are all accepted treatments.

183. In both decompression and epicondylectomy, the ulnar nerve is not disturbed from its bed and, therefore, is not put at vascular risk by partial skeletonization. Additionally, anterior transposition risks kinking the nerve.

184. Simple decompression can fail to expose or treat the site of actual compression of the ulnar nerve. In addition, the nerve continues to course behind the medial epicondyle and is stretched when the elbow flexes. Epicondylectomy has been criticized for removing the osseous protection of the ulnar nerve afforded by the medial epicondyle.

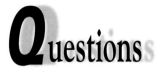
# Questions

185. A 54-year-old librarian has a 2-month history of her arms "giving out and falling asleep" during work. She spends the majority of her time shelving books (often overhead as she is 5'1" tall) and performing keyboard activities. She also notes that for about the past 3 weeks, her ring and small fingers have been tingling. How would you distinguish between thoracic outlet syndrome and cubital tunnel syndrome through clinical testing?

186. A 48-year-old female telephone operator was released to return to work 4 weeks after a left carpal tunnel release, when she suddenly developed severe burning pain in her hand. Her incision appeared well-healed with no signs of inflammation. Her hand was mildly edematous, and she was very apprehensive about moving her fingers. Is this a case of not wanting to work? How would you handle it?

187. What are the stages of progression of RSD?

188. A 51-year-old man developed painless, fluctuant swelling over his left posterior olecranon after an 800-mile automobile trip. He recalls that he frequently used the driver's side armrest. He has full ROM and no neurologic symptoms. What is his problem?

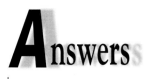

**185.** Thoracic outlet syndrome typically produces sensory changes in a C8-T1 dermatomal distribution, involving the medial aspect of the **arm**, hand, and the little finger. In contrast, the sensory changes associated with cubital tunnel syndrome are confined to the ulnar aspect of the hand and ulnar 1½ digits. A careful assessment of the arm may implicate TOS if sensory changes are present. Vascular changes such as pallor, cyanosis, or edema also occasionally occur in TOS, but not in cubital tunnel syndrome.

Thoracic outlet syndrome may be aggravated by postural changes such as drooping shoulders and overhead activities, whereas cubital tunnel syndrome is worsened by sustained elbow flexion. An examiner may discern the presence of such aggravating activities from a patient's history, or attempt to reproduce her symptoms by provocative tests. Lastly, Tinel's sign may be present at the elbow with cubital tunnel, but not with TOS. Adson's and overhead exercise tests are positive in TOS but not in cubital tunnel.

**186.** This patient probably has reflex sympathetic dystropy (RSD), which a three-phase bone scan can usually confirm. Early diagnosis and treatment are critical to improving the outcome with this diagnosis. Approach the patient with a firm, positive attitude, providing support while encouraging independence. She should be involved in supervised physical therapy sessions and a structured home program. Management includes edema control, pain management, early motion, ADL, and total body conditioning. Carlson and Watson described a stress-loading program consisting of active exercises that alternate compression and traction of the upper extremity; the patient performs a steady "scrubbing" for 3 to 10 minutes t.i.d. and carries a weighted bag whenever standing or walking. Drug therapy and/or stellate ganglion blocks may hasten the resolution of symptoms.

**187.** The **acute stage**, lasting up to 3 months, is characterized by burning pain and soft edema. Early vasomotor reflex spasm produces vasoconstriction and cool, pale, clammy skin. The body later responds by "shutting down" sympathetic function, evidenced by warm, reddened, dry skin. Increased hair and nail growth occur during this stage, and the skin appears glossy.

The **dystrophic stage**, from 3 to 9 months, includes pain occurring with motion and brawny edema. The patient experiences hyperesthesia to touch, progressive stiffness, decreased sweating, trophic skin changes, and osteoporosis.

The **atrophic stage**, from 10 months onward, is accompanied by decreasing pain, but there is fibrosis, joint ankylosis, and irreversible functional loss. The involved area becomes pale, dry, and cool.

**188.** This man developed olecranon bursitis from sustained compression and/or blunt trauma over his elbow. This condition should respond well to conservative treatment, including rest, cold compression, and NSAIDs.

# Chapter 5

# Hand and Wrist

TIMOTHY S. LOTH, MD

CAROLYN T. WADSWORTH, MS, PT, OCS, CHT

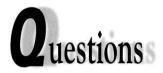

# Questions

1. Identify the labeled structures on the representation of the lateral and dorsal views of the finger in Figure 5-1.

**Figure** 5-1  A. Radial side of the left middle finger

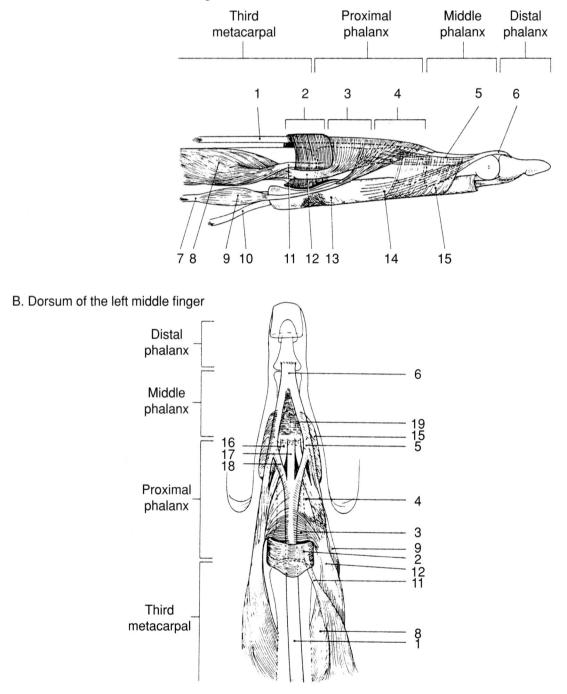

B. Dorsum of the left middle finger

2. What is the origin, insertion, and function of the sagittal bands?

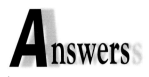**A**nswers

1. (1) extensor digitorum communis tendon; (2) sagittal bands; (3) transverse fibers of the intrinsic muscle apparatus; (4) oblique fibers of the intrinsic muscle apparatus; (5) conjoined lateral band; (6) terminal tendon; (7) flexor digitorum profundus tendon; (8) second dorsal interosseous muscle; (9) lumbrical muscle; (10) flexor digitorum sublimis tendon; (11) medial tendon of the superficial belly of the interosseous muscle; (12) lateral tendon of the deep belly of the interosseous muscle; (13) flexor pulley mechanism; (14) oblique retinacular ligament; (15) transverse retinacular ligament; (16) medial band of the oblique fibers of the intrinsic expansion; (17) central slip; (18) lateral slips; and (19) triangular ligament.

2. The origin is the extensor tendon over the metacarpophalangeal (MCP) joint, passing superficial to the MCP joint capsule and the phalangeal attachment of the medial tendon of the superficial head of the interosseous muscle and deep to the lateral tendon of the deep head of the interosseous muscle. The insertion is the volar proximal phalanx and edge of the volar plate. The sagittal bands extend the proximal phalanx, stabilize the extensor tendon in the midline, and prevent dorsal bowstringing of the extensor tendon.

3. Why is it necessary to splint the MCP joints in flexion (as pictured in Figure 5-2) in order to allow the extensor digitorum communis (EDC) muscle to extend the proximal interphalangeal (PIP) joints after an ulnar nerve injury?

**Figure** 5-2

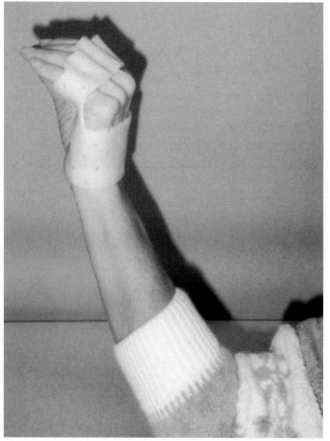

4. Describe the anatomy of the EDC distal to the MCP joint.

5. Describe the interosseous hood (interosseous aponeurotic expansion, dorsal expansion, and dorsal aponeurosis).

6. What is the function of the transverse portion of the interosseous hood?

7. Describe the origin, insertion, function, and pathophysiology of the oblique and transverse retinacular ligaments.

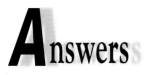

# Answers

3. If MCP joint hyperextension is not prevented, most of the excursion and force of the EDC muscle is expended in proximal phalangeal extension through the sagittal bands, preventing the distal action that could extend the PIP joints.

4. It trifurcates over the proximal one half of the proximal phalanx. The central slip inserts on the base of the middle phalanx joined by the interosseous medial band. The lateral two slips join the interossei and lumbricals, forming the conjoined lateral bands.

5. All dorsal and volar interossei insert into the interosseous hood, which runs from the proximal portion of the proximal phalanx to the insertion at the base of the middle phalanx. The proximal portion of the hood contains transverse fibers that run dorsally over the common extensor tendon and help flex the MCP joint. Oblique fibers of the distal interosseous hood joined by the lumbrical tendons insert into the lateral tubercles through the medial bands at the dorsal base of the middle phalanx. They assist in PIP joint extension. Lateral slips from the common extensor tendon combine with fibers from the extensor hood to create the conjoined lateral bands distally.

6. MCP joint flexion.

7. The oblique retinacular ligament (ORL) originates from the volar lateral aspect of the proximal phalanx coursing dorsally, volar to the axis of the PIP joint to terminate in the terminal extensor tendon. It links motion of the distal interphalangeal (DIP) and PIP joints. With PIP joint flexion, the ligament is relaxed, allowing DIP joint flexion. Proximal interphalangeal joint extension tightens the ligament facilitating DIP joint extension. Pathologic contracture of the ORL, e.g., Dupuytren's disease or a burn injury, may produce a boutonniere deformity, with PIP joint flexion and DIP joint extension. Conversely, stretching of the ORL may allow the finger to assume a swan-neck and/or mallet deformity with PIP joint extension and DIP joint flexion. The ligament may be reconstructed to correct a swan-neck or mallet finger deformity.

   The transverse retinacular ligament prevents dorsal shift of the lateral bands. It attaches to the edge of the flexor sheath at the level of the PIP joint and attaches dorsally to the lateral aspect of the conjoined lateral bands. Swan-neck deformity results from attenuation of the transverse retinacular ligament, allowing dorsal translation of the lateral bands. Boutonniere deformity develops as a result of tightening of the transverse retinacular ligament in association with disruption of the central slip and triangular ligament, allowing volar displacement of the lateral bands associated with transfer of extensor power to the DIP joint, which becomes hyperextended.

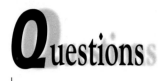
# Questions

8. How do you test to confirm a contracture in the ORL?

9. Describe the insertions of the interosseous muscles.

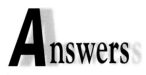

8. With the PIP joint in full extension, measure passive DIP joint flexion (see Figure 5-3, A); then allow the PIP joint to flex and again measure passive DIP joint flexion (see Figure 5-3, B); if DIP joint flexion increases in the second measurement, then the ORL is contracted. (Note: If DIP joint flexion decreases in the second measurement, then the conjoined lateral bands may be contracted; if DIP joint flexion is limited but unchanged by the position of the PIP joint, there probably is a DIP joint contracture.)

**Figure** 5-3   A

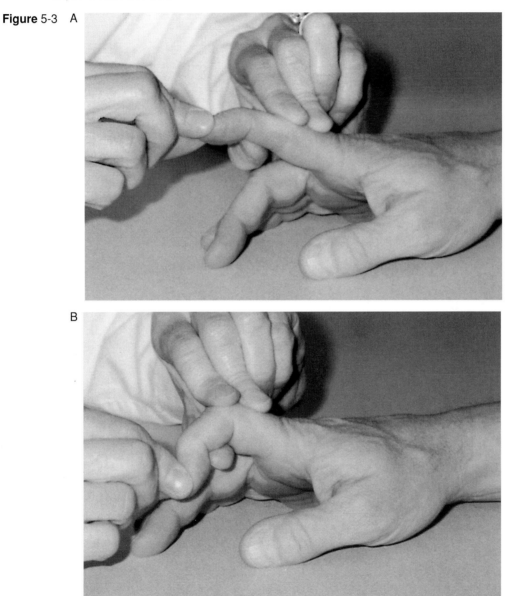

9. The first, second, and fourth dorsal interossei have two muscle bellies. The superficial one courses deep to the sagittal bands through its medial tendon and inserts at the base of the proximal phalanx. The deep head courses superficial to the sagittal bands through the lateral tendon and inserts into the dorsal aponeurosis. The three volar and the third dorsal interosseous muscles each have only one tendon that inserts into the dorsal aponeurosis.

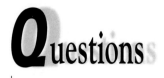**Q**uestions

10. Describe the origins, insertions, and functions of the lumbrical muscles.

11. What does a positive Bunnell-Littler test indicate?

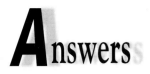

10. The first and second lumbricals originate from the radial aspect of the index and long finger flexor digitorum profundus (FDP) tendons in the palm, pass volar to the transverse metacarpal ligament, volar to the axis of MCP motion, and insert into the radial lateral band over the midproximal phalanx. The third and fourth lumbricals arise from contiguous FDP tendons of the long and ring, and ring and small fingers, respectively. They insert into the radial lateral bands over the midproximal phalanx. In addition to producing PIP and DIP joint extension, they contribute to MCP joint flexion and coordinate balance and precision within the hand.

11. The Bunnell-Littler test is performed by attempting to passively flex the PIP joint, first with the MCP joint passively extended (see Figure 5-4, A), then with the MCP joint passively flexed (see Figure 5-4, B). If more PIP joint flexion occurs with the MCP joint flexed, then tightness exists in the intrinsic muscles—a positive test.

**Figure** 5-4   A

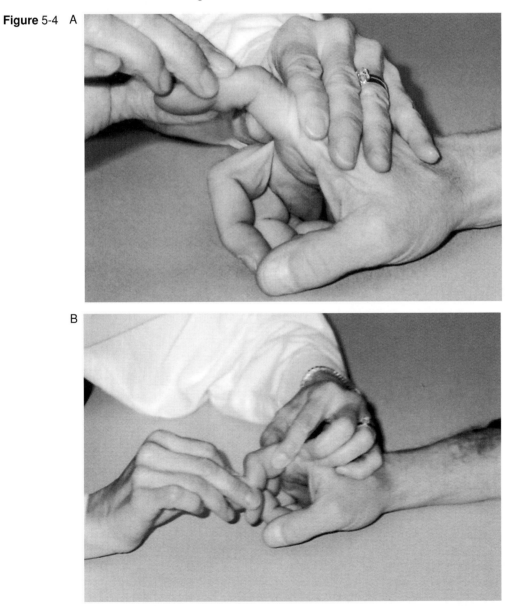

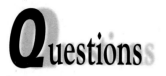

# Questions

12. Describe the origin, insertion, and function of the adductor pollicis muscle.

13. What does a positive Froment's sign indicate?

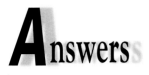

# Answers

12. The adductor pollicis muscle has two heads of origin (oblique and transverse). The transverse head originates from the distal two thirds of the palmar long finger metacarpal. The oblique head originates from the capitate, the bases of the index and long metacarpals, the palmar ligaments of the carpus, and the flexor carpi radialis (FCR) sheath. The two heads converge and insert into the ulnar sesamoid, the ulnar base of the proximal phalanx, and the dorsal hood. The adductor pollicis muscle adducts the first metacarpal and extends the distal phalanx.

13. Froment's sign occurs when, during attempted key (lateral) pinch, the thumb interphalangeal (IP) joint collapses into flexion (see left hand in Figure 5-5). It results because the flexor pollicis longus (FPL) muscle has overpowered the extensor mechanism, typically revealing ulnar nerve involvement, with weakness in the deep head of the flexor pollicis brevis (FPB) and the adductor pollicis muscles, which contribute to the thumb's dorsal hood and assist extension. Occasionally it may signify radial nerve involvement with weakness in the extensor pollicis longus (EPL) muscle. A positive test may also result from median nerve involvement with weakness in the superficial head of the FPB and the abductor pollicis brevis (APB) muscles, which also contribute to the thumb's dorsal hood.

**Figure** 5-5

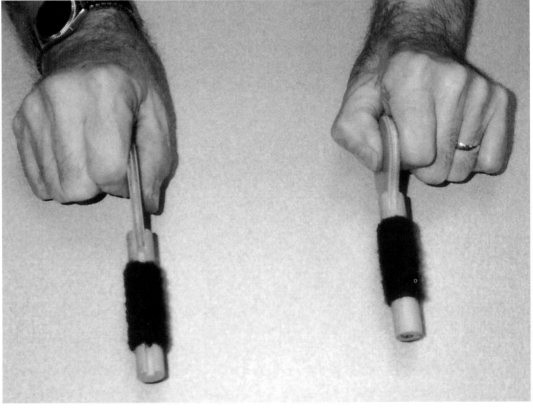

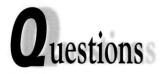

**14.** Describe how to isolate the flexor digitorum sublimis (FDS) muscle when testing PIP joint flexion. Describe how to isolate the intrinsic muscles when testing PIP joint extension. Explain why active motion (in an open chain situation) "anchors" a muscle proximally, and passive motion "anchors" it distally.

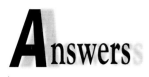 **A**nswers

**14.** Either the FDS muscle or the FDP muscle can flex the PIP joint; to isolate the FDS muscle, you must "anchor" the FDP muscle distally by passively extending all fingers except the one being tested (this maneuver pulls the FDP tendons distally "en masse" so that no one tendon can contract individually). The patient then attempts to flex the PIP joint, which is only possible if the FDS is functional (see Figure 5-6, A). Similarly, either the EDC muscle or the intrinsic muscles can extend the PIP joint; to isolate the intrinsic muscles instruct the patient to actively extend his MCP joint, "anchoring" the EDC muscle proximally (see Figure 5-6, B); the patient then attempts to extend his PIP joint, which is only possible if the intrinsic muscles are functional (see Figure 5-6, C).

**Figure** 5-6   **A**

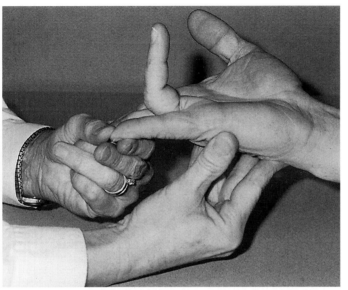

**B**

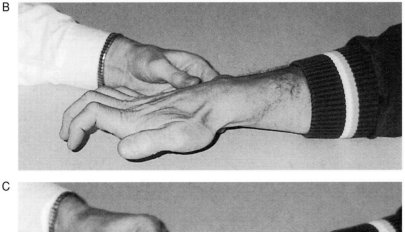

**C**

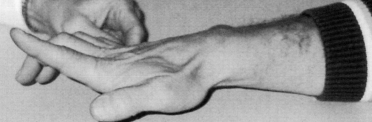

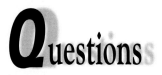

15. The interdependence of the PIP and DIP joints during flexion and during extension is essential to hand function. Explain the mechanics that facilitate the simultaneous flexion of both joints and the simultaneous extension of both joints.

16. If an examiner was unable to passively flex a patient's MCP joint beyond 50° when the PIP joint was concurrently flexed, but could flex the MCP joint to 90° when the PIP joint was extended, what would be causing the restriction?

17. How should acute open and closed ruptures of the central slip be treated?

18. What are the pathologic conditions causing boutonniere deformity of the PIP joint?

19. How is a chronic boutonniere deformity prepared for surgical reconstruction?

20. What is the most disabling element of the boutonniere deformity?

21. What causes limitation of flexion of the DIP joint in a boutonniere deformity?

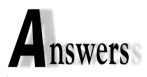

# Answers

15. Through insertions into the bases of the middle and distal phalanges, the FDS and FDP muscles flex the PIP and DIP joints respectively. During flexion, the volar shift of the lateral bands at the PIP joint allows more DIP joint flexion than if the lateral bands were fixed dorsally. Also, as the PIP joint flexes, the extensor mechanism is pulled distally through the central slip insertion so that it offers less resistance to DIP joint flexion.

    The extrinsic and intrinsic extensor motors both have dual insertions into the bases of the middle and distal phalanges through which they extend the PIP and DIP joints. In addition, as the PIP joint extends, the ORL is tightened and contributes to DIP joint extension; this extra force helps overcome the passive tension that develops in the FDP muscle as the PIP joint extends.

16. Passive insufficiency of the EDC, in which the tendon lacks enough extensibility to allow both joints to achieve full range of motion (ROM) simultaneously.

17. An open rupture is directly repaired and treated with Kirschner wire (K-wire) fixation and splinting of the PIP joint in extension for 6 to 8 weeks, leaving the DIP joint free. After K-wire removal, a night splint is used for 2 months (see Figure 5-7). If extensor lag persists after 4 months, tendolysis of the extensor mechanism may help. A closed tear is treated with a splint to hold the PIP joint in extension for 8 weeks with the DIP joint free, after which the splint is gradually removed and replaced by night splinting for 2 months.

**Figure** 5-7

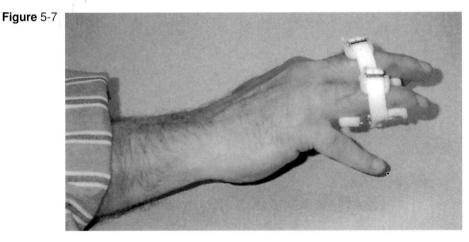

18. (1) An insufficient central slip; (2) tear or attenuation of the triangular ligament; (3) migration of the lateral bands volarly; (4) flexion contracture of the PIP joint; (5) hyperextension of the DIP joint from tension by the shortened lateral bands; and (6) contracture of the ORL.

19. The preoperative goal is to obtain full passive extension of the PIP joint. A dynamic splint is applied until the PIP joint reaches neutral, followed by static splinting of the PIP joint in neutral with the DIP joint flexed to stretch the contracted ORL for 4 weeks. If the PIP joint cannot be splinted to neutral, a persistent volar capsular contracture is present. Volar release may be necessary. This usually produces good intraoperative ROM that unfortunately is rarely maintained after extensor reconstruction.

20. Limitation of DIP joint flexion.

21. A tenodesis effect caused by volar displacement of the lateral bands and contracture of the oblique retinacular ligaments. Central slip disruption causes a transfer of extensor power to the DIP joint, which further contributes to contracture development.

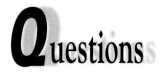

**22.** What reconstructive options are available for a chronic boutonniere deformity with full passive ROM?

**23.** Identify the zones of extensor tendon injury in Figure 5-8.

**Figure** 5-8

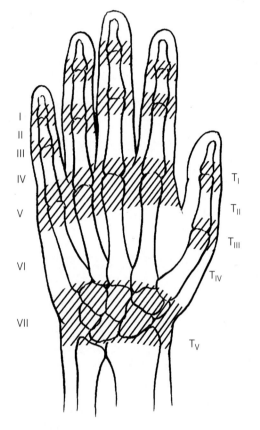

**24.** What is the approximate duration of protection for tendon repairs in each zone?

**25.** Describe the treatment of an extensor tendon laceration at the level of the MCP joint.

# Answers

22. (1) Oblique or stepcut tenotomy of the lateral bands distal to the central slip insertion over the proximal metaphysis of the middle phalanx (Dolphin, Fowler, or Nalebuff); (2) dorsal transposition and suture of the lateral bands (Littler); (3) transposition of the lateral bands to the central slip (Matev and Littler); and (4) V-Y plasty of the central slip to achieve appropriate tension.

23. Zone I—DIP joint and distal phalanx
    Zone II—middle phalanx
    Zone III—PIP joint
    Zone IV—proximal phalanx
    Zone V—MCP joint
    Zone VI—metacarpal
    Zone VII—wrist
    Zone $T_I$—thumb IP joint and distal phalanx
    Zone $T_{II}$—thumb proximal phalanx
    Zone $T_{III}$—thumb MCP joint
    Zone $T_{IV}$—thumb metacarpal
    Zone $T_V$—wrist

24. Zones I and II require 8 weeks.
    Zones III and IV require 6 weeks.
    Zones V, VI, and VII require 4 to 6 weeks.

25. Repair by direct suture. Postoperatively place the patient in a volar forearm-hand splint with the wrist in 45° of extension, the MCP joint in 50° flexion, and the IP joints in extension for 4 weeks (see Figure 5-9). Start AROM at 4 weeks and light resistive flexion and extension at 6 weeks. Postoperative protocols for dynamic extension splinting, which allow early mobilization of the interphalangeal joints, and protected ROM of the MCP joints are also successful.

**Figure** 5-9

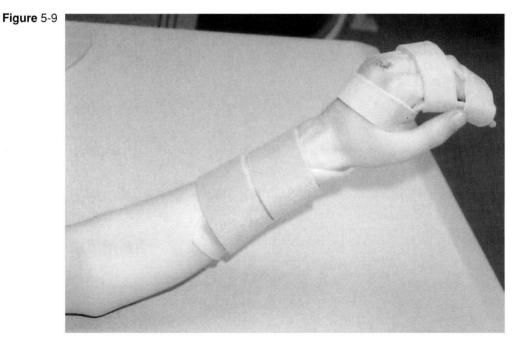

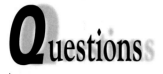

**26.** Name the structures on the dorsum of the hand in Figure 5-10.

**Figure** 5-10

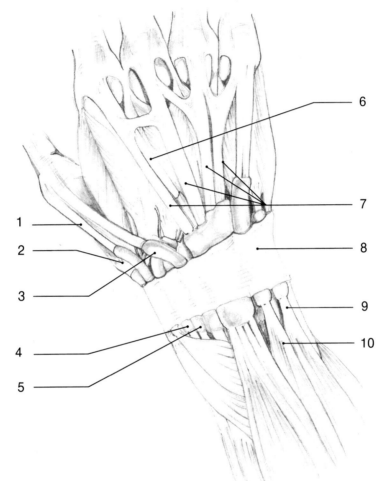

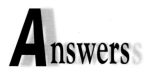

**26.** (1) Extensor pollicis brevis; (2) abductor pollicis longus; (3) extensor pollicis longus; (4) extensor carpi radialis longus; (5) extensor carpi radialis brevis; (6) extensor indicis proprius; (7) extensor digitorum communis; (8) extensor retinaculum; (9) extensor carpi ulnaris; and (10) extensor digiti minimi.

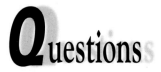

**27.** Describe the finger pulley system (Doyle and Blythe) in Figure 5-11.

**Figure** 5-11

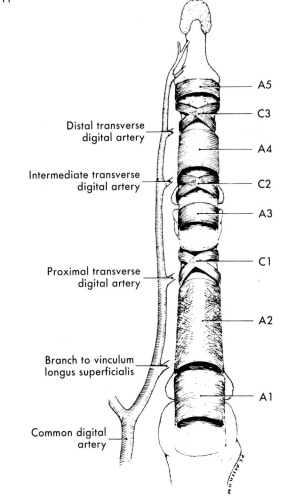

A5
C3
A4
C2
A3
C1
A2
A1

Distal transverse digital artery

Intermediate transverse digital artery

Proximal transverse digital artery

Branch to vinculum longus superficialis

Common digital artery

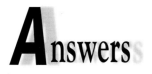
# Answers

27. Odd-numbered annular (A) pulleys overlie joints: A1—MCP, A3—PIP, and A5—DIP joint. Even-numbered pulleys overlie bone: A2—proximal phalanx, A4—middle phalanx. Cruciate (C) pulleys lie between: C1—A2 and A3, C2—A3 and A4, and C3—A4 and A5.

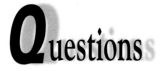

**28.** Identify the zones of flexor tendon injury in Figure 5-12.

**Figure** 5-12

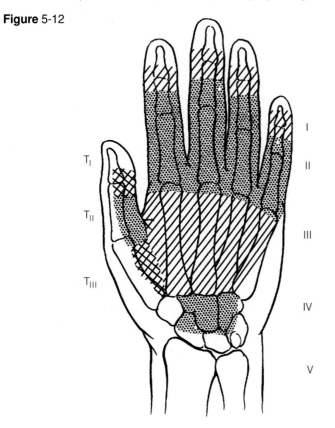

**29.** What are the two principal mechanisms of tendon healing in flexor zone II?

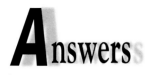

# Answers

28. Zone I is the area between the FDP tendon insertion and the FDS tendon insertion; zone II is the area between the FDS tendon insertion and the proximal edge of the fibro-osseous tunnel (level of the distal palmar skin crease); zone III is the area between the proximal flexor tendon sheath and the distal edge of the carpal tunnel; zone IV is the carpal tunnel; and zone V is the area between the proximal carpal tunnel and the volar forearm. Zone $T_I$ is the insertion area of the FPL tendon; zone $T_{II}$ is the area between the IP joint and the proximal edge of the flexor tendon sheath; zone $T_{III}$ is the area of the thenar muscles.

29. Tendon healing occurs through extrinsic healing, which is mediated through fibroblast ingrowth and is dependent upon adhesion formation between the tendon and surrounding tissue. The adhesions do provide blood supply to the healing tendon; however, they may interfere with smooth gliding within the tendon sheath. The other process is intrinsic tendon healing, which (as its name implies) occurs through tenocyte mediated joining of apposed tendon ends. Theoretically, this type of healing produces fewer adhesions. Blood supply for the healing tendon is provided through intact vincular systems, and further nutrition is provided through synovial fluid bathing the healing site.

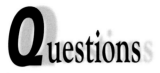

# Questions

30. Describe the rehabilitation protocol following surgical repair of flexor tendon lacerations.

**Figure** 5-13

A

B

C

D

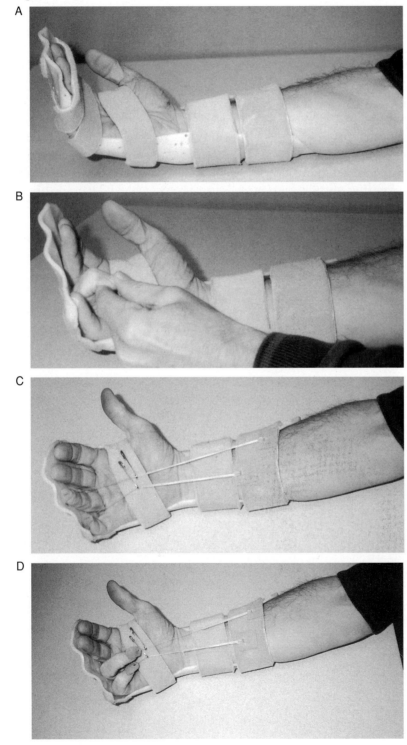

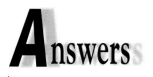

**30.** The goals of a postoperative flexor tendon rehabilitation program are to:
- protect the healing tendon from excessive forces
- increase tensile strength within the tendon as it heals
- prevent adhesions that limit the tendon's excursion

Numerous protocols have been advocated to achieve these goals. Success has been reported from varying techniques, such as controlled passive motion (see Figure 5-13, A and B), dynamic flexion (see Figure 5-13, C and D), and early active motion in a wrist tenodesis splint (see Figure 5-13, E and F).

The common objective of all protocols is to achieve tendon gliding through digit motion within a protected range. This is achieved by placing the patient in a dorsal blocking splint. The wrist angle of the splint varies according to the specific program. Increasing wrist flexion relaxes the repaired flexor tendons, but increases tension in the opposing extensor tendons. Thus, positioning in wrist flexion is desired during rest (Figure 5-13, E), but positioning in wrist extension may be preferred if active flexion (place and hold) is to be performed in order to decrease resistance from the extensor tendons (Figure 5-13, F). The MCP joints are positioned in flexion to maintain collateral ligament length and to prevent excessive tension on the tendon repair site. The IP joints are allowed to move from full extension to full flexion to prevent joint contracture and promote tendon gliding. The patient may actively extend the digits within the confines of the splint, but is cautioned to avoid active flexion. Flexion is obtained either through dynamic traction, passively, or place and hold methods.

Approximately 4 to 6 weeks after surgery, the splint is discontinued, and the patient is instructed to initiate active flexion. The program then progresses through isolated tendon excursion and blocking and strengthening exercises.

**Figure** 5-13 continued

E

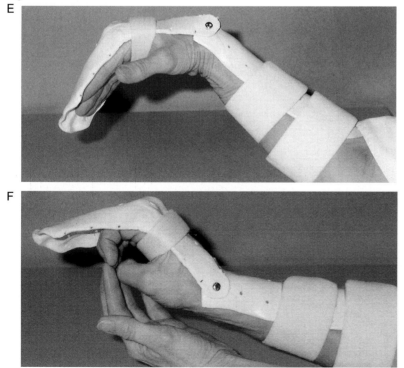

F

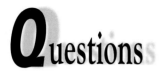

# Questions

31. Describe the mechanics of the thumb carpometacarpal (CMC) joint.

32. Relate the anatomical configuration of the MCP joints to the position in which they should be immobilized.

33. Describe the ligament and joint capsule anatomy of the extended and flexed MCP joint.

34. Why is the PIP joint splinted in a position close to full extension after a stable hyperextension sprain?

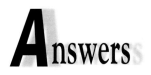

31. The thumb CMC joint is a saddle articulation between the reciprocally-shaped articular surfaces of the trapezium and the first metacarpal. It permits thenar extension to 55°, in which the concave metacarpal surface moves on the convex trapezial surface; abduction to 50°, in which the convex metacarpal surface moves on the concave trapezial surface; and axial rotation of 17° when in a loose-packed position. Circumduction occurs through a combination of flexion, extension, abduction, and adduction. In addition to the wide ROM made possible by the CMC joint, the thumb rests in a plane that forms an 80° angle with the plane of the palm, providing opposition for grip and pinch.

32. Strong collateral ligaments run obliquely from the dorsal metacarpal heads to insert volarly on the phalangeal bases (see Figure 5-14, A). Because of their eccentric placement and the cam-shaped metacarpal heads (which become wider toward the volar surface), the ligaments are taut in flexion (see Figure 5-14, B). Thus flexion is the desired position of immobilization to maintain the full length of the collateral ligaments. Conversely, immobilization of the MCP joint in extension allows the ligament to shorten, increasing the risk of associated joint extension contractures.

**Figure** 5-14

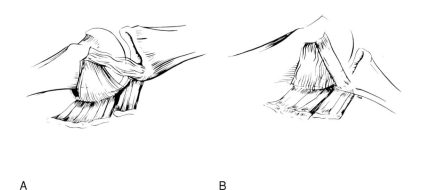

A                                   B

33. With MCP joint extension, there are loose collateral ligaments and joint capsule and a large intrasynovial capacity. The joint abducts and adducts easily. With MCP joint flexion, the collaterals are tight and the intracapsular volume is decreased.

34. Unlike the MCP joint, in which the collateral ligaments are taut in flexion, the PIP joint collateral ligaments are taut in extension. Since the PIP joint is vulnerable to flexion contracture, you should splint it in no more than 20° of flexion to avoid shortening of the collateral ligaments, capsule, and the volar supporting structures, which become redundant as flexion increases.

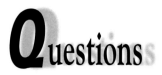

35. A 20-year-old carpenter injured his right small finger when a drill bit entangled his glove. In addition to a laceration over the volar aspect of his proximal phalanx, he sustained a dorsal dislocation of the PIP joint. Radiographs revealed a 2-mm bony avulsion of the volar plate from the base of the middle phalanx. There was no evidence of tendon or collateral ligament injury. Following closed reduction he was initially immobilized in a hand-based ulnar gutter splint that maintained his ring and small finger MCP joints in 85° of flexion and his IP joints in 25° of extension. Two weeks postinjury, how would you achieve "controlled motion" in this initially unstable dislocation?

36. When performing joint mobilization, you typically mobilize a **concave** joint surface in the direction of the limb motion desired, and a **convex** joint surface opposite the direction of the limb motion desired. Applying this principle, describe the appropriate mobilization techniques for increasing flexion of: (a) the radiocarpal joint; (b) the MCP joint; and (c) the PIP joint.

37. What is the most common finger infection?

38. What are the synovial changes associated with rheumatoid arthritis?

39. What joint changes occur in rheumatoid arthritis?

40. What are the indications for surgery in rheumatoid arthritis?

41. Describe the wrist deformities seen in rheumatoid arthritis.

35. A dorsal block splint, allowing PIP joint flexion from 25° to 110°, permits motion in an acceptable range while still protecting the injury (see Figure 5-15, A and B). Controlled motion helps prevent adhesions between the gliding tissue planes surrounding the flexor and extensor tendons. After 7 days in the splint, if the joint is stable, the splint is discontinued, but the injured finger is "buddy taped" to an adjacent finger to provide protection while allowing functional motion.

**Figure** 5-15

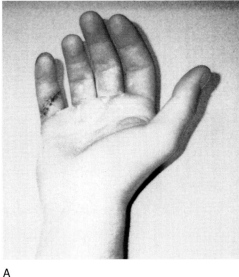
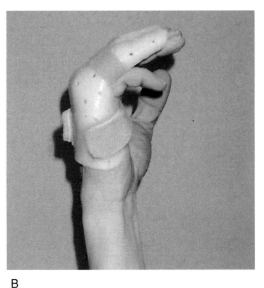

A                                                                      B

36. (a) To increase flexion of the radiocarpal joint, stabilize the radius and mobilize the carpals in a dorsal direction. (b) To increase flexion of the MCP joint, stabilize the metacarpal and mobilize the proximal phalanx in a volar direction. (c) To increase flexion of the PIP joint, stabilize the proximal phalanx and mobilize the middle phalanx in a volar direction.

37. A paronychia, which involves the tissue around the nailbed.

38. Inflammation, hyperemia, increased synovial fluid production, and proliferation of synovial lining; also rheumatoid pannus (a vascular granulation tissue) produces collagenase that is activated by plasma and is destructive to cartilage, ligaments, tendons, and bone.

39. Increased joint pressure from an increase in synovial fluid production leads to interference with nutrition and distention of the capsule and ligaments. Lysosomal enzymes from the inflamed synovium erode articular cartilage and weaken tendons and ligaments. Painful inhibition within muscles produces atrophy and contractures. Periarticular osteoporosis, cysts, and spurs also develop. The wrist and finger joints may be considered as links in a system that is constantly exposed to external forces while undergoing internal destruction. Joint laxity and mechanical imbalance form a cycle in which collapse deformities are self-perpetuating.

40. The indications for surgery include severe pain and chronic synovitis not responding to good medical therapy, nerve entrapment, tendon ruptures, and deformity resulting in functional loss. Some patients with rheumatoid arthritis can have horrible-looking hands that function well without much pain. It is better not to operate until the patient meets the aforementioned criteria.

41. Ulnar translocation of the carpus, erosion of the carpus and radial metacarpal shift, supination and volar dislocation of the carpus beneath the radius, rupture or attenuation of the radial wrist extensors, and dorsal subluxation or dislocation of the distal ulna. The wrist usually becomes flexed and radially deviated.

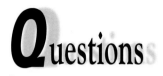

# Questions

42. What are the potential causes of triggering of the finger in rheumatoid patients?

43. What are the most frequent tendon ruptures seen in rheumatoid arthritis?

44. Describe rheumatoid arthritic MCP joint deformities.

45. What are the principles of treatment of early MCP joint disease in rheumatoid arthritis?

46. What is the most common deformity of the PIP joint in rheumatoid arthritis?

47. Describe the pathomechanics of boutonniere deformity in rheumatoid arthritis.

48. Describe the pathomechanics of the rheumatoid arthritic boutonniere thumb (Nalebuff type I deformity).

# **A**nswers

**42.** There are several sites for triggering in rheumatoid arthritic hands: (1) the A1 pulley (as with conventional trigger finger); (2) the FDS decussation (may require excising the slip of the FDS or an intratendinous nodule); and (3) a nodule in the FDP tendon near A2 can cause the finger to lock into extension—this requires tenosynovectomy and nodule excision.

**43.** In order of occurrence: ruptures of the ring and small finger extensor tendons, the EPL, other extensor tendons, the FPL, and other flexor tendons.

**44.** Initially there is enlargement and swelling of the knuckles; later, volar subluxation of the joint, ulnar displacement of the extensor tendons, and ulnar deviation of the fingers. Contributing factors include ulnar inclination of the metacarpal heads, the ulna-volar force of the extrinsic flexor tendons, contracture or spasm of the intrinsic muscles, and "zig-zag" of intercalated segments.

**45.** Conservative care consisting of maximal medical management, intraarticular steroid injections, and instruction in joint protection techniques using resting and functional splints and adaptive devices. Hydrotherapy or fluidotherapy may be used in conjunction with gentle active and isometric exercises to decrease pain and edema and to preserve joint and muscle function. Synovectomy and soft tissue reconstructive procedures (intrinsic releases, extensor realignment, and crossed intrinsic transfer) are considered if the articular surfaces of the MCP joints are mildly involved.

**46.** The swan-neck deformity is most common.

**47.** Dorsal synovitis, capsular distention, and attenuation of the central slip and triangular ligament allow PIP joint extension lag and palmar displacement of the lateral bands. As both the extrinsic and intrinsic extensors are lost, PIP joint flexion is unopposed. Extensor pull is transferred to the distal phalanx, causing DIP joint hyperextension. Joint destruction and fixed contracture gradually develop.

**48.** The deformity involves flexion of the MCP joint and hyperextension of the IP joint. Dorsal synovitis of the MCP joint causes attenuation of the capsule and extensor apparatus (EPB) with associated volar displacement of the EPL and intrinsic tendons. With attempted extension of the MCP joint, there is hyperextension of the interphalangeal joint. The proximal phalanx subluxates volarly. Disease in this deformity is primarily at the MCP joint (see Figure 5-16).

**Figure** 5-16

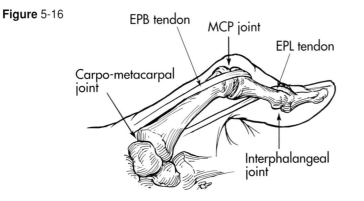

EPB tendon   MCP joint

EPL tendon

Carpo-metacarpal joint

Interphalangeal joint

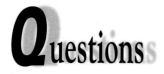

# Questions

49. Describe the pathomechanics of a thumb swan-neck (Nalebuff type III) deformity in rheumatoid arthritis.

50. Describe Dupuytren's disease.

51. Other than the palmar surface of the hand, what other areas can be affected by Dupuytren's?

52. What is the inheritance pattern of Dupuytren's?

53. What other conditions are associated with Dupuytren's?

54. How should dorsal dislocation of the thumb MCP joint be reduced?

55. How should hyperextension volar plate injuries of the thumb MCP joint be treated?

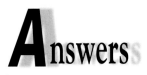

**49.** Hyperextension of the MCP joint and flexion of the interphalangeal joint develop as a result of dorsoradial subluxation-dislocation of the thumb metacarpal base on the trapezium. Hyperextension of the MCP joint results from stretching of the volar plate secondary to MCP synovitis and extension forces concentrated at the joint. The primary pathology is at the thumb CMC joint (see Figure 5-17).

**Figure** 5-17

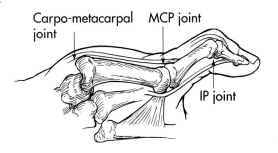

Carpo-metacarpal joint  MCP joint  IP joint

**50.** Palmar nodules and cords associated with flexion contractures of the MCP, less frequently the PIP, and occasionally the DIP joints caused by disease of the palmar aponeurosis and its digital prolongations. The disease most commonly affects the ring and little fingers.

**51.** The knuckle pads (Garrod's nodes), the dorsum of the penis (Peyronie's disease), and the plantar fascia (Lederhosen's disease).

**52.** Autosomal dominant, variable penetrance; most frequent in persons of northern European descent; male to female ratio = 8:1.

**53.** Epilepsy, alcoholism, diabetes, trauma (can aggravate it, but is probably not a primary cause).

**54.** Avoid traction reduction because pulling the phalanx back into position may interpose the volar plate in the joint, thereby creating a complex dislocation. Instead, hyperextend the proximal phalanx on the metacarpal with the thumb interphalangeal joint and wrist flexed, then push the base of the phalanx over the metacarpal head to affect reduction.

**55.** In a thumb spica cast for 3 to 4 weeks with the MCP joint in 15° to 20° of flexion. May require protective splinting for an additional 2 weeks.

# Questions

56. Following open reduction of a complex finger MCP joint dorsal dislocation, how is the patient treated?

57. How is dislocation of the thumb CMC joint treated?

58. What are the prerequisites for tendon transfers?

59. Describe the postoperative care for tendon transfers.

60. In radial nerve palsy, which functions should be restored through tendon transfer?

61. Which functions should be restored through tendon transfer in low median nerve palsy?

62. Which functions require restoration in high median nerve palsy?

63. True or false? Ulnar clawing is worse in low ulnar nerve palsy than in high ulnar nerve palsy.

64. In low ulnar nerve palsies, what hand functions should be reconstructed with tendon transfer?

# **A**nswers

**56.** Place the patient in a dorsal block splint with his MCP joint flexed 60° (50° if the collateral ligaments required repair) for 3 weeks; the patient may perform AROM within the confines of the splint (see Figure 5-18, A and B). Discontinue the splint after 3 weeks, but "buddy tape" for protection for an additional 3 weeks. Instruct the patient to perform full AROM and progress to pain-free resistance.

**Figure** 5-18

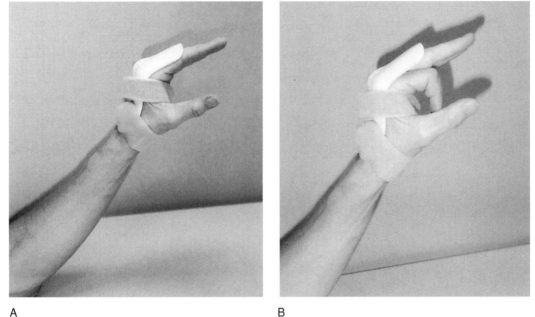

A          B

**57.** This is controversial, with advocates of both closed reduction and open repair. Because the joint is very unstable after reduction, pronation of the thumb combined with closed pinning followed by 6 weeks of immobilization is recommended in closed treatment. Open repair of the ligament and capsule combined with wire fixation of the joint in a reduced position is again followed by 6 weeks of immobilization.

**58.** Bony stability, no edema or inflammation, an adequate soft tissue bed, mobile joints; adequate strength, sufficient excursion, and expendable donor muscle; and potential for proper direction of pull or pulley.

**59.** Protect the transfer by placing the patient in a static splint that relieves tension on the involved tendon for 3 to 4 weeks, then begin active ROM exercises. Continue protective splinting for an additional 3 to 6 weeks for sleeping or activities in which excessive force could occur.

**60.** Thumb extension and abduction; finger and wrist extension.

**61.** Thumb abduction and opposition.

**62.** Thumb opposition and DIP and PIP joint flexion of the index and long fingers.

**63.** True. The clawing tends to be worse with low ulnar nerve palsies because the ulnar profundus motors are intact in low ulnar nerve palsy, thereby enhancing the flexion deformity.

**64.** MCP joint flexion and IP joint extension of the ulnar digits, thumb adduction, and index finger abduction.

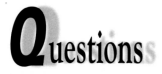

# Questions

65. In high ulnar nerve palsy, which muscle functions often require replacement?

66. Following intravenous injections in the cubital fossa, a drug addict complains that his hand appears "flat" at rest. His thumb lies in the plane of his palm, and he is unable to oppose it to his other fingers. He also has difficulty flexing his index and long fingers. What is his problem?

67. What features distinguish pronator syndrome from carpal tunnel syndrome?

68. What are the four potential sites of compression of the median nerve in pronator syndrome?

69. Describe the findings in anterior interosseous syndrome.

70. What are the possible sites of compression in anterior interosseous syndrome?

71. Describe the course of the radial nerve from its origin in the brachium through the arm.

72. Describe the sites of compression in radial tunnel syndrome.

73. Describe the most common physical and electrodiagnostic findings in radial tunnel syndrome.

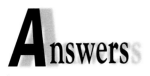

65. In addition to those described above for low ulnar nerve palsy, there is loss of the FDP muscles of the ring and small fingers. Although there is a loss of flexor carpi ulnaris (FCU) muscle function, this does not require reconstruction.

66. This patient has a median nerve injury.

67. A positive Tinel's sign in the forearm, reproduction of symptoms with nerve compression in the proximal forearm, frequently a negative Phalen's test, and pain with resisted pronation are present in pronator syndrome. In addition, you may see forearm pain with resisted flexion of the PIP joints of the ring and long fingers in pronator syndrome, but not in carpal tunnel syndrome. Advanced cases of pronator syndrome may demonstrate weakness in the FPL muscle, FDS muscles, and FDP muscles of the index and long fingers.

68. (1) Beneath the supracondylar process and ligament of Struthers; (2) the lacertus fibrosus; (3) the pronator teres muscle; and (4) at the arch of the FDS muscle.

69. The patient typically describes achy forearm pain followed by weakness or loss of function affecting the FPL muscle, and the FDP muscles to the index and long fingers. The pronator quadratus muscle is also affected in this syndrome. Patients frequently complain of the inability to flex the thumb at the IP joint, and attempts to make a circle with the thumb and index finger result in the pathognomic "flat pinch." Sensation is not affected.

70. The proximal one third of the forearm, related to tendinous bands at the deep head of the pronator teres muscle; the origin of the FDS muscle of the long finger; the origin of the FCR muscle; secondary to accessory muscles, e.g., FDS connected to FDP, Gantzer's muscle (accessory head to the FPL), palmaris profundus, and flexor carpi radialis brevis; or an enlarged bicipital bursa. Anterior interosseous nerve palsy has also been associated with fractures or thrombosis of the ulnar collateral vessels.

71. The radial nerve is a branch of the posterior cord of the brachial plexus that runs posteriorly, leaving the axilla through the "triangular space." This "space" is bordered superiorly by the inferior part of the teres major muscle, laterally by the humeral shaft, and medially by the long head of the triceps muscle. The radial nerve is then accompanied by the profunda brachii artery as it passes obliquely across the posterior humerus between the lateral and medial heads of the triceps muscle. It then travels in a shallow groove (radial groove), deep to the lateral head of the triceps muscle. It penetrates the lateral intermuscular septum, proximal to the elbow, then enters the anterior compartment of the arm. Here it is bordered medially by the brachialis muscle and laterally by the brachioradialis muscle proximally and the extensor carpi radialis longus (ECRL) muscle distally. The radial nerve divides into the superficial branch and posterior interosseous nerve at approximately the level of the lateral epicondyle of the humerus.

72. Fibrous bands lying anterior to the radial head, radial recurrent vessels (leash of Henry), tendinous margin of the extensor carpi radialis brevis (ECRB) muscle, the Arcade of Frohse, and fibrous bands within the supinator.

73. Pain over the radial nerve in the area of the mobile wad. The patient complains of aching in the extensor-supinator area. Maximal tenderness in radial tunnel syndrome is usually 4 to 8 cm distal to the lateral epicondyle in the supinator muscle. Sensory changes are usually absent. The patient's pain is characteristically distal to the lateral epicondyle and should not be confused with lateral epicondylitis. Resisted long finger MCP joint extension, resisted forearm supination, or passive hyperpronation will often localize the pain in the radial tunnel and can be helpful in this diagnosis. Electrodiagnostic studies of the radial nerve are usually negative.

# Questions

74. A 55-year-old physical education teacher complains of dorsal radial wrist pain with numbness affecting the dorsal thumb, index, and long fingers. The symptoms do not waken the patient at night. They are intermittent but intense at times. Upon physical examination, the median nerve compression test (Phalen's test) and Tinel's over the median nerve from the elbow to the wrist were negative. Two-point discrimination was normal. The patient complained of shooting pains when the radial styloid was percussed. What is this patient's diagnosis and how should he be treated?

75. The brachioradialis reflex, elicited at the distal, lateral forearm, is mediated primarily through which nerve root?

76. What are the sites of compression in posterior interosseous nerve palsy?

77. A 65-year-old steelworker is referred for intermittent pain along the medial proximal forearm and numbness in the small and ring fingers. He is awakened intermittently at night with numbness in the hand and pain in the arm. Motor and sensory testing are within normal limits. Adson's test is negative. There is tenderness over the medial elbow 3 cm distal to the medial epicondyle. There is a positive Tinel's sign in this area radiating to the ring and small fingers. The elbow flexion test is positive. Nerve conduction velocity and electromyogram (EMG) for the median and ulnar nerves were normal. What is his diagnosis? How should this patient be treated?

78. What are the sites of compression of the ulnar nerve in cubital tunnel syndrome?

79. What are the surgical options for treatment of cubital tunnel syndrome?

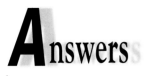

**74.** The patient most likely has Wartenberg's syndrome, also known as cheiralgia paresthetica. This is a neuritis of the superficial branch of the radial nerve. It usually occurs near the radial styloid where the nerve becomes subcutaneous, and can be caused by compression between the ECRL and brachioradialis tendons. It may be posttraumatic or have no specific cause. You should ask about tight watchbands or bracelets, which might irritate the nerve. Anomalous muscles have also been described as producing neuritic symptoms. If removal of the jewelry is not effective in improving the patient's symptoms, a thumb spica splint may be effective with care to mold the splint so that there is no pressure over the irritable nerve. Surgical neurolysis may be considered if conservative means are ineffective.

**75.** The brachioradialis reflex is mediated through C6.

**76.** Usually the arcade of Frohse, although compression also has been described in the middle or distal aspect of the supinator muscle. Specific causes are ganglia, lipoma, fibroma, or rheumatoid arthritis of the radiohumeral joint.

**77.** The patient has cubital tunnel syndrome. Although positive electrodiagnostic studies are helpful in confirming the diagnosis, mild cases frequently will have negative findings on EMG and nerve conduction velocity. The vast majority of the patients present with normal two-point discrimination and motor tests. Prolongation of two-point discrimination and muscle atrophy and weakness are usually very late signs. Initial care should be conservative, consisting of precautions in elbow posturing such as avoidance of a flexed elbow position or resting on the elbow and forearm. An elbow pad can be used to avoid direct trauma, depending upon how irritable the nerve is. In addition, a 30° to 45° elbow splint can be applied to rest the elbow either full-time or at night only, in an attempt to decrease nerve irritability (see Figure 5-19). Nonsteroidal antiinflammatory drugs (NSAIDs) or a course of iontophoresis may help as well. If conservative care is unsuccessful, then surgical options may be considered.

**Figure** 5-19

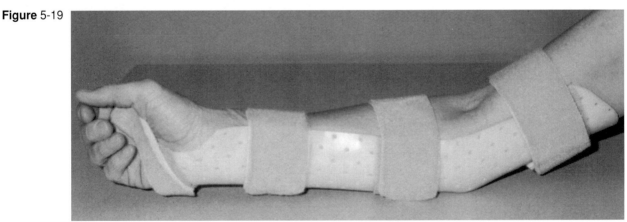

**78.** The cubital tunnel, arcade of Struthers, anconeus epitrochlearis, medial head of the triceps muscle, aponeurosis of the FCU muscle, and others including osteophytes, ganglia, or lipomas, and hypermobility of the ulnar nerve.

**79.** Simple in situ decompression of the ulnar nerve, anterior transposition of the ulnar nerve (subcutaneous, submuscular, or intramuscular), and medial epicondylectomy.

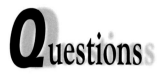

80. A 39-year-old laborer at an industrial plant complains of lateral proximal forearm pain that developed spontaneously without specific injury approximately 2 months earlier. He complains of weakness in the extremity with heavy use of the hand but denies numbness, tingling, or paresthesias. He is not tender over the lateral epicondyle, but has moderate tenderness at a point 6 cm distal to the lateral epicondyle and pain with resisted long finger extension. There is no motor weakness. Resisted wrist extension produces minimal pain, but resisted supination is extremely painful at the aforementioned site of tenderness. Radiographic films of the elbow were normal. What is the patient's differential diagnosis?

81. How is radial tunnel syndrome treated?

82. A 25-year-old gymnast fell from the parallel bars, landing on his dorsiflexed wrist. Since this episode, he complains of intermittent numbness and tingling in the ulnar two digits. Upon physical examination, there is pain in the ulnar palm with mild swelling. Digital ROM and two-point discrimination are normal. The intrinsics of the hand measure 5/5 on motor testing. Allen's test demonstrates excellent flow to the hand through the radial artery. There is no filling through the ulnar artery. What is the differential diagnosis?

83. How is Allen's test performed?

84. What are the borders of Guyon's canal?

85. Where does the deep motor branch of the ulnar nerve separate from the main nerve trunk?

86. An 18-year-old man sustained a deep laceration over his hypothenar area while fending off a knife attack. He underwent surgical repair of the ulnar artery and nerve just distal to the pisiform. How should he be managed?

87. Seven weeks after injury, the patient in question 86 complains of excessive sweating over the ulnar side of his hand and that his small finger "sticks out." He fears that his surgery has failed. What should you do?

88. Describe Wallerian degeneration.

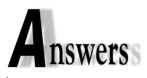

**A**nswers

80. Differential diagnosis for nontraumatic lateral proximal forearm pain includes lateral epicondylitis (tennis elbow), osteochondritis dissecans, radial tunnel syndrome, and cervical radiculitis. Of these, the most likely diagnosis is radial tunnel syndrome because of the localized pain distal to the lateral epicondyle, pain with resisted middle finger extension and forearm supination.

81. Nonoperative treatment consists of rest, NSAIDs, and wrist splinting in 30° extension and/or elbow splinting in 90° flexion for a period of 4 to 6 weeks. Surgical release of the radial tunnel is indicated when conservative care fails to alleviate the symptoms. Following surgery, immobilize the elbow in 90° flexion for 3 weeks with the forearm neutral, then start ROM exercises, progressing to resistance.

82. Sensory changes may be due to irritation of the ulnar nerve and may represent a contusion to the nerve, with or without carpal fracture or CMC dislocation. What is more likely in this case, because of the abnormal vascular filling from the ulnar artery, is that the patient has sustained an ulnar artery thrombosis. This can be confirmed through Doppler evaluation or an arteriogram. Radiographs of the wrist are helpful and EMG and nerve conduction studies can rule out ulnar nerve compromise in Guyon's canal.

83. The patient is asked to make a tight fist and straighten the fingers completely three consecutive times while the examiner occludes the radial and ulnar arteries just proximal to the wrist. After the third fist, the patient is asked to relax the hand. The investigator then releases the ulnar artery, maintaining compression over the radial artery. If there is a complete superficial palmar arch, all of the fingers will pink up with release of the ulnar artery within 5 seconds. The test is then repeated, this time maintaining compression over the ulnar artery and releasing pressure over the radial artery to check its patency.

84. Guyon's canal is a triangular-shaped area. The roof is formed by the volar carpal ligament, the lateral wall by the hook of the hamate and the insertion of the transverse carpal ligament (TCL), and the medial wall by pisohamate ligament and the pisiform bone.

85. Within Guyon's canal. It then passes distally and radially around the distal end of the base of the hook of the hamate to enter the deep midpalmar fat (retroflexor fat) with the deep branch of the ulnar artery. This branch continues radially to innervate the deeper intrinsics of the hand.

86. The patient should be placed in a forearm-hand ulnar gutter splint with his wrist in slight flexion to minimize tension on the repair site. The splint should also hold the MCP joints of the ring and small fingers in 70° to 90° of flexion to prevent clawing; the IP joints are left free of the splint. The patient starts active exercise as soon as healing permits. The splint may be modified to being hand-based and is worn until clawing is no longer evident.

87. These symptoms are normal and, in fact, are an indication of progression of healing. The sweating indicates return of sympathetic function. The abducted small finger (Wartenberg's sign) is resulting from function of the abductor digiti minimi muscle, which is imbalanced at this time due to loss of the volar interosseous muscles. As the nerve continues to regenerate distal to the repair site, additional intrinsic muscle function should return, and he will be able to adduct his small finger.

88. Schwann cells digest fragmented myelin in the endoneurial tubules distal to axonal interruption and in the proximal axonal zone of injury. The debris is removed by 2 to 8 weeks, and then there is progressive shrinkage in the fascicular cross-sectional area. Shrinkage may reach a maximum as early as 3 months after injury. The fascicular cross-sectional area may be only 17% of normal by 2 years.

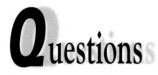

# Questions

89. When does proximal axonal budding occur?

90. What is the usual sequence of healing following laceration of a peripheral nerve?

91. What effect does nerve degeneration have on the skeletal muscle it supplies?

92. Is electrical stimulation of denervated muscle effective in delaying deterioration of the motor end plates?

93. What are the three periods of regeneration delay seen after peripheral nerve injury as the nerve begins to grow?

94. Although there are numerous normal variations and considerable overlap of sensory territories of the nerves supplying the hand, certain areas are considered to be solely innervated by each nerve. Where are the "pure" areas for cursory testing of median, ulnar, and radial nerve sensation?

95. Describe the splints used following median, ulnar, and radial nerve injuries.

96. A 16-year-old football player reports that while holding the jersey of an opposing player who was pulling away, he felt a sudden snap in his ring finger. He then had a burning pain sensation, swelling in the distal finger, and was unable to actively flex his DIP joint. What was his injury?

97. How should the patient in question 96 be treated?

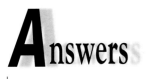

# Answers

89. About 4 days after injury. It may be delayed 14 to 21 days in severe crush or avulsion injuries.

90. The perikaryon (cell body) responds to injury by increasing its metabolic activity by the fourth day. Anywhere from 15% to 80% of the cell bodies die following section of the nerve trunk. Another factor that may prevent full recovery following nerve injury is that the injured axon segment, which must be regenerated, may be too long. It may, in a sense, exceed the cell body's capacity for repair. The axon distal to severance undergoes Wallerian degeneration. While the axon and myelin sheath degenerate, the Schwann cells and macrophages remove the necrotic debris. Unmyelinated axons degenerate within 1 week. The fascicular cross-sectional area also decreases with time. Wallerian degeneration also occurs over a shorter distance in the proximal stump in the zone of injury. Ninety-six hours after a sharp traumatic injury, axonal sprouting begins. In extreme trauma, axonal sprouting may be delayed as long as 3 weeks. Schwann cells form tubules for the regenerating axons. The new nerve fibers pass down new endoneurial tubules. This may result in a loss of specificity of the nerve fibers as some of the sensory and motor fibers pass into tubules for end organs for which they were not intended.

91. Muscle atrophy develops with progressive destruction of motor end plates. The motor end plates begin to deteriorate by the third month after denervation.

92. Measurements of capacity for work of muscle after denervation, as well as histologic evaluation of denervated human muscle with and without electrical stimulation, have not shown significant differences.

93. (1) Neuronal survival (4 to 20 days); (2) axonal traversing of the suture line or area of injury (3 to 50 days); and (3) end-organ connection (axon grows down the distal end of the neural tube at approximately 1 mm/day).

94. Branches of the three major peripheral nerves carry sensation from the hand in the following manner: the median nerve transmits sensation from the lateral portion of the palm and thenar surface and the volar aspect of the lateral 3½ digits (including the fingertips dorsally to the PIP joints); innervation is purest at the tip of the index finger. The ulnar nerve supplies the ulnar side of the hand and medial 1½ digits (both dorsal and volar surfaces); innervation is purest at the tip of the little finger. The radial nerve innervates the dorsum of the hand lateral to the fourth metacarpal and the dorsal surfaces of the lateral 3½ digits as far distally as the PIP joints; innervation is purest at the dorsal web space between the thumb and index finger.

95. The objective of splinting after nerve loss is to maintain functional hand position and prevent deformities resulting from muscle imbalance. Although splint requirements differ according to individual needs, there are some common factors. Median nerve involvement requires a splint that at a minimum maintains thumb abduction; a tenodesis attachment may also be used to assist index and long finger flexion. Ulnar nerve loss typically produces clawing from loss of the intrinsic muscles in the fourth and fifth digits; a splint must counteract hyperextension of the MCP joints. Radial nerve lesions eliminate active wrist extension, so a cock-up splint is necessary to position the hand in a functional position. An outrigger to accommodate for loss of MCP joint extension may be added if needed.

96. This athlete sustained an avulsion of the FDP tendon from the distal phalanx.

97. Avulsion of the FDP is the third most common closed tendon injury in sports (after distal extensor tendon and central slip injuries). It requires surgical reattachment with a pull out wire suture or bone anchor suture. Rehabilitation follows the flexor tendon repair protocol.

98. The chief of general surgery at your hospital asks you to look at his right dominant long finger that he just jammed into a stretcher while transferring a patient. From the time of the accident, he has been unable to actively extend the DIP joint. Profundus function is intact, and the skin is intact. There is tenderness over the dorsal aspect of the DIP joint, and he has a 50° extension lag. Radiographic films of the finger demonstrate no bony injury. What is the diagnosis, and how would you manage this aggressive surgeon who wishes to continue operating?

99. A 35-year-old symphony conductor injured her right long finger approximately 2 months earlier, but she does not recall the mechanism of injury. She complains of DIP joint pain and an inability to extend the distal phalanx. Opon physical examination, she has a characteristic mallet finger deformity with no bony changes noted on radiographic films. How should this problem be treated?

100. The conductor from question 99 underwent a period of splinting for 12 weeks and subsequently underwent a therapy program to wean from the splint and to commence ROM exercises. She returns to her physician with a 45° extension lag at the DIP joint with an associated swan-neck deformity of the finger. Passive ROM is normal and free of pain. What are her surgical options?

101. What are the options for treatment for a 58-year-old woman with deformity and pain from idiopathic osteoarthritis of the DIP joint?

102. A 68-year-old man has noted progressive loss of motion in his ring and small fingers associated with thick cords in the palm. What is his diagnosis, and what are your recommendations regarding his treatment? (See Figure 5-20.)

**Figure** 5-20

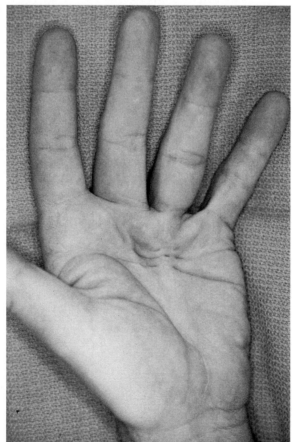

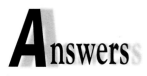

**98.** The patient has a mallet finger. The mallet finger results from either an avulsion of bone from the base of the distal phalanx with the attached terminal extensor tendon, or rupture of the terminal extensor tendon. Treatment of a tendinous mallet finger is full-time splinting of the DIP joint in full to slight hyperextension for 6 to 8 weeks with a period of weaning from the splint. The splinting must be continuous; otherwise, the tendon will heal in a lengthened position resulting in a residual extension lag. To allow the patient to continue operating, extra splints may be fabricated that could be gas sterilized and applied with sterile tape or Velcro following surgical scrub. Another option for treatment would be pinning the DIP joint in full extension with a transarticular K-wire for 6 weeks. The latter treatment risks damage to the articular surface by the K-wire, as well as increases the potential for infection and nail deformity.

**99.** This patient has a chronic mallet finger. Even as late as 3 months, patients have been treated with extension splinting over a period of 8 to 12 weeks with correction of the mallet deformity. The finger should be splinted in full extension to slight hyperextension as described in question 98, except that the duration should be extended 2 to 6 weeks.

**100.** There are several methods of reconstructing a mallet finger with associated swan-neck deformity. One of the better techniques is a release of the central slip over the PIP joint, which rebalances the extensor mechanism. Patients are allowed active ROM shortly after the operation, with intermittent splinting of the PIP and DIP joints in an extension gutter over a 3-week period to prevent extensor lag at the PIP joint. This treatment has proved effective in correcting the swan-neck and mallet deformities. Other corrective techniques include surgically shortening the terminal extensor tendon or spiral oblique ligament reconstruction.

**101.** Conservative measures include intermittent splinting, NSAIDs, and local corticosteroid injections. Surgical options include DIP joint replacement arthroplasty versus DIP joint arthrodesis. Arthrodesis is favored because it is long-lasting and has fewer complications than joint replacements.

**102.** The patient has Dupuytren's disease with contractures of the ring and small fingers. Surgery is recommended for 20° to 30° contractures of the MCP joint and any contracture of the PIP joint. Following surgical fasciectomy, the dressings are removed in 2 to 5 days and AROM initiated. Extension splints are used between exercises and at night for 4 to 6 weeks and then the patient is weaned to night splinting for 6 to 12 weeks (see Figure 5-21).

**Figure** 5-21

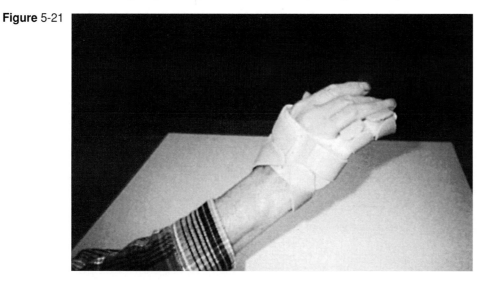

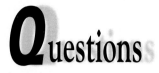
# Questions

103. A 52-year-old, right-hand dominant waste management worker lacerated his left thumb on a windshield wiper 5 days earlier. Over the past 3 days, he has noted increasing pain and swelling in the thumb with intermittent purulent drainage and inability to sleep because of throbbing pain. Upon physical examination, there is fusiform swelling of the thumb. It is tender volarly from the tip into the palm. Active motion was minimal because of pain. The IP joint is held in mild flexion, and passive extension of the thumb IP joint caused severe pain. There is a 1.5-cm oblique laceration over the flexion crease of the thumb IP joint with purulent material draining from it. What is the patient's diagnosis, and how should he be treated?

104. A 45-year-old factory worker complains of right, dominant wrist pain of 3 weeks duration. His condition is aggravated by using snipping shears and handling tools. Palpation reveals localized tenderness and mild swelling just distal to the radial styloid process. Finkelstein's test is positive. What is his diagnosis and how is it treated conservatively?

105. If conservative treatment in question 104 is not successful, what are other treatment options?

# 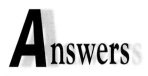nswers

103. The patient has FPL septic tenosynovitis. With the infection present at least 3 days, he will require incision and drainage with resection of the flexor tendon sheath between the flexor pulleys. The purulent material should be cultured and gram stained and the patient started on IV antibiotics, including coverage for gram-negative organisms because of his occupation. The wound should be left open and allowed to close secondarily or with a delayed primary closure once the infection has adequately resolved. Active and passive ROM exercises should be initiated early to prevent adhesions.

104. This patient has deQuervain's syndrome, i.e., tenosynovitis of the APL and EPB in the first dorsal compartment. Resisted thumb extension and passive thumb flexion produce acute pain. Conservative treatment includes NSAIDs, corticosteroid injection into the first dorsal compartment, and/or rest in a forearm-thumb spica splint (see Figure 5-22). Application of cold every 2 to 3 hours is another useful modality. When his acute symptoms subside in 1 to 2 weeks, the patient should be instructed to begin AROM, progressing to pain-free resistance. He should also be instructed in activity modification to prevent recurrence.

**Figure** 5-22

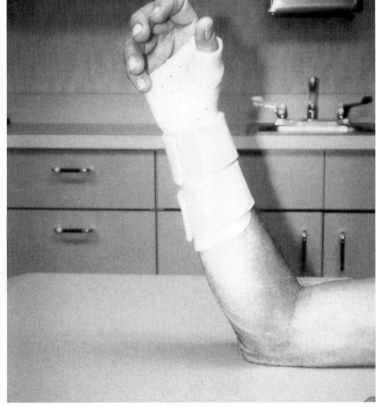

105. Surgical incision of the compartment usually relieves symptoms. Postsurgical rehabilitation involves initiating active exercises of the thumb and wrist in the early postoperative period (1 to 3 days). The patient is instructed to progress to light resistive exercise and functional activities as symptoms permit. Some prefer a wrist cock-up splint in 10° of extension for two weeks to prevent volar tendon prolapse.

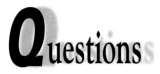

**106.** A 26-year-old, right-hand dominant man presents to the emergency room 1 hour after a severe crush injury to the right hand as a result of being trapped in a printing press. The hand is covered with green ink and markedly swollen with lacerations at the level of the distal flexion creases of all of the fingers. There is a linear laceration running along the axis of the long finger from the PIP joint to the base of the palm, which then runs ulnarward at the wrist flexion crease. Another 270° laceration runs across the base of the thumb, leaving a 2-cm skin bridge dorsally, 1 cm proximal to the MCP joint. All of the fingers have two-point discrimination greater than 15 mm, but sharp and dull discrimination are intact. Intrinsic muscle function is absent. Extrinsic muscle function is intact although extremely limited because of pain and swelling. Radiographic films demonstrate a dislocation of the trapezial-metacarpal joint. Once the ink was cleaned from the tips of the fingers, capillary refill was noted to be less than 5 seconds. How should this injury be treated?

**107.** At the delayed primary closure, it is noted that the patient's fingers are extremely stiff and have assumed a position of MCP joint extension and IP joint flexion. What can be done intraoperatively to help improve finger motion and correct this abnormal hand posture?

**108.** During the delayed closure surgery, it is not possible to maintain the hand in a "safe position" (the fingers spring back into a claw position). If the well-fitted dressing with splints does not maintain the "safe position," what else can be done to maintain adequate position of the fingers?

**109.** Despite a conscientious program of postoperative therapy with edema control and splinting in excellent position, the patient develops a flexion contracture of the long finger. This appears to be related to a linear scar, which was the result of one of the palmar lacerations he sustained in the original accident described in question 106. He lacks 30° of PIP joint and 45° of DIP joint extension. How should this problem be corrected?

**110.** Approximately 3 months following the crush injury, you find that although full composite passive flexion of the index finger can be achieved, the patient lacks ¾" of touching his proximal palmar crease actively. What is probably causing this differential in active and passive ROM?

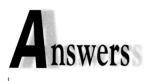

**A**nswers

**106.** The major concerns in this case are as follows:

(1) *Compartment syndrome of the intrinsic muscles*. With severe crushing injury, there must be a high index of suspicion for compartment syndrome. In the hand, the intrinsic muscles are divided into multiple compartments, each of which would require decompression in this type of injury. The diagnosis of compartment syndrome can be confirmed through intracompartmental pressure determination. In this case, the dorsal and palmar interossei, the thenar, hypothenar, and adductor compartments required release. The thenar musculature was completely destroyed, requiring extensive debridement.

(2) *Contaminated, open, crushing injury*. Although neurapraxia can account for the sensory deficit, assuming that all of the deficit is produced by the crush injury can give a false sense of security, and lead to missing the diagnosis of a lacerated nerve. Simultaneous with the complete debridement of devitalized and heavily contaminated tissue, lacerations should be explored to rule out repairable nerve injuries. For this type of injury, it would be appropriate to release the carpal and ulnar tunnels to decompress the nerves at these potential sites of compression.

(3) *Skeletal injury*. The thumb trapezial-metacarpal joint was found to be completely unstable. The thenar musculature was largely destroyed, and the thumb metacarpal was dislocated. A repair of the volar-oblique ligament and the joint capsule was carried out, and the trapezial-metacarpal joint was pinned in a reduced position with a .062 K-wire for 6 weeks.

(4) *Rehabilitation*. To facilitate rehabilitation of the hand, the digits were placed in a "safe position"; 70° to 80° of MCP joint flexion with the IP joints in nearly full extension. The skin was left open because of the significant swelling, and the patient was returned to the operating room 5 days postoperatively for delayed primary closure.

**107.** Manipulation of the digits under anesthesia can often dramatically increase ROM of the fingers and help facilitate better positioning. Placing the hand in a well-fitted compression dressing that maintains a safe position with strict postoperative elevation should help.

**108.** Temporary K-wire fixation of the MCP joints in 70° to 90° of flexion is a useful technique for maintaining the "safe position" in the face of marked swelling from crush injury or severe burns to the hand.

**109.** Flexion contractures of the digits can result from a number of causes. A linear scar crossing a joint palmar to the axis of rotation of the finger can produce limitation of extension. Flexor tendon shortening or adhesions can produce limited extension. At the PIP joint, thickening of the check rein ligaments can produce a flexion contracture at this joint, as can capsular contractures as a result of significant joint injuries. The initial approach to this problem would be an aggressive program of therapy including dynamic and static splinting in attempt to achieve full extension. If this is not effective, Z-plasty of the scar with sequential release of any other sites of limitation is necessary. This may require tenolysis, check rein ligament release, possibly collateral ligament release, and skin grafting.

**110.** Given that the patient has full PROM, you could rule out the presence of contractures within the joints, or the structures crossing the joints dorsally. Therefore, the lack of AROM can be attributed to inadequacy of the flexor mechanism—either weakness or loss of tendon gliding. With no evidence of neurological involvement, and with partial active flexion of the PIP and DIP joints, you could assume that the neuromuscular structures are intact. The lack of full AROM must be due to tendon adhesions within the flexor sheath.

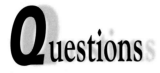

111. Following a crush injury with widespread vascular and soft tissue injury, there is a marked tendency toward fibrosis and adhesion formation throughout the hand. Describe an exercise program that would maximize tendon gliding.

112. A 26-year-old woman complains that the fingers in both of her hands feel cold, numb, and tingly, and her symptoms are aggravated by exposure to cold. She has noticed hand color changes consisting of white, followed by painful red digits. At times the fingers have remained white for over an hour, and this condition has caused her a great deal of pain. Upon physical examination, her fingers are pink but cool to the touch. Allen's test demonstrates good flow both from the radial and ulnar arteries. What is her most likely diagnosis?

113. How should this patient be initially worked up?

114. The patient's noninvasive vascular studies confirmed vasospastic disease without obstructive lesions. Based on these findings, what are the treatment recommendations?

115. What is a digital sympathectomy?

116. A 43-year-old secretary complains of gradual onset of progressive difficulty in writing. She denies any previous history of trauma or any neurologic conditions in her family history. She is otherwise healthy and takes no medications. She denies any paresthesias or muscular weakness. Her physical examination demonstrates normal motor and sensory function in the extremity. Her deep tendon reflexes are 2+ and bilaterally equal. When asked to write, she is noted to grasp the pen awkwardly and write in an extremely slow and labored manner. After 45 seconds, she is unable to write any further because of inability to effectively hold the pen. What is this patient's most likely diagnosis, and how can it be confirmed?

117. What are the characteristic EMG findings in the patient with focal dystonia?

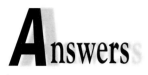

**111.** Continuous passive motion (CPM) is a useful adjunct but has to be applied selectively in order not to jeopardize healing fractures, tendons, etc. Active movement should be performed in a variety of fist positions to enhance excursion of the FDS and FDP tendons together and separately (see Figure 5-23). Also the MCP and PIP joints can be blocked individually to encourage tendon "pull through" at different sites in the finger. Passive stretching and dynamic or static progressive splinting are useful in stretching adhesions and remodelling scar tissue.

**Figure** 5-23

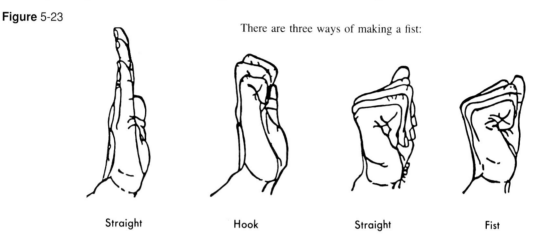

There are three ways of making a fist:

Straight        Hook        Straight        Fist

**112.** Raynaud's disease.

**113.** History and serologic testing should be directed toward ruling out connective tissue disease. Rheumatoid factor (RF), antinuclear antibodies (ANA), complete blood count (CBC), and erythrocyte sedimentation rate (ESR) are helpful initial screening tests. Noninvasive vascular studies are also helpful to confirm vasospastic disease through cold immersion stress testing of the digits. Doppler studies may suggest fixed arterial lesions.

**114.** The patient is instructed to keep her hands warm at all times. Mittens are more effective in keeping the digits warm than gloves, because mittens prevent cold air from surrounding each digit. Chemical hand warmers are also an effective supplement to keep the fingers from getting cold. If these measures are ineffective, pharmacologic treatment consisting of calcium channel blockers, such as nifedipine, have been effective in managing the patient with vasospastic disease. The patient is instructed to cease smoking and caffeine intake.

**115.** A digital sympathectomy is adventitial stripping of sympathetic fibers over a segment of the digital artery in the palm and fingers. In patients with a vasospastic component to their ischemic disease, digital sympathectomy interrupts the sympathetic outflow that causes constriction of the digital vessels.

**116.** The patient most likely has "writer's cramp," also known as focal dystonia. The diagnosis can be confirmed through EMG studies.

**117.** There is excessive co-contraction of the antagonist and agonist muscles consisting of abnormally prolonged bursts of electrical activity.

118. What are the treatment recommendations for the patient with "writer's cramp" (focal dystonia)?

119. An 18-year-old pole-vaulter missed the landing pit, falling on his extended right wrist. He had immediate pain and swelling and came to the emergency room where radiographic films were obtained. What do these films show? (See Figure 5-24, A and B.)

**Figure** 5-24    A

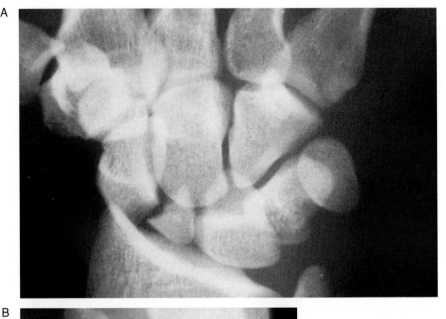

B

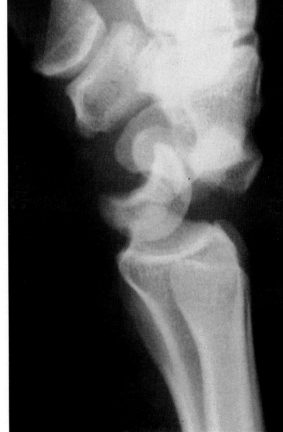

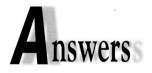

**118.** The treatment of this condition has generally been frustrating. An initial approach consists of changing the hand posture during writing and adjusting the writing implement, using different types of pen diameters and other types of writing devices. The patient is analyzed with attention to body posturing and proper writing techniques. Biofeedback may be effective. Medical management with oral or IV beta blockers and anticholinergics has had limited success. A new promising technique involves the injection of botulinum toxin into the most active dystonic muscles (identified by EMG while the patient is writing). These injections have facilitated temporary weakening of the muscles injected, resulting in a temporary functional improvement through selective weakening of the overactive muscles. A significant drawback is the need for maintenance injections on a monthly to bimonthly frequency.

**119.** The anteroposterior (AP) and lateral radiographic films of the right wrist show a dorsal transscaphoid perilunate dislocation.

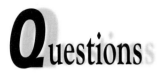

120. What are the common complications of lunate dislocation?

121. You are treating a patient who is 4 weeks postlunate dislocation. She was splinted for 3 weeks, then was referred to you to begin ROM. On her second visit, you note edema over the dorsum of her hand. In spite of her hand feeling cool and clammy to you, she complains of burning pain. What do you suspect is producing her symptoms?

122. What is a DISI deformity?

123. What is a VISI deformity?

124. List seven general indications for surgery in metacarpal and phalangeal fractures.

125. A 25-year-old, right-hand dominant man fell while skateboarding, sustaining an injury to his right thumb. His radiographic film (see Figure 5-25) demonstrates an intraarticular fracture of the base of the thumb metacarpal. Describe the management of this patient.

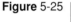 **Figure** 5-25

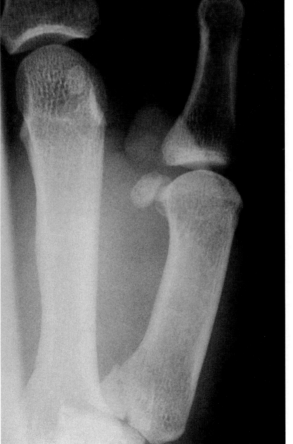

126. How are stable phalangeal fractures treated?

127. What is the average time of clinical union of closed unstable phalangeal fractures?

128. Describe the technique of extension block splinting for dorsal fracture-dislocation of the PIP joint.

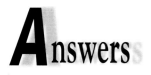

# Answers

**120.** The patient presents acutely with a painful, swollen wrist. Motion is restricted by pain and deformity. He may experience symptoms of median nerve compression. Chronic complications include wrist instability, deformity, avascular necrosis of the lunate, and wrist arthrosis.

**121.** This may be the onset of reflex sympathetic dystrophy (RSD). Diagnostic criteria include diffuse pain, decreased hand function, and sympathetic dysfunction. Following early vasomotor reflex spasm, the hand may later become warm, reddened, and dry. The patient experiences pain out of proportion to her injury, progressive stiffness, and trophic changes in the later stages of this condition.

**122.** A DISI (dorsal intercalated segment instability) deformity refers to palmar migration of the lunate with dorsal tilt of its distal articular surface, with associated palmar flexion of the distal pole of the scaphoid. It is usually associated with a scapholunate angle greater than 70° and a capitate-lunate angle greater than 15°. A DISI deformity is associated with scapholunate instability and scaphoid nonunion.

**123.** In the VISI (volar intercalated segment instability) deformity, the lunate assumes a dorsal position in the wrist relative to the capitate and its distal articular surface faces palmarward. There is a decreased scapholunate angle. This condition is associated with ulnar-side carpal instability such as lunotriquetral tears, as well as ligamentous laxity of the wrist.

**124.** (1) Open fractures; (2) displaced intraarticular fractures; (3) malrotation, seen most often in spiral and short oblique fracture patterns; (4) displaced phalangeal neck fractures; (5) fractures with bone loss; (6) multiple hand and wrist fractures associated with significant soft tissue injury; and (7) multitrauma with associated hand fractures.

**125.** This intraarticular fracture of the base of the metacarpal is displaced approximately 1 mm. In assessing whether a patient would benefit from surgical intervention, a surgeon considers whether significant clinical improvement can be obtained through surgery. An attempt at closed treatment should strongly be considered. Tomograms obtained in a thumb spica cast demonstrated minimal displacement. If additional displacement were to be noted on thumb tomograms, surgery would be indicated.

**126.** "Buddy taping." If there is any doubt regarding stability, use 10 to 14 days of splinting, then "buddy taping."

**127.** From 3 to 4 weeks. After immobilization for 3 weeks, phalangeal fractures can be treated with "buddy taping" to protect them for an additional 2 to 3 weeks.

**128.** Following closed reduction, confirmed by radiography, the hand is placed in a splint or short arm cast with an aluminum splint outrigger with the PIP joint flexed adequately to maintain reduction (usually 60°). A radiograph of the hand in the splint is obtained. If reduction is not maintained, external fixation, open reduction and internal fixation, or volar plate arthroplasty may be necessary. If satisfactory reduction is maintained, the PIP joint is allowed to flex and extend in the splint within the limits of the extension block. The proximal portion of the finger must be stabilized to the splint so that extension of the finger is blocked in the splint. (See Figure 5-15, A and B on page 239.) Flexion is reduced 15° per week so that full extension may be achieved by 4 to 6 weeks. At this time, the splinting is removed and "buddy taping" is used for 2 to 3 weeks. This technique is not applicable to unstable fracture-dislocation (greater than 40% of articular surface).

129. A 25-year-old laborer inadvertently caught his long finger in a router at work, sustaining a complex nail bed injury involving complete avulsion of the nail with a laceration extending in a stellate manner from the midportion of the sterile matrix proximally through the germinal matrix. There is a comminuted fracture of the distal phalanx at its midportion with an associated tuft fracture. How should this fracture and nail bed injury be managed?

130. A 12-year-old boy fell from a skateboard, injuring his ring and small fingers. Upon evaluation, he has swelling and tenderness at the bases of the proximal phalanges and has rotational deformity of the ring finger (see Figure 5-26, A, B, and C). What is the nature of the injury, and how should he be treated?

**Figure** 5-26

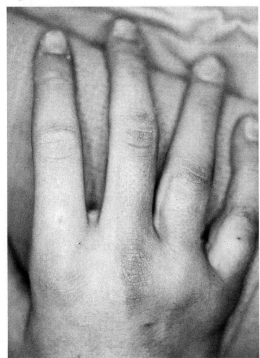

A

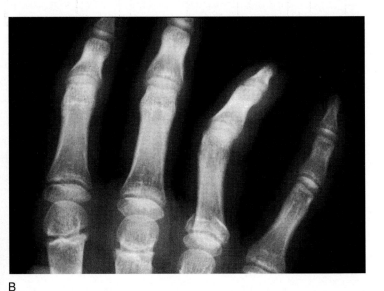

B

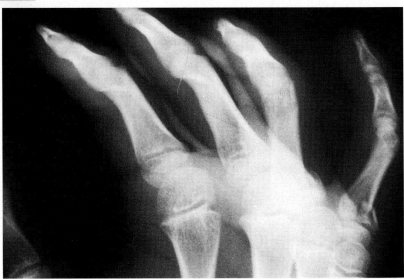

C

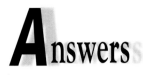
# Answers

129. Acutely, the best management consists of judicial debridement of the wounds, removal of any residual nail to fully expose the nail bed, and meticulous repair of the nail bed using fine absorbable sutures, such as 6-0 or 7-0 Vicryl. The fracture should be reduced and, if necessary, stabilized with K-wires. Even if rigid bony fixation is not achieved, the K-wires can impart additional soft tissue stability, which aids wound healing. If the fingernail is intact following cleansing, it can be replaced to prevent scar formation between the germinal matrix and the nail fold. Alternatives to keep the nail fold open include Xeroform gauze and Silastic nail splints, left in place for 2 weeks. The digit is then splinted, and ROM of the free joints pursued in 3 to 5 days.

130. These are Salter-Harris II fractures of the bases of the ring and small finger proximal phalanges with associated rotational and angular deformities. Closed reduction under hematoma block anesthesia is usually effective in facilitating a stable reduction. The hand is placed in a "safe position," or intrinsic plus, splint from the tips of the fingers to the mid forearm. AROM is initiated in 3 to 4 weeks with "buddy taping" to adjacent uninjured fingers. PROM can be started at 4 to 6 and strengthening 6 to 8 weeks after injury. It is rare that operative intervention is required in this type of injury. The fractures typically go on to union in 3 to 6 weeks.

131. A 28-year-old soccer goalie was kicked in the hand while attempting a save. Physical exam demonstrates ulnar deviation and radial rotation of the small finger. This digit is swollen and tender with limited motion because of pain (see Figure 5-27, A). Radiographic films (see Figure 5-27, B and C) of the hand demonstrate a fracture of the proximal phalanx. Describe treatment of this injury.

**Figure** 5-27

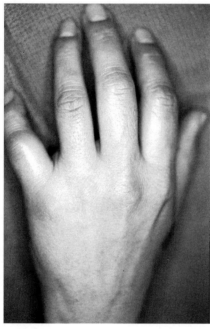

A

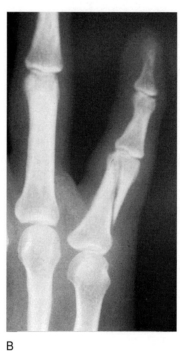

B

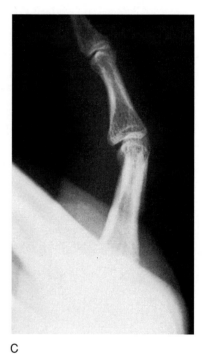

C

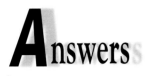

# **A**nswers

131. Closed reduction should be performed following adequate anesthesia (ulnar nerve block and hematoma or metacarpal block). If reduction can be held with "buddy taping" and splinting, closed treatment should be continued. This particular fracture proved unstable, requiring closed pinning (see Figure 5-28). If after pinning the fracture no motion is detected under fluoroscopy, early active ROM with protective splinting between exercises can be initiated.

**Figure** 5-28

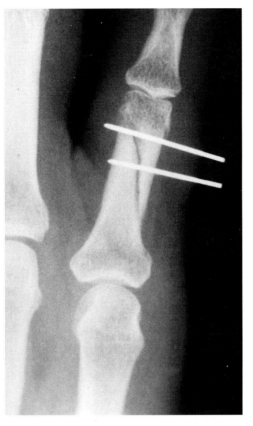

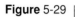

132. A 32-year-old mechanic injured his thumb while playing football. The thumb was caught in another player's face guard and jerked radially. The thumb was swollen and markedly tender over the ulnar aspect. He demonstrated no end point of his ulnar collateral ligament (UCL) when stress testing the MCP joint. The radiographic film is demonstrated in Figure 5-29. What is his diagnosis, and what should the treatment involve?

**Figure** 5-29

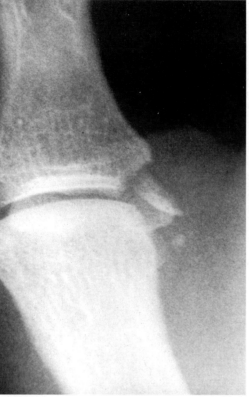

133. Describe the splinting and exercise protocols following a nondisplaced metacarpal shaft or neck fracture that is in good alignment.

134. What is a Stener lesion?

135. What are clinical indications for repair of the ulnar collateral ligament of the thumb?

**132.** The patient has an avulsion injury of the ulnar base of the proximal phalanx of the thumb. Treatment of a fragment displaced to this degree would require open reduction and internal fixation (see Figure 5-30).

**Figure** 5-30

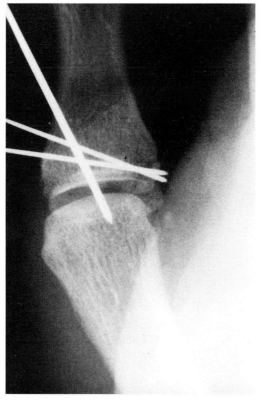

**133.** Place the patient in a dorsal forearm-hand splint, Galvston MC brace, P1 block, ulnar gutter splint, or short arm cast with dorsal molding over the volar metacarpal head that positions the wrist in 35° of extension and the MCP joints in 75° of flexion, leaving the other joints free. Instruct the patient to perform active flexion and extension within the confines of the splint. Manage edema with elevation and retrograde massage as necessary. Discontinue the splint after 2 to 3 weeks and begin full AROM; add resistance at 4 to 6 weeks.

**134.** The Stener lesion was described by Bertil Stener following exploration of 39 cases of complete rupture of the UCL of the thumb MCP joint. In 25 cases, he found interposition of the adductor aponeurosis between the base of the proximal phalanx (where the collateral ligament had been avulsed) and the retracted stump of the collateral ligament. The adductor apparently becomes interposed between the torn ligament end, and the base of the phalanx as the thumb is widely abducted during the injury. With the adductor interposed between the ligament and its site of attachment, prognosis for a stable thumb is poor if left to "heal" in this position.

**135.** Clinical stress testing can be helpful in distinguishing partial from complete ruptures. In acute injuries, it is often helpful to block the area with an anesthetic agent, performing either a digital block or a pericapsular block. The MCP joint should be stressed in positions of 0° and 30° of flexion. If no end point is identified with stress testing, it is clear that the collateral ligament is completely ruptured and should be repaired.

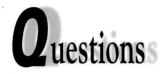

**136.** What are some of the radiographic techniques used to determine the need for repair of the UCL of the thumb MCP joint?

**137.** How is treatment of radial collateral ligament (RCL) injury of the thumb MCP joint different from that of the UCL?

**138.** What is the rehabilitation protocol for partial or complete tears of the UCL of the thumb MCP joint?

**139.** A patient with a bony "gamekeeper's thumb" returns to the office 6 weeks after operative repair. K-wires have been removed 4 weeks postoperatively. Upon examination, the patient is still swollen and tender over the UCL. The MP joint is stiff. The radiographic films demonstrate an absence of bony healing between the fragment and the base of the proximal phalanx. What should be done about this bony "nonunion"?

**140.** The patient returns 3 weeks after initiation of the rehabilitation program, and stress testing of the UCL demonstrates moderate pain and persistent instability. What are the treatment options at this point?

**141.** An 18-year-old football player caught his small finger in another player's shoulder pads, snapping the finger. Tendon function appeared to be intact except for an inability to adduct the finger. There was swelling around the MCP joint, and tenderness localized primarily over its radial aspect. Radiographic films were normal. What is the differential diagnosis for this injury?

**142.** How can the diagnosis of a torn RCL of the MCP joint be made?

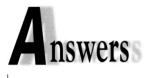

# Answers

136. Some of the radiographic techniques include the following: (1) Plain radiographic films may demonstrate a displaced and rotated fragment of the base. (2) Stress radiographic films of the MCP joint will indicate that surgery is recommended if there is greater than 10° to 15° of instability noted compared with the opposite uninjured side or if there is greater than 30° stressed abduction arc. (3) A thumb MCP joint arthrogram, as described by Bowers, can demonstrate a displaced or trapped UCL tear. (4) Magnetic resonance imaging (MRI) is another promising, though expensive, imaging technique. Most complete tears can be identified clinically.

137. There is very little difference between the two. For complete ruptures, operative repair is recommended. For partial tears of the RCL, 4 weeks of immobilization is recommended.

138. Both nonoperative treatment of partial tears, and surgical ligamentous repairs require 4 to 6 weeks of immobilization in a short arm, or glove, thumb spica cast. Following cast removal, the patient is instructed in AROM for the CMC, MCP, and IP joints of the thumb. The patient must take care to avoid abduction and extension at the MCP joint, and initially avoid forceful pinching activities. Gradual progression to resistive exercises in a pain-free range is allowed after 6 to 8 weeks. Maintaining stability should take precedence over regaining full mobility. A protective thumb post splint (allowing CMC and IP joint movement, while stabilizing the MCP joint) can be worn during activities that place his thumb at risk for re-injury for up to 3 months.

139. Not all avulsion fractures of the base of the proximal phalanx of the thumb MCP joint go on to bony union, but they can develop an asymptomatic fibrous union. A stress test of the UCL should be performed. If the joint is stable, you should proceed with a gradual rehabilitation program. After 2 to 3 weeks, the patient is reevaluated. Because of joint stiffness from recent immobilization, you can be misled into believing that the collateral ligament is stable. Once postimmobilization stiffness is worked out, the collateral ligament stability should be reassessed.

140. The presence of significant instability at this point indicates a treatment failure. Additional cast immobilization will not be effective in "tightening up" the repair. The repair should be explored and a repeat repair performed. If the tissue is inadequate for simple open reduction and internal fixation (ORIF), the bony fragment may be excised and the ligament advanced into the base of the proximal phalanx, or a ligament reconstruction may be performed similar to those utilized in chronic UCL injuries.

141. Pain around the radial aspect of the MCP joint with associated swelling and an inability to adduct the finger are highly suggestive of an injury to the RCL of the MCP joint. Capsular tear, chondral fracture of the metacarpal head, and a ruptured interosseous muscle are other diagnostic considerations.

142. Although there are a number of sophisticated diagnostic tests available, including MRI, the simplest and least expensive is a stress test of the RCL. This is performed by placing the MCP joint in a position of 90° of flexion and applying an abduction stress to the joint. This must be compared with the opposite, unaffected hand in order to take into account idiosyncratic ligamentous laxity. If there is a significant difference in laxity, the diagnosis is made.

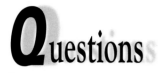

143. How should an RCL tear be treated?

144. Although ulnar positive variance is associated with ulnar impaction syndrome, ulnar negative variance is associated with what wrist condition?

145. What is Kienböck disease?

146. What is the etiology of Kienböck disease?

147. What is the most popular treatment for Lichtman's stages II and III Kienböck disease with ulnar neutral or negative variance?

148. A 37-year-old teaching tennis pro presents with an insidious onset of right-dominant wrist pain approximately 6 months ago. The pain is dull and aching in nature and is becoming worse. His symptoms are aggravated by forceful gripping, serving, and overhead shots. The patient reports occasional clicking in his wrist during pronation. Physical examination reveals tenderness over the medial wrist area but no deformity. Forearm and wrist ROM are full. There are no sensory changes. Grip strength equals the uninvolved hand. Radiographs reveal an ulnar positive variance. How would you proceed?

149. Describe the TFCC. What is its role?

150. A 65-year-old woman presents with complaints of catching at the PIP joint of her ring finger. She describes the PIP joint becoming locked into flexion and is able to demonstrate it in your office. She says it is much worse in the morning—she frequently awakes with the digit held in a locked position. What is the diagnosis and how should she be treated?

151. What physical findings would you expect with a trigger finger?

# Answers

143. Incomplete ligament tears can usually be treated with splint or cast immobilization with the MCP joint at about 45° of flexion for 3 to 4 weeks. Once acute tenderness subsides, "buddy taping" the digits for an additional 3 to 4 weeks is recommended.

    The acute management of complete RCL tears of the MCP joints is controversial. Nonoperative treatment can be successful; however, the percentage of failures is much lower using direct surgical repair. The nonoperative treatment for complete tears is similar to the treatment of incomplete tears with immobilization in a cast or splint for 4 to 6 weeks and with subsequent "buddy taping." Index finger RCL repair is mandatory because of the need for MCP radial stability for pinch.

144. Ulnar negative variance is most frequently associated with Kienböck disease.

145. Kienböck disease is an avascular necrosis of the lunate.

146. Although controversial, most experts believe that the avascular necrosis is the result of a posttraumatic insult to a susceptible wrist (i. e., ulnar negative variance and single vessel perfusing the lunate). Occult lunate fractures have been identified in early Kienböck disease and are felt to represent a traumatic sequelae.

147. Distal radial shortening or ulnar lengthening. The rationale for either of these treatments is to achieve a better distribution of force at the level of the radioulnar interface with the lunate. Of the two procedures proposed, the radial shortening is less technically demanding.

148. This patient most likely has a degenerative lesion of the triangular fibrocartilage complex (TFCC). He can be treated conservatively with long arm cast immobilization with the elbow at 90° and the forearm in neutral rotation for 4 to 6 weeks. If his symptoms persist, the diagnosis should be confirmed with arthrographic or arthroscopic examination. Central TFCC perforations can be debrided arthroscopically with an early return to activity. Peripheral detachments require open or arthroscopic repair. Ulnar impaction can be treated by arthroscopic or open arthroplasty, or ulnar shortening osteotomy.

149. The TFCC is comprised by a confluence of structures, including the articular disc, UCL, extensor carpi ulnaris (ECU) sheath, meniscus homologue, and dorsal and volar radioulnar ligaments. It contributes to stability of the distal radioulnar joint and transmits force across the wrist to the ulna. Normally the ulna bears 20% of the axial load of the forearm. Forceful grasp increases the load on the distal radioulnar joint; repetitive loading may produce degenerative changes in the disc.

150. This most likely is a trigger finger. Treatment would consist of an injection of the flexor tendon sheath with a mixture of steroid and anesthetic, which is frequently curative. Alternative treatments include splinting programs to maintain the MCP joint in extension. The last option is surgical release of the A-1 pulley, reserved for cases in which conservative treatment was not successful.

151. The most obvious finding is having the patient demonstrate the triggering. This usually can be elicited by asking the patient to make a tight fist and then to extend the digits. The affected finger will be maintained in flexion at the PIP joint and then suddenly snap into extension as the thickened part of the flexor tendon passes under the A-1 pulley. Sometimes the patient has to manually straighten the finger to overcome the locking. Typically, the patient will have marked tenderness overlying the A-1 pulley and nodular enlargement of the flexor tendon in this area.

152. A 52-year-old woman with rheumatoid arthritis complains of spontaneous long finger catching. She recalls no injury. Upon physical examination, she has full flexion of the digits; however, when she attempts to extend the fingers, she is unable to obtain full extension of the long finger MCP joint. There is dorsal swelling and tenderness around this area. She lacks 30° active extension at the MCP joint. In addition, the digit deviates 20° ulnarly at the MP joint with attempted digital extension. With passive assistance, however, the digit can be brought into full extension and held in this position. Radiographic films were unremarkable for revealing a pathologic condition at this joint. Likewise, the wrist is minimally involved with the rheumatoid disease. What is the diagnosis, and how should she be treated?

153. A 35-year-old cook is referred by his company doctor for "locking" of the long finger MCP joint. There is no history of trauma, and upon physical examination, there is no swelling noted. The digital ROM demonstrates near normal flexion, but there is a 40° lack of active and passive extension at the MCP joint. His extensor tendon feels intact, and his neurosensory exam is intact. Apart from slight enlargement of the radial condyle of the metacarpal head, there are no radiographic abnormalities. What is this patient's diagnosis and treatment?

154. A 32-year-old banker complains of a mass at the base of the thumb that has worsened over the past few weeks. He notices intermittent tingling in the thumb that is aggravated by bowling. Physical examination demonstrates a firm 10 mm x 2 mm mass palpable on the ulnar aspect of the thumb at the level of the MCP joint. Rolling and percussion of the mass produces paresthesias in the thumb tip. What is this patient's diagnosis?

155. Describe treatment of "bowler's thumb."

156. A 3-month-old boy is brought to his physician's office because the parents noted that he is unable to fully extend his thumb. There is no history of congenital abnormalities in the family. Figure 5-31 demonstrates the extent of passive extension of the thumb. Actively, the thumb will extend no farther than 30° short of neutral. There is no other evidence of congenital problems. Apart from the loss of extension of the IP joint, physical examination demonstrates good flexion of the thumb. The remaining digits are normal. He has a fullness in the flexor tendon overlying the volar MCP joint. What is the diagnosis?

**Figure** 5-31

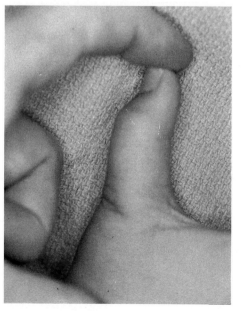

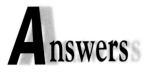

# Answers

**152.** Trigger finger in a patient with rheumatoid disease may be caused by a number of problems ranging from the classical triggering at the A-1 pulley to other entities, such as nodular involvement of the flexor tendons at various levels. In this particular case, the patient is experiencing locking because of subluxation of the extensor mechanism over the long finger MCP joint as a result of attritional rupture of the radial sagittal band. Although nonoperative treatment can be successful through a program of splinting, a more reliable treatment is operative repair or reconstruction of the sagittal band.

**153.** A locking MCP joint is usually associated with a metacarpal head osteophyte or prominence, which catches on the collateral ligament or volar plate producing limitation of full extension. Although gentle manipulation can be attempted, forceful attempts at unlocking the joint should not be made. Given time, the joint will sometimes unlock spontaneously. Injection of the joint with a mixture of steroid and anesthetic will facilitate reduction of inflammation, which may be responsible for the previously well-tolerated bony metacarpal head prominence, causing impingement on an edematous volar plate or collateral ligament. If after several weeks the joint is not unlocked, then operative intervention is warranted with exploration of the joint with removal of the impinging source. Some patients will experience unlocking of the joint with an interval of symptom-free motion followed by a relocking of the joint. In this event, early operative intervention is recommended.

**154.** This patient has "bowler's thumb," which is perineural fibrosis of the ulnar digital nerve of the thumb caused by repeated pressure of the bowling ball against the nerve. This condition is usually seen in fairly avid bowlers, and upon further questioning, the patient admitted that he was a tournament-level player. Varying degrees of this condition can occur, ranging from intermittent pain and numbness to constant sensory changes along the ulnar aspect of the thumb.

**155.** Although surgical decompression with neurolysis and epineurectomy may be performed, the best results have come from early recognition and conservative treatment. If recognized early, the elimination of the repeated trauma through cessation of bowling, adjustment of the bowling ball grip through redrilling the thumb hole, or application of accommodative padding have been helpful. A shield or splint can sometimes be a helpful adjunct for those patients who will not give up bowling.

**156.** This condition most likely represents congenital trigger thumb, wherein there is enlargement of the flexor pollicis longus tendon at the level of the A-1 pulley in the thumb. Its incarceration would account for the lack of extension at the IP joint of the thumb.

**157.** How should this patient be treated?

**158.** A 35-year-old man sustained a closed humeral fracture as pictured in Figure 5-32, A in a motor vehicle accident. When he came to the emergency room, he was asked to extend his wrist and fingers. He had complete loss of MCP and wrist extension as seen in Figure 5-32, B. What is his problem referable to the hand, and how should it be managed?

**Figure** 5-32

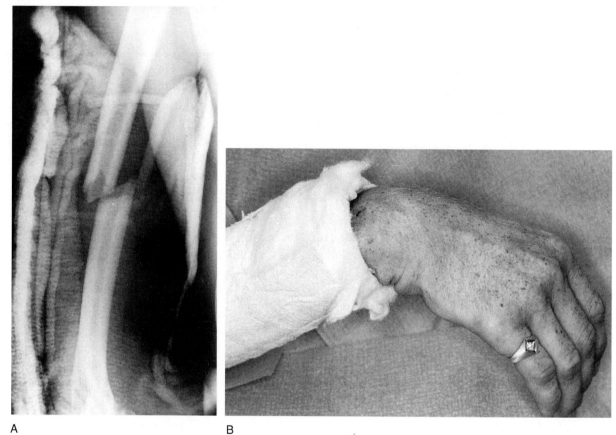

A                                    B

**159.** Four months later the fracture has healed, but the patient in question 158 shows no clinical signs of recovery of his radial nerve function. What should be done now?

**160.** A 51-year-old golfer complains of spontaneous onset of medial elbow pain 3 months earlier that has progressively worsened. He is tender over the medial epicondyle and has pain with resisted pronation and wrist flexion. Radiographic films are normal. Describe your management of this patient.

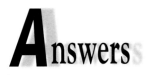

# Answers

**157.** There is controversy regarding treatment of congenital trigger thumb and trigger fingers. Some practitioners favor passive stretching by the parents and splinting, and others favor benign neglect with the expectation that some patients will spontaneously unlock their digits. Other orthopedists recommend surgical release upon diagnosis because of reports in literature of a low percentage of spontaneous correction. A reasonable, middle-of-the-road approach is surgical release at 9 to 12 months of age if the digit has not spontaneously unlocked.

**158.** This humeral fracture is associated with a radial nerve palsy, which accounts for lack of MCP extension of the digits and loss of wrist extension. Because he has a closed injury with the nerve palsy already in effect, you would expect a high likelihood of spontaneous nerve recovery without exploration—over 90% of patients experience spontaneous recovery. Management would consist of a splint, fracture brace, or cast for the humeral fracture and a cock-up wrist splint and physical therapy to maintain mobility of the digits.

**159.** Repeat electrodiagnostic studies should be obtained and compared to those obtained early in the clinical course (3 to 4 weeks after injury). In the absence of any clinical or electrodiagnostic improvement, exploration is indicated after 3½ to 4 months of observation in closed injuries.

**160.** Initial nonsurgical management of medial epicondylitis consists of rest and NSAIDs. Patients are instructed to avoid provocative activities. Corticosteroid injection and counterforce bracing are often beneficial. After symptoms have subsided, a rehabilitation program consisting of progressive stretching and multi-angle isometric exercises, followed by resisted concentric and eccentric exercises can be initiated. Equipment and/or activity modifications are often indicated. Surgery is reserved for cases unresponsive to conservative care.

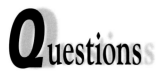

# Questions

161. The illustration shown (Figure 5-33) is the lateral view of a 10-year-old child's wrist. The patient's mother noticed this lump with the wrist in a flexed posture. The mass is 1 cm x 1 cm in size, pain-free, and readily transilluminates. What are the treatment options?

**Figure** 5-33

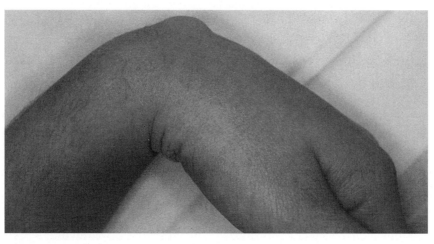

162. Describe the site of origin of most dorsal carpal ganglion cysts.

163. A 10-year-old girl has deformities of her left hand that have become progressively painful. A radiographic film is shown (Figure 5-34). What is the patient's diagnosis, and how should this problem be approached?

**Figure** 5-34

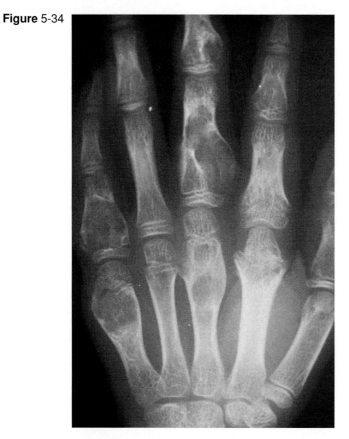

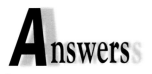

# Answers

161. A dorsal wrist mass in this area that is pain-free and transilluminates is most likely a dorsal carpal ganglion cyst. Other diagnostic possibilities include a giant cell tumor, extensor tenosynovitis, exostosis, or a soft tissue tumor. Because the wrist is a fairly characteristic location for a dorsal carpal ganglion cyst, treatment recommendations depend on the patient's degree of symptomatology. If the mass changes significantly in size or character, biopsy should be considered. An asymptomatic patient can be followed as needed. If the parent or the patient expresses symptoms with activities that do not respond to a period of splinting, surgical excision or mass aspiration may be considered.

162. The typical location of the base of the stalk of a dorsal carpal ganglion cyst is the dorsal scapholunate capsule and ligament.

163. This patient has multiple enchondromatosis. In a patient with symptomatic enchondromata with significant thinning of the cortex, a physician should consider excision.

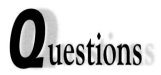

**164.** A 50-year-old secretary slammed her finger in a cabinet drawer at work 1 week earlier and went to her physician with swelling of her affected index finger. Upon physical examination, there is lobulated nodular swelling dorsally and palmarly overlying the middle phalanx. The skin demonstrates no significant changes. Neurosensory examination is intact. Her digital ROM is near normal. A radiograph is shown (Figure 5-35). She wants to know whether her proposed operation will be covered under workers' compensation. What is your response?

**Figure** 5-35

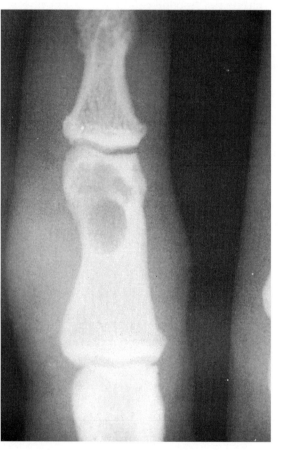

**165.** What is the diagnosis?

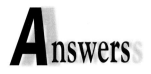

# Answers

164. The radiographic changes seen are consistent with a long-standing process of more than 1 week's duration. It is likely that slamming her finger in a cabinet had nothing to do with the process that has produced enlargement of the digit and erosion of the bone.

165. The most likely cause of gradual erosion of the middle phalanx (suggested by the rounded appearance and sclerotic margins of the defect), with associated soft tissue enlargement in several lobulated areas in the digit, is a giant cell tumor of the tendon sheath.

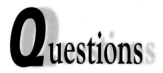

**166.** A 14-year-old girl complains of right wrist pain after a fall in gymnastics class. The wrist has remained symptomatic, and she complains of a dorsoulnar prominence with deformity. Careful questioning reveals that this deformity had been present prior to her injury. A radiographic film of the right wrist is shown (Figure 5-36). What is the diagnosis?

**Figure** 5-36

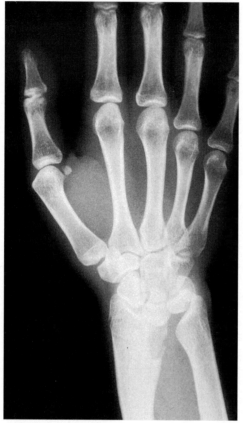

**167.** How would you confirm this diagnosis?

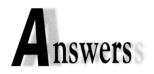

# Answers

**166.** Madelung's deformity.

**167.** Often radiographic films of the opposite wrist will demonstrate a similar deformity. A radiographic film of the left wrist is illustrated (Figure 5-37). Characteristic radiographic changes include decreased radial length with triangular shape, usually associated with early fusion of the ulnar half of the distal physis. There is often an area of lucency at the ulnar border of the distal radius, with ulnar and volar angulation of the distal radial articular surface. The ulna is shortened with enlargement of the ulnar head, associated with dorsal subluxation. The carpus tends to be wedge-shaped with the apex located proximally.

**Figure** 5-37

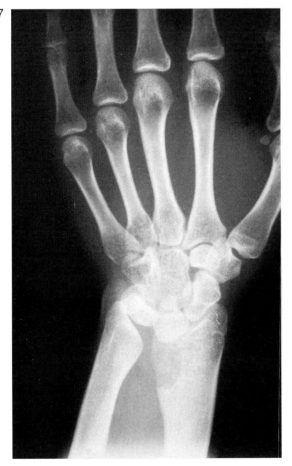

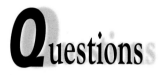

**168.** A 68-year-old woman has had recalcitrant pain at the base of the thenar eminence. Her examination demonstrates fairly good ROM of the thumb; however, she has significant trapeziometacarpal grind. A radiographic film is shown (Figure 5-38). What is her diagnosis?

**Figure** 5-38

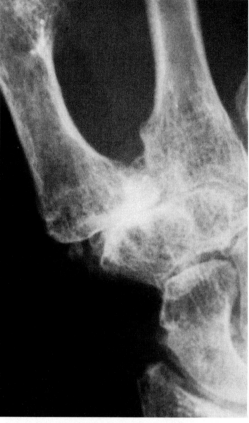

**169.** What are the recommended treatments for this problem?

**170.** The scaphoid is the most frequently fractured bone in the wrist. How does its intercarpal location place it at risk for injury?

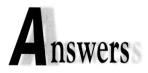

**168.** This is advanced trapeziometacarpal arthrosis.

**169.** Despite severe radiographic appearance, many of these patients can be managed with a program of NSAIDs and intermittent splint usage. Occasionally, intraarticular steroid injection can reduce acute inflammation and alleviate severe symptoms. Surgical options include trapeziometacarpal arthrodesis or one of the many trapeziometacarpal arthroplasties, using tendon suspension and prosthetic replacement.

**170.** Although the scaphoid lies in the proximal row of carpal bones, its distal pole spans the midcarpal joint, exposing it to shearing forces through the waist. A fall on the outstretched, supinated hand is the typical mechanism that produces a scaphoid fracture.

171. A 23-year-old college soccer player injured his wrist last season and has had the diagnosis of scaphoid fracture made. He played the majority of the season in an athletic splint so that he could continue to participate; he spent the rest of the off season in a cast. He returned home for summer vacation and presents at his physician's office for follow-up care. He has been in a short-arm, thumb spica cast with an electrical stimulator applied for the past 3 months. He wants to be ready to play the coming season starting in September. A radiographic film is shown (Figure 5-39). This radiographic film shows no change from those taken 3, 6, and 9 months earlier. How should this patient be treated?

**Figure** 5-39

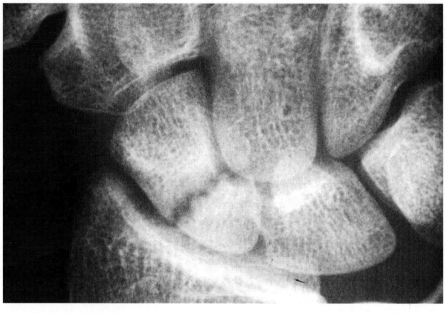

172. What is the clinical significance of the blood supply of the scaphoid?

173. A 28-year-old factory worker is sent to your office by his company because of bilateral hand complaints. He states that during the course of his shift, his hands became clumsy and weak, and he has difficulty with dropping objects. He has noted problems with holding the newspaper and driving the car. When he goes to bed at night, he is intermittently awakened by his hands falling asleep—he has to shake his hands to obtain relief. What is his differential diagnosis, and what is the most likely diagnosis?

174. Assuming this is carpal tunnel syndrome, what clinical tests should you perform to confirm the diagnosis?

175. Assuming the patient has clinical evidence of carpal tunnel syndrome but has no interest in surgical intervention, what conservative measures would you suggest that might help decrease his symptoms?

176. What factors would lead to recommendation of carpal tunnel release as opposed to conservative care?

177. Are there advantages to an endoscopic carpal tunnel release versus an open release?

178. What are the functions of the hand's arches? How does the carpal arch differ from the others, and what additional functions does it have?

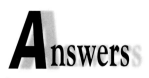**nswers**

171. To have this patient ready for the next season, with no change in the radiographic appearance of his fracture over a 9-month period, either a closed pinning of the fracture or ORIF and bone grafting should be performed.

172. Because of the distal-to-proximal direction of flow, fractures in the proximal portion of the scaphoid are more liable to cause interruption of the blood supply and lead to avascular necrosis of the scaphoid proximal pole and nonunion.

173. The most likely diagnosis is carpal tunnel syndrome. The differential diagnosis for this patient includes compressive neuropathies including cervical radiculopathy, thoracic outlet syndrome, pronator syndrome, cubital tunnel syndrome, radial tunnel syndrome, and, most frequently, ulnar tunnel and carpal tunnel syndromes. You would also have to consider the possibility of nerve trauma as seen with hypothenar hammer syndrome and vascular disorders such as Raynaud's phenomena.

174. The most frequently used tests to confirm diagnosis of carpal tunnel syndrome include Phalen's test, reversed Phalen's test, median nerve compression test, Tinel's sign over the median nerve at the level of the wrist, as well as motor testing of the APB, inspection for atrophy of the APB, and abnormalities in vibratory and monofilament sensation, and two-point discrimination (threshold changes precede innervation density changes) in the distribution of the median nerve.

175. The use of wrist splints, carpal tunnel injection with corticosteroid, modification of work activities, vitamin B6 therapy, and NSAIDs have all been employed with varying degrees of success.

176. A history of constant sensory loss, atrophy of the thenar musculature with weakness, or prolongation of two-point discrimination compared with the opposite hand are factors that indicate that conservative care is not likely to be successful. In these patients, operative release is appropriate.

177. At this time, there is no evidence that supports improved functional recovery relative to either technique. Proponents of the endoscopic release claim there is less postsurgical morbidity, but after 6 weeks, most patients are able to resume functional and job-related activities following both techniques. The endoscopic technique carries a higher risk of inadvertent arterial and nerve injury and incomplete release of the transverse carpal ligament, but would appear to produce less scarring.

178. Three volarly concave arches emerge from the arrangement of the wrist and hand skeleton to enhance prehensile function. The longitudinal arch spans the hand lengthwise, and two lateral arches run transversely, one at the level of the metacarpal heads and the other at the carpus. The longitudinal arch accommodates finger flexion. The flexible metacarpal arch is controlled by action of the intrinsic muscles, particularly the thenar and hypothenar muscles; it assists grasping and pinching functions. The relatively stable carpal arch forms a base for the fingers; it is also the floor of the carpal tunnel, which serves as a conduit for the nine extrinsic flexor tendons and the median nerve.

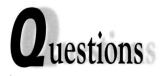

**179.** When testing grip strength with a Jamar dynamometer, how are the values from the five handle positions normally distributed when graphed?

**180.** What are the clinical ramifications of the "multijoint" muscles crossing the wrist and hand?

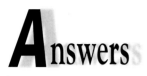
# Answers

**179.** The values form a bell-shaped curve, peaking in the second handle position.

**180.** Wrist ROM is influenced by finger position because the length of the extrinsic tendons only permits a given amount of motion, i.e., wrist flexion is less when the fingers are simultaneously flexed than when they are extended. Conversely, the wrist's position also affects finger ROM, i.e., finger flexion is less when the wrist is simultaneously flexed than when it is extended. Thus, a therapist should consider: (1) the importance of maintaining a constant position of all other joints, when measuring any one particular joint; (2) identifying hand position when measuring strength; and (3) incorporating tenodesis into treatment planning, such as using wrist extension to enhance grasp in a C6 spinal cord injured patient, or wrist flexion to enhance finger extension in a patient with cerebral palsy.

# Chapter 6

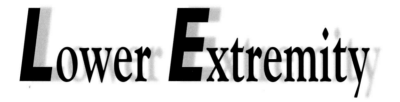

# Lower Extremity

TIMOTHY S. LOTH, MD

STAN DYSART, MD

KENNETH KOVAL, MD

WILLIAM BANDY, PhD, PT, SCS, ATC

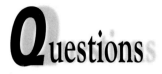
# Questions

1. What gait abnormalities are observed in a patient with degenerative disease of the hip joint?

2. In a patient with fixed flexion deformities of the hips, what compensatory posture does the lumbar spine assume?

3. While performing a Thomas test for the hip, the patient presents with a positive test when pulling the right limb into flexion, and a negative test when pulling the left limb into flexion. What problem is indicated?

4. A 62-year-old overweight individual complains of right groin pain with ambulation. Radiographic films demonstrate degenerative arthritis of the hip. What nonoperative measures might be considered before performing a total joint replacement?

5. A 75-year-old man has been referred for a hip replacement because of complaints of groin pain when ambulating and because of radiographic films that demonstrate degenerative arthritis. Additional history reveals that he has bilateral thigh and calf pain when walking distances greater than one block, and that discomfort is relieved by sitting. What additional evaluation should be considered prior to performing a total joint replacement?

6. A 26-year-old heavy laborer has extensive posttraumatic hip arthritis and concentric joint space loss. He has failed nonoperative therapy and would like to proceed with operative therapy. He would like to continue in his current occupation after the procedure. What surgical option is best?

7. A 35-year-old office manager has been diagnosed with traumatic hip arthritis and has progression of pain and limitation of activities of daily living despite adequate nonoperative management. Radiographic films show extensive involvement of the joint. The patient has a history of low back pain that is chronic and has required one previous hospital admission. What is the best surgical option for this young patient?

8. What is the effect of hip arthrodesis on oxygen consumption and gait efficiency when compared to the normal hip? Is energy consumption greater when compared to a total hip replacement?

9. In clinical experience, does use of a larger head size in total hip arthroplasty lead to a lower incidence of hip dislocation?

10. In patients who undergo total joint replacement of both the hip and the knee on the same side, how much total combined hip and knee flexion is required to easily climb stairs and get out of a chair?

11. What is the force in terms of body weight across the patellofemoral joint while walking on a level surface?

12. When going up and down stairs, the force across the patellofemoral joint increases. What is the increased force in terms of body weight?

13. What effect does squatting have on the force experienced through the patellofemoral joint?

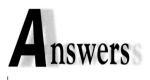
# Answers

1. There will often be shortening of the stance phase of the affected limb (secondary to pain), decreased step length on the unaffected side, and increased step length on the affected side. There is also displacement of the body over the affected hip (Trendelenburg gait) in an attempt to decrease the muscle contraction forces across the joint.

2. The patient will generally develop a hyperlordotic posture of the lumbar spine with a prominence of the buttocks with ambulation.

3. This patient's flexion contracture affects the left hip. The Thomas test is used to assess a hip flexion contracture. The supine patient holds the flexed hip and knee to the chest, while the other leg remains straight. If no hip flexor tightness exists, the hip being tested (the straight leg) will remain on the examining table. If hip flexor tightness is present, the patient's straight leg will raise off the table.

4. Activity modification, use of nonsteroidal antiinflammatory drugs (NSAIDs), weight reduction, and use of a cane in the left (opposite) hand when ambulating. Use of a cane in the contralateral hand reduces hip compressive force. Hip replacement is reserved for failure of nonoperative therapy.

5. The patient's differential diagnosis includes spinal stenosis and vascular claudication. An evaluation of the lumbar spine with radiographs, computerized tomography (CT), and magnetic resonance imaging (MRI) should be considered. Also an examination for vascular compromise is indicated, because symptoms of leg pain with ambulation may be caused by vascular claudication.

6. Hip arthrodesis is the option most likely to produce pain-free function of long duration. Although hip replacement is an option for the younger individual with degenerative arthritis, it is not recommended in the individual who is a heavy laborer. A patient engaged in heavy labor or with extensive degenerative changes is a poor candidate for femoral osteotomy.

   The positioning of the hip is important for maximal postoperative function. Neutral rotation, neutral abduction and adduction, and 30° of hip flexion are considered ideal. Internal rotation and hip abduction are to be avoided. Slight hip adduction (10°) and up to 5° of external rotation are well tolerated.

7. A total joint replacement is the best option for this patient. The patient's history of low back pain contraindicates hip arthrodesis. A successful hip arthrodesis exposes the lumbar spine and ipsilateral knee to increased stress. Long-term follow-up of successful hip arthrodesis demonstrates ipsilateral knee and back pain in 60% of patients. A femoral osteotomy would be appropriate in the patient with more localized arthrosis.

8. In a study of energy expenditure after hip arthrodesis, mean oxygen consumption was 32% more than normal, gait efficiency was 53% of normal, and energy consumption was greater than that reported after total hip replacement.

9. No. Dislocation after total hip arthroplasty is truly a multifactorial problem. Factors such as previous surgery, surgical approach, component position, soft tissue reconstruction, and patient compliance have a much greater influence on clinical dislocation rates.

10. Combined hip and knee flexion of 190° or more is generally required.

11. The force is 1 to 1.5 times body weight.

12. The force is 3 to 4 times body weight.

13. Squatting may markedly increase the force across the patellofemoral joint up to 7 times body weight.

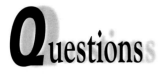
14. What is the most likely cause of long-standing problems in a patient with pain distributed diffusely across the anterior knee, no instability on clinical testing, increased parapatellar pain during resisted knee extension, and localized tenderness on palpation of the borders of the patella?

15. Define the Maquet procedure for the knee.

16. What is the major mode of failure seen in total knee arthroplasty (TKA)?

17. What is the leading cause of revision in most series of TKA?

18. What is the major determinant of postoperative knee flexion in condylar TKA?

19. What factors are associated with patellar instability after TKA?

20. What are the differences in infection and loosening rates in constrained knee designs when compared to unconstrained prosthetic designs?

21. What effect does CPM have on wound healing and incidence of thromboembolism in the immediate postoperative period after a total knee replacement?

22. What is the benefit of CPM in patients undergoing TKA?

23. What is the most common cause of death in the patient undergoing total hip or knee arthroplasty?

24. What risk factors are associated with thromboembolic disease?

25. During rehabilitation of a patient following a total knee arthroplasty, what signs and symptoms would lead you to be concerned about deep vein thrombosis?

26. What are the benefits of open synovectomy of the knee in the patient with rheumatoid arthritis?

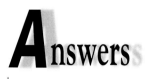

14. Patellofemoral dysfunction. The patient should be evaluated for patellar alignment or patellar tracking problems and muscle imbalance in the quadriceps and hamstrings.

15. It is a surgical procedure for patellofemoral dysfunction in which the tibial tubercle is elevated with a bone plug from the ilium in an effort to decrease patellofemoral pressure. The anterior displacement of the tibial tubercle reduces the force vector across the patella and thereby reduces compressive forces on the patella.

16. Implant loosening. This can result from improper implant positioning, poor surgical technique, and the use of constrained implants that increase stresses at the bone implant interfaces.

17. Patellar failure is the leading cause of revision.

18. Preoperative knee flexion is the major determinant of postoperative knee flexion. This has been found to be more of a determinant than use of continuous passive movement (CPM), the use of a cruciate retaining rather than cruciate sacrificing prosthesis, or preoperative or postoperative knee alignment.

19. The factors are excessive internal rotation of the femoral component, excessive internal rotation of the tibial component, and preoperative valgus limb alignment.

20. When compared to unconstrained designs, a constrained knee prosthesis has increased loosening and infection rates.

21. There appears to be no significant effect compared to patients not receiving postoperative CPM.

22. Controlled evaluations have shown that CPM results in a decreased rate of manipulation to achieve motion. There is no evidence that CPM results in increased motion or in increased quadriceps muscle strength at long-term follow-up. Hospital stay is also not decreased.

23. Pulmonary embolism is the most common cause of death.

24. Three general categories of risk factors attributed to Virchow are venous stasis, injury, and hypercoagulability. Associated with venous stasis are heart failure, immobility, and previous thrombosis. Obesity is considered by some to be a secondary risk factor. Endothelial injury is attendant with many orthopaedic procedures and orthopaedic trauma. Hypercoagulable states are associated with adenocarcinoma, any congenital or acquired deficiencies of endogenous anticoagulant proteins (including antithrombin III and heparin cofactor II), and congenital abnormalities or deficiencies of plasminogen or fibrinogen.

    There is a significant association of venous thromboembolism and patients undergoing total hip or total knee replacement. If prophylaxis is not used, deep vein thrombosis has been documented to occur in 40% to 60% of patients undergoing total hip or knee arthroplasty. Prolonged venous stasis and endothelial injury are associated with intraoperative limb positioning in total hip arthroplasty. Venous stasis and potential venous endothelial injury are associated with use of the thigh tourniquet and with intraoperative manipulation in those patients undergoing total knee arthroplasty.

25. Clinical findings that would lead to concern include persistent calf pain, leg cramps, painful leg movements, and excessive swelling in the leg.

26. The benefits of open synovectomy of the knee in rheumatoid arthritis include diminished pain and swelling and no change or a slight decrease in range of motion (ROM) of the knee. There is usually no increase in ROM postoperatively, and there is no appreciable prevention of joint deterioration.

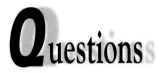

27. An arthrodesis of the knee should be accomplished in what position?

28. The sartorius muscle is innervated by which nerve?

29. The gluteus medius and minimis muscles are primary abductors of the hip. They are innervated by which nerve?

30. Evaluation of a 30-year-old woman with "hip pain" indicates the following: passive ROM is pain-free and full; she experiences pain with resisted hip extension and resisted knee flexion; and she has pain over the ischial tuberosity. The problem is most likely with which tissue?

31. Evaluation of the gait of a 65-year-old homemaker reveals lateral lean of the trunk to the right when the right lower extremity is in stance phase. Provide the name of this gait deviation, two possible causes for such a deviation, and the muscle that should be tested to differentiate between the two causes.

32. What is the function of the popliteus muscle?

33. What is the function of the semimembranosus muscle?

34. How should acute complete ruptures of the quadriceps tendon be treated?

35. How should partial quadriceps tendon ruptures be treated?

36. Describe the three grades of quadriceps muscle contusion.

37. What is the blood supply to the patella, and what segment of the patella can undergo avascular necrosis (AVN) after transverse fracture?

38. Describe the clinical findings in a patellar ligament rupture.

39. A 32-year-old accountant was playing racquetball and felt severe infrapatellar pain when he abruptly changed direction to make a shot. Since that episode, he has been unable to walk on the leg. Upon physical examination, there is swelling in the area of the patellar ligament with tenderness. There is a palpable defect in the patellar ligament. He is unable to actively extend the knee. What is the diagnosis and how should this problem be treated?

40. A 16-year-old girl was playing soccer and had severe pain in her knee as she fell to the ground. She has been able to ambulate on the leg, although there is pain throughout her knee. Physical examination demonstrates the knee to be in a slightly flexed position with the patella laterally dislocated. What factors predispose to dislocation of the patella?

41. How should this patient be treated?

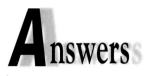

**27.** In 10° to 15° of flexion and 5° to 10° of valgus.

**28.** The femoral nerve.

**29.** The superior gluteal nerve.

**30.** The hamstring muscles. Given that resisted movement caused pain and passive movement was pain-free, most likely the tissue involved is muscle. Given that the action of the hamstring muscles is both hip extension and knee flexion, and that the hamstring muscles originate from the ischial tuberosity (the site of pain with palpation), the most likely muscles to be involved are the hamstrings.

**31.** The gait deviation is termed Trendelenburg gait. Possible causes include a weak gluteus medius muscle on the right or intraarticular hip joint pain on the right. Muscle testing of the right gluteus medius muscle would help to clarify the cause of the problem and provide direction for appropriate intervention.

**32.** Internal rotation of the tibia on the femur.

**33.** Flexion and internal rotation of the tibia.

**34.** Operative repair, sometimes using a reinforcing Scuderi flap.

**35.** In a cylinder cast in either extension for 5 to 6 weeks or in a cast brace.

**36.** Grade 1—mild pain and swelling, knee flexion ROM greater than 90°, recovery in 2 to 25 days. Grade 2—moderate pain and swelling, knee flexion ROM between 45° and 90°, recovery between 30 and 100 days. Grade 3—severe pain and swelling, discoloration possible, knee flexion ROM less than 45°, recovery may be extended to 180 days. Myositis ossificans, the formation of heterotrophic bone within the muscle, may be a complication of repeated contusions.

**37.** A patellar plexus that enters in the central portion, but does not supply the patella until it reaches the distal pole. In transverse fractures, the proximal pole may undergo AVN.

**38.** The patient complains of pain about the knee with inability to extend the knee. There may be a palpable defect in the patellar ligament and the patella will be in an abnormally proximal position.

**39.** This patient has ruptured his patellar ligament. These injuries usually occur in patients under the age of 40. Surgical repair should be performed if the patient is unable to extend the knee against gravity. It is possible to treat these injuries nonoperatively, if the retinacular attachments of the vastus medialis and lateralis muscles are intact, thus allowing some extension of the knee. However, a surgical repair should be performed if there is any evidence of proximal migration of the patella. Knee flexion will frequently demonstrate a high-riding patella, whereas if the knee is held in extension, this may not be obvious.

**40.** Predisposing factors include hypermobility of the patella due to poor muscle tone, genu valgum, attenuation of the medial support structures, weakened vastus medialis muscle, patella alta, shallow patellofemoral groove, increased femoral neck anteversion, excessive external tibial torsion, excessive pronation, laterally inserted patellar tendon, and genu recurvatum, which causes laxity in the extensor mechanism.

**41.** Reduction of the dislocated patella through knee extension and medially directed pressure on the patella. For first-time dislocators, if no articular fractures are present, a cylinder cast or knee immobilizer may be used for 4 to 6 weeks. Quadriceps muscle exercises should be performed after the acute tenderness of the dislocation subsides.

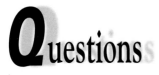

**42.** List possible therapeutic interventions that may aid in the facilitation of vastus medialis oblique (VMO) muscle firing.

**43.** What are the complications associated with dislocation of the patella?

**44.** What is the main reason for obtaining radiographs following reduction of a patellar dislocation?

**45.** When performing a tibial tubercle transfer to correct a laterally dislocating patella, in which direction is the tibial tubercle moved?

**46.** What problems result from common peroneal nerve palsy?

**47.** What deformities develop with palsy of the tibial nerve?

**48.** What is the only muscle that, when transferred, will have sufficient strength to produce active plantar flexion in the presence of a paralyzed triceps surae muscle?

**49.** What functional difficulties do patients have with femoral nerve palsy?

**50.** What is the recommended muscle transfer for a femoral nerve palsy?

**51.** What is the normal end feel for knee extension?

**52.** An 18-year-old man has had recurrent locking of the knee. He has a history of previous patellar dislocations. What is the most likely diagnosis and how should he be treated?

**53.** Describe the most common location of osteochondritis dissecans (OCD) in the knee.

**54.** What is the best management for nondisplaced osteochondritis dissecans of the medial femoral condyle identified in a skeletally immature boy?

**55.** Define the abrasion arthroplasty procedure for the knee.

**56.** Describe the pathologic changes in Osgood-Schlatter's disease.

**57.** Define apophysitis.

**58.** At what age is Osgood-Schlatter's disease most common?

**59.** What is the natural history of Osgood-Schlatter's disease?

**60.** In the presentation of Osgood-Schlatter's disease, what study is mandatory to rule out other possible pathologic conditions such as tumors?

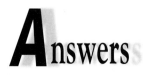# Answers

42. Interventions include: (1) positioning the femur in external rotation to relax the tension from lateral structures and put the VMO on stretch; (2) utilizing the hip adductors (since the VMO arises from the tendon of the adductor magnus, firing the adductors will facilitate VMO contraction); and (3) attempting to control effusion as even minimal swelling of the knee will inhibit VMO contraction.

43. (1) Recurrent dislocation; (2) osteochondral fractures; (3) chondromalacia patella; and (4) degenerative joint disease.

44. To look for osteochondral fracture fragments.

45. Distally and medially. Moving the tibial tubercle distally and medially essentially tightens the structures of the knee medial to the patella by aligning the pull of the quadriceps muscle through the patellar tendon.

46. Loss of dorsiflexion and eversion of the foot.

47. A cavus foot from plantar fascia contracture; the Achilles tendon becomes elongated and the calcaneus is rotated into dorsiflexion.

48. The tibialis anterior muscle. This muscle can be transferred through the interosseous membrane.

49. These patients ambulate well on level surfaces. They are unable, however, to effectively climb stairs or inclined surfaces.

50. The biceps femoris muscle is transferred to the extensor mechanism.

51. Bone to bone. End feel is the sensation that the examiner feels in a joint as it reaches the end of its ROM passively. A proper evaluation of end feel assists the examiner in the assessment of the pathology.

52. This patient most likely has loose bodies that are causing the knee to lock. These are the result of shearing of osteochondral fragments with the previous knee dislocations. Treatment is knee arthroscopy. A less likely diagnosis is meniscal tear. Arthroscopy helps to clarify the diagnosis.

53. The lateral aspect of the medial femoral condyle.

54. Activity modification and a short period of immobilization supplemented with isometric strengthening exercises of the knee.

55. Abrasion arthroplasty is a surgical procedure in which a full thickness defect in articular cartilage is abraded past the tidemark into subchondral bone.

56. Apophysitis of the tibial tubercle secondary to repetitive microtrauma resulting in inflammation and new bone formation at the tendon-bone junction.

57. It is inflammation of an apophysis. An apophysis is a cartilaginous structure (growth plate) near the end of a bone that is subjected primarily to tensile forces. Apophysitis is a common disorder in adolescents as a result of repetitive microtrauma at musculo-tendinous origins and insertions, especially around the pelvis.

58. Age 13 to 14 years in boys, 10 to 11 in girls.

59. In the majority of cases, there is complete resolution 1 to 2 years after onset.

60. AP and lateral radiographs of the knee.

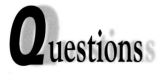

# Questions

61. Which of the following treatment modalities is contraindicated in Osgood-Schlatter's disease—rest and immobilization, isometric knee exercises, knee pads, or steroid injections?

62. Describe the most common cause and location of Baker's cyst in childhood.

63. Describe the natural history of Baker's cyst in childhood.

64. A patient complains of pain in the back of the knee. Standing toe raises cause slight pain. Examination indicates no joint instability. Static resisted knee flexion at 90° was found to be strong and painless. Static resisted plantarflexion with the knee extended was painless, but passive dorsiflexion of the ankle was painful. There was palpable tenderness over the posterior knee. What problem do you suspect?

65. Name the two phases of the normal gait cycle and provide the approximate percentage of time attributed to each.

66. Name the subdivisions (intervals) of stance phase.

67. Toe-off signals which phase?

68. Provide the average percentage of time spent in each interval of gait.

69. Describe the function of efficient gait.

70. In the normal gait cycle, when is hip flexion maximized?

71. Describe the position of the knee at heel strike.

72. Describe the position of the knee at mid single limb stance.

73. Describe the relationship of shoulder girdle rotation to pelvic rotation during gait.

74. Describe the characteristics of gait in a 1-year-old child.

75. At what age is the adult gait pattern achieved?

76. What are the characteristics of antalgic gait?

77. Describe the position of the ground reaction force vector in relation to the hip, knee, and ankle at the beginning of weight acceptance and the resultant torque created at each of the three joints.

78. Describe the gait deviations that would be seen in a patient with a severed left common peroneal nerve at the level of the fibular head.

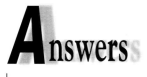

61. Steroid injections, because they can induce weakening of the patellar tendon and subcutaneous fat necrosis.

62. Synovial popliteal cysts that arise between the semimembranosus and gastrocnemius tendons are most commonly idiopathic lesions.

63. There is spontaneous resolution within 2 to 5 years.

64. First-degree strain of the gastrocnemius muscle near its insertion. Given that toe raises caused pain suggests a plantarflexion muscle. No pain with resisted plantar flexion suggests that the resistance applied was not sufficient to stress a minor strain to the plantarflexors, a common occurrence in an examination. Pain with passive movement in the opposite direction of the muscle (dorsiflexion) also suggests the gastrocnemius muscle. The area of pain with palpation was consistent with the insertion of the gastrocnemius muscle, the posterior femoral condyle.

65. Stance phase, 60%; swing phase, 40%.

66. (1) Weight acceptance; (2) single limb stance; and (3) weight release.

67. Swing phase.

68. Weight acceptance, 11%; single limb stance, 39%; weight release, 11%; and swing phase 39%.

69. Forward body progression allowing only small oscillations in the center of gravity in three planes.

70. At foot strike, hip flexion approximates 40°.

71. 10° of flexion.

72. 0° of flexion.

73. A reciprocal transverse rotation occurs through the vertebral column.

74. Slower velocity, shorter step length, and increased cadence are accompanied by lack of reciprocal swing of the upper and lower limbs and a wider base of support.

75. Gait characteristics are similar to those of an adult by age 7.

76. Decreased stance phase time on the affected limb, with a shorter swing phase in the contralateral limb; lateral trunk displacement toward the affected side during ipsilateral stance.

77. At the beginning of weight acceptance, the ground reaction force vector falls anterior to the hip, creating a hip flexion moment that is counteracted by eccentric activity of the gluteus maximus, hamstring, and adductor magnus muscles. The vector is posterior to the knee, creating a flexion moment that is controlled by eccentric activity of the quadriceps femoris muscle. At the ankle, the ground reaction force is posterior to the center of the joint, creating a plantar flexion moment that is counteracted by eccentric activity of the ankle dorsiflexor muscles.

78. Severing the common peroneal nerve at the level of the fibular head would eliminate innervation to the tibialis anterior, extensor hallucis longus, extensor digitorum longus, extensor digitorum brevis, peroneus longus, peroneus brevis, and peroneus tertius muscles. The resulting gait deviations would include contact with the forefoot and lateral side of the foot at initial contact, "foot slap" or lack of controlled plantar flexion at loading response, and problems with floor clearance during mid and terminal swing—all on the left side. Typically, the patient deals with problems of floor clearance by increasing hip and knee flexion during swing, the so-called "steppage" gait, or by vaulting on the contralateral lower extremity or circumducting the ipsilateral hip.

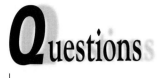
**79.** Name the labeled structures on the posterior thigh (see Figure 6-1).

**Figure** 6-1

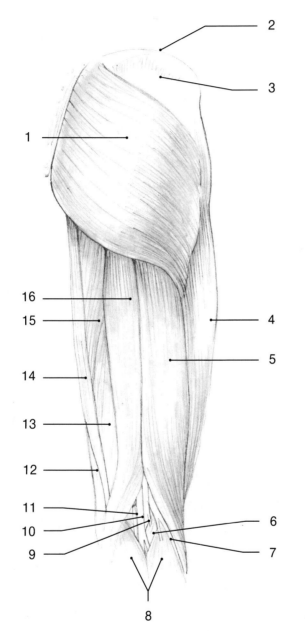

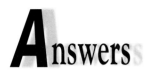
**A**nswers

**79.** (1) Gluteus maximus muscle; (2) iliac crest; (3) fascia over gluteus medius muscle; (4) iliotibial tract; (5) biceps femoris muscle, long head; (6) plantaris muscle; (7) common peroneal nerve; (8) gastrocnemius muscle, medial and lateral heads; (9) tibial nerve; (10) popliteal vein; (11) popliteal artery; (12) sartorius muscle; (13) semimembranosus muscle; (14) gracilis muscle; (15) adductor magnus muscle; and (16) semitendinosus muscle.

80. Name the structures in the deep aspect of the buttock (see Figure 6-2).

**Figure** 6-2

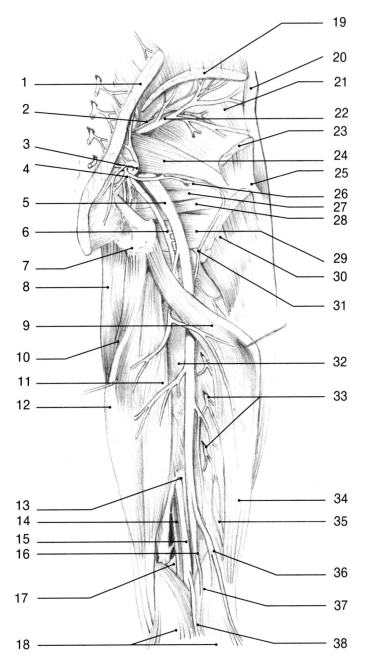

1
2
3
4
5
6
7
8
9
10
11
12
13
14
15
16
17
18

19
20
21
22
23
24
25
26
27
28
29
30
31
32
33
34
35
36
37
38

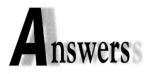

**A**nswers

80. (1) Gluteus maximus muscle (cut); (2) superior gluteal artery; (3) inferior gluteal nerve; (4) inferior gluteal artery; (5) sciatic nerve; (6) posterior femoral cutaneous nerve; (7) ischial tuberosity; (8) gracilis muscle; (9) biceps femoris muscle, long head; (10) adductor magnus muscle; (11) semimembranosus muscle; (12) semitendinosus muscle; (13) adductor hiatus; (14) popliteal artery; (15) popliteal vein; (16) tibial nerve; (17) adductor tubercle of femur; (18) gastrocnemius muscle, medial and lateral heads; (19) gluteus medius muscle (cut); (20) tensor fasciae latae muscle; (21) gluteus minimus muscle; (22) superior gluteal nerve; (23) gluteus medius muscle (cut); (24) piriformis muscle; (25) greater trochanter; (26) superior gemellus muscle; (27) obturator internus muscle; (28) inferior gemellus muscle; (29) quadratus femoris muscle; (30) gluteus maximus muscle (cut); (31) medial femoral circumflex artery; (32) adductor magnus muscle; (33) perforating arteries; (34) biceps muscle, long head (retracted); (35) biceps muscle, short head; (36) common peroneal nerve; (37) medial sural cutaneous nerve; and (38) lesser saphenous vein.

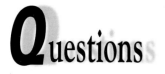

**81.** Name the medial thigh structures (see Figure 6-3).

**Figure** 6-3

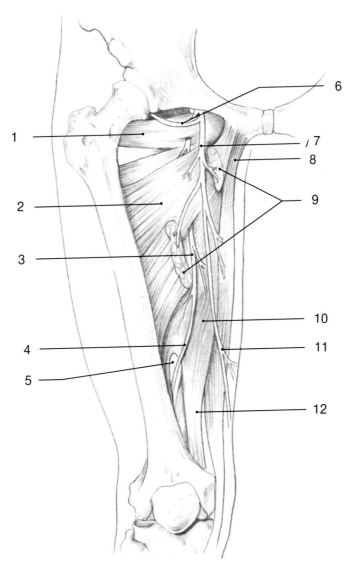

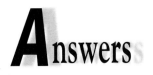

81.  (1) Obturator externus muscle; (2)adductor brevis muscle; (3) posterior branch of obturator nerve; (4) articular branch of (knee) obturator nerve; (5) hiatus of adductor canal; (6) articular branch of (hip) obturator nerve; (7) anterior branch of obturator nerve; (8) gracilis muscle; (9) adductor longus muscle (cut); (10) adductor magnus muscle; (11) cutaneous branch of obturator nerve; and (12) adductor magnus tendon.

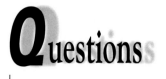

82. Identify each labeled structure on the anterior leg (see Figure 6-4).

**Figure** 6-4

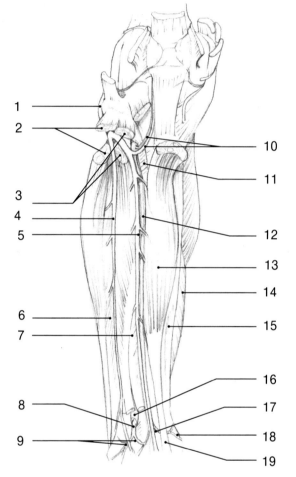

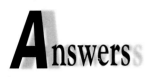

**A**nswers

82. (1) Common peroneal nerve; (2) peroneus longus muscle (cut); (3) extensor digitorum longus muscle (cut); (4) superficial peroneal nerve; (5) deep peroneal nerve; (6) peroneus brevis muscle; (7) extensor hallucis longus muscle; (8) perforating branch of peroneal artery; (9)anterior lateral malleolar arteries; (10) anterior tibial recurrent artery and recurrent articular artery; (11) interosseus membrane; (12) anterior tibial artery; (13) tibialis anterior muscle; (14) soleus muscle; (15) tibia; (16) interosseous membrane; (17) anterior medial malleolar artery; (18) medial malleolus; and (19) tibialis anterior tendon.

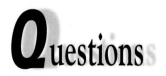

**Q**uestions

83. How does the mechanical axis of the lower limb differ from the anatomic axis of the lower limb? What is the average angle between the anatomic axis and mechanical axis in men and women?

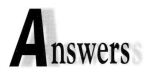

## Answers

83. The mechanical axis (H-O-C) of the normal limb passes through the center of the femoral head, just medial to the center of the knee and center of the tibial plafond. The anatomic axis passes through the midshaft of the femur and the midshaft of the tibia. The mechanical axis coincides with the tibial shaft axis, but forms an acute angle of approximately 6° with the femoral shaft axis. The average angle between the anatomic axis and mechanical axis in men is 5° of valgus; in women it is 7° of valgus. The obtuse angle of 170° to 175° between the anatomic axes of the femur and the tibia is known as physiologic valgus (see Figure 6-5).

**Figure** 6-5

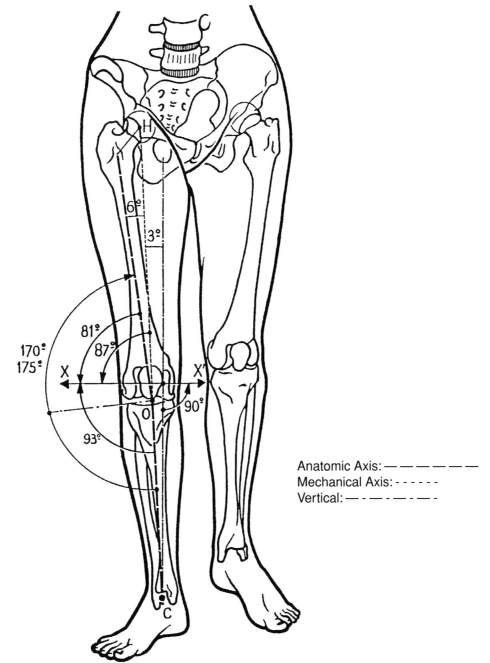

Anatomic Axis: — — — — — —
Mechanical Axis: - - - - - -
Vertical: — - — - — - — -

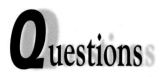

84. Describe the primary vascular supply to the hip.

85. True or false? In adults, the artery within the ligamentum teres provides a significant blood supply to the femoral head.

86. Describe the attachments of the hip joint capsule onto the femoral neck.

87. How should a 40-year-old woman with a fracture at the base of the right femoral neck and other injuries be treated?

88. What are the indications for prosthetic replacement after femoral neck fracture?

89. When used for stabilization of an intertrochanteric hip fracture, what is the advantage of a sliding hip screw over a rigid nail plate?

90. What is the most common complication associated with hip fractures in geriatric patients?

91. What is the treatment of choice for femoral shaft fractures?

92. What are the biomechanical advantages of an intramedullary femoral nailing versus a femoral plating?

93. Which meniscus is more mobile?

94. Which meniscus is peripherally attached to the knee joint capsule?

95. What are the functions of the menisci?

96. A patient complains of knee pain and occasional "catching." Upon examination of the knee, you find all static resisted movements to be strong and painless. The patient is unable to fully extend the knee and presents with a positive Steinmann's test. What may be the problem?

97. What tests would be confirmatory of a torn meniscus?

# Answers

84. The profunda femora artery divides into the medial and lateral femoral circumflex arteries. The ascending branch of the lateral circumflex artery and the medial circumflex artery form an extracapsular ring at the base of the femoral neck. This ring gives rise to ascending cervical arteries that traverse the femoral neck proximally to form a second ring at the base of the femoral head. Branches from this second ring penetrate the femoral head and provide its primary blood supply.

85. False. In adults, the artery within the ligamentum teres has only a limited role in providing blood supply to the femoral head.

86. Anteriorly, the capsule attaches to the femoral neck at the intertrochanteric line; posteriorly, the capsule attaches to the midportion of the femoral neck.

87. Urgent closed reduction and pinning.

88. Prosthetic replacement should be considered in elderly patients with a displaced femoral neck fracture when an adequate reduction cannot be obtained or when severe posterior comminution precludes stable internal fixation.

89. The sliding hip screw allows controlled impaction of the fracture. In addition, the sliding hip screw is load sharing compared with the rigid nail plate, which is load bearing.

90. Venous thrombosis is seen in 40% to 90% of patients in whom no prophylaxis has been given.

91. Surgical stabilization with an intramedullary nail is the treatment of choice.

92. Biomechanically, intramedullary femoral nails offer several advantages over plates, screws, and external fixation: (1) The intramedullary canal is closer to the center of gravity of the body than the plate position on the lateral surface of the bone; consequently, intramedullary nails are subjected to smaller bending loads than plates and are thus less likely to result in fatigue failure. (2) Intramedullary nails act as load-sharing devices in fractures that have cortical contact of the major fragments. If the nail is not locked at both the proximal and distal ends, it will act as a gliding splint and allow continued compression as the fracture is loaded. (3) Stress shielding with resultant cortical osteopenia, commonly seen with plating, is avoided with intramedullary implants. (4) Refracture after implant removal is rare with the use of intramedullary devices, secondary to the lack of cortical osteopenia and the minimum number of stress risers created in the bone. (5) In midshaft femoral fractures, large diameter intramedullary devices that fill the medullary canal automatically reestablish the bony alignment.

93. The lateral meniscus.

94. The medial meniscus. The lateral meniscus is not attached to the capsule at the popliteus hiatus.

95. Menisci functions are shock absorption, knee stability, and articular cartilage nutrition.

96. A history of "catching" may indicate meniscus or patellar pathology. Inability to fully extend the knee may be due to something blocking full extension, such as a torn meniscus. Steinmann's test indicates meniscal involvement when there is point tenderness and pain at the joint line that appears to move anteriorly when the knee is extended and posteriorly when the knee is flexed.

97. A positive McMurray test, an Apley grind test demonstrating pain during compression and relief during distraction, radiologic studies, an MRI or an arthrogram, and arthroscopy (indicated urgently only if mechanical locking of the knee is present).

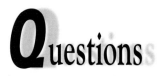

98. What is the best treatment for a peripheral one-third tear of the medial meniscus, extending greater than 1 cm in length that can be displaced into the joint when probed in a 20-year-old athlete with no other injury?

99. Describe the shapes of the medial and lateral tibial plateaus.

100. Through what compartment does the majority of the load pass in the normal knee during weight bearing?

101. What is the mechanism of injury for tibial plateau fractures?

102. How are knee dislocations classified?

103. What is the mechanism of injury in anterior knee dislocation?

104. Which ligament is the primary stabilizer of the knee against posterior movement of the tibia on the femur?

105. For rehabilitation after a posterior cruciate ligament (PCL) injury, strengthening of which muscle group should be emphasized early?

106. What tests are used to evaluate damage to the PCL?

107. List possible mechanisms for injury to the ACL.

108. A patient presents with a history of hyperextension injury during running. He "felt a pop" and experienced immediate swelling. On initial evaluation in the emergency room, joint aspiration reveals hemarthrosis. What is the most likely diagnosis?

109. What is the most sensitive test for anterior knee instability?

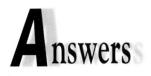

# Answers

98. Arthroscopic repair. There is a high success rate of repair in this type of lesion and total meniscectomy increases the risk of degenerative joint disease.

99. The lateral plateau is convex, and the medial plateau is concave.

100. Sixty percent of the load passes through the medial compartment.

101. Tibial plateau fractures result from indirect coronal or direct axial compressive forces, or both. Fracture fragment size, location, and displacement are determined by the magnitude, direction, and location of the generated force, the bone quality, and the degree of knee flexion at the moment of impact. The interplay of varus and compression results in medial plateau fractures, whereas the interaction of valgus and compression produces lateral fracture patterns. The prevalence of lateral plateau fractures is related to the valgus inclination of the anatomic axis and the usual lateral direction of the applied force.

102. Knee dislocations are classified by the relationship of the tibia to the femur. The five major types are anterior, posterior, lateral, medial, and rotatory. Anterior dislocations result from hyperextension of the knee. Posterior dislocations result from a posterior-directed force on the anterior aspect of the tibia. Medial and lateral dislocations result from varus and valgus stress, respectively. Rotary dislocations occur with combined anterior/posterior and medial/lateral forces.

103. Knee hyperextension can tear the posterior capsule and rupture the PCL and anterior cruciate ligament (ACL).

104. The PCL (that arises from the posterior margin of the tibia and courses superior, anterior, and medial to insert into the lateral wall of the medial femoral condyle) provides approximately 85% to 95% of the total restraining force to posterior displacement of the tibia.

105. The quadriceps muscle, because it can assist in stabilization of the knee by preventing posterior displacement of the tibia, a movement that can further damage the PCL. Caution should be used when exercising the hamstring muscles early in rehabilitation, since contracting the hamstring muscles will pull the tibia posteriorly and potentially damage the PCL.

106. Tests for the stability of the PCL include: (1) Godfrey's (or posterior sag) test—the examiner holds the feet of the supine patient with the hips and knees at 90° and views the knee from the lateral side; a positive test occurs when a posterior sag of the tibia is observed. (2) Posterior sag (or gravity drawer) test—with the patient supine, the hips flexed to 45°, the knees flexed to 90°, and the feet flat on the table, viewing the knee from the lateral side reveals a lack of tibial tubercle prominence (due to gravitational force). (3) Posterior drawer test—with the patient supine, knees flexed to 90°, and feet flat on the table, the tibia is pushed posteriorly by the examiner.

107. Mechanisms include a blow to the knee, a change of direction, and knee hyperextension.

108. Anterior cruciate ligament rupture. Associated pathologic findings such as a torn meniscus may be present in a significant percentage of cases.

109. The Lachman test. With the patient in a supine position and the knee in approximately 15° of flexion, the distal femoral condyle is gripped in one hand, thereby stabilizing the femur. The proximal tibia is drawn anteriorly with the other hand. Abnormal tests demonstrate anterior displacement of the tibia without a firm end point compared to the uninjured knee.

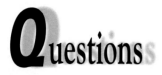

110. What is the best treatment for functional ACL insufficiency in an athletically active 20-year-old patient with symptoms persisting after rehabilitation?

111. Differentiate between an autograft and an allograft in reference to graft material that can be used to surgically reconstruct the ACL.

112. When does the vascularization of the patellar tendon autograft used in ACL reconstruction occur?

113. List the advantages of closed kinetic chain exercises for the patient after ACL reconstruction.

114. List one test for knee stability that would be positive for a patient who has sustained a second-degree sprain of the medial collateral complex of the right knee.

115. What is the best treatment for an isolated acute tear of the medial collateral ligament?

116. Rank the following knee problem/surgeries from longest (first) to shortest (last) rehabilitation, assuming no complications: second degree medial collateral ligament sprain (nonsurgical), ACL reconstruction using a patellar tendon graft, meniscectomy.

117. How should the injury shown in Figure 6-6 be treated?

**Figure** 6-6

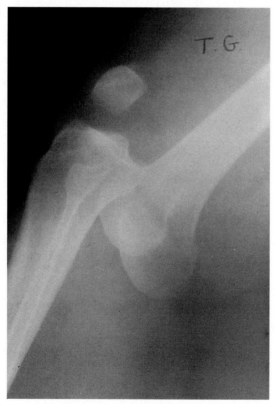

118. What is the Salter-Harris classification?

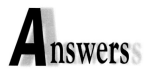 **nswers**

110. Reconstruction of the ACL using autologous material such as bone-patellar tendon or bone-hamstring tendon grafts. Repair of intersubstance tears of the anterior cruciate has shown unreliable results. A patient with less demanding expectations may return to asymptomatic daily activities with a rehabilitation program and brace support for noncompetitive sports.

111. Autograft is tissue transferred from one part of a patient's body to another. Allograft is tissue transferred from the same species. A common graft used for reconstruction of the ACL is the patellar tendon.

112. Vascularization occurs from the sixth to twelfth week; the graft may be at its weakest point during this time.

113. Closed kinetic chain exercises occur with the distal segment fixed so that movement at one joint results in simultaneous movement of all other joints in the kinetic chain (such as a squat). Advantages include: (1) compressive forces of the body on the knee decrease anterior translation of the tibia on the femur; (2) closed chain activity of the lower extremity causes a co-contraction of the hamstring and quadriceps muscles, with the hamstring contraction acting to decrease anterior translation; and (3) the movement is more functional than open chain activity.

114. Valgus stress to the right knee in 30° of knee flexion. The examiner applies a valgus stress (pushes the knee medially) at the knee while the ankle is stabilized.

115. A cast brace with early protected ROM exercises.

116. Although the length of rehabilitation will vary depending on surgical technique and philosophy of treatment, in general the procedures rank as follows: (1) ACL reconstruction—6 to 9 months; (2) second-degree medial collateral ligament sprain (nonsurgical)—3 to 6 weeks; and (3) meniscectomy—2 to 3 weeks.

117. Immediate closed reduction and splinting in slight flexion is the treatment of choice. A thorough neurovascular examination is mandatory. Anterior dislocations can cause a traction injury to the popliteal artery, resulting in an acute intimal tear or intraluminal thrombus. Arteriography should be performed in all patients. Ligamentous repair or reconstruction or both is recommended to allow early ROM to avoid knee stiffness.

118. It is a classification of fractures involving the epiphyseal plate that are classified as type I through type V, depending on severity and fracture morphology.

119. What is the treatment of choice for this closed tibial/fibular fracture shown in Figure 6-7, A and B, without other injuries?

**Figure** 6-7

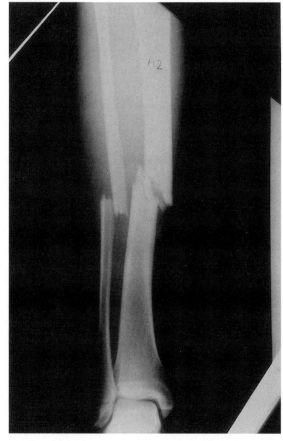
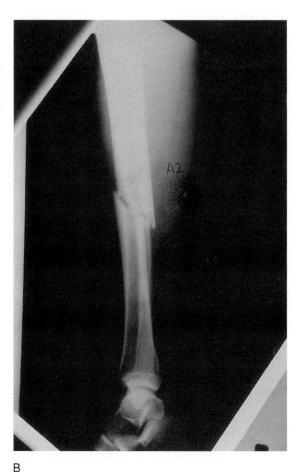

A

B

120. With early weight bearing, can this fracture be expected to shorten?

121. Describe the possible factors that can result in a fracture becoming a nonunion.

122. Describe the contents of the compartments of the lower leg (shank).

123. What is the most reliable sign or symptom of a compartment syndrome?

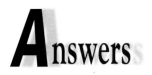

# Answers

119. Closed reduction and application of a long leg cast is the treatment of choice.

120. No, tibial shaft fractures do not usually shorten more than the amount measured on the initial radiographic film.

121. The factors that can result in a fracture becoming a nonunion are excessive motion, fracture gap, infection, and failure of revascularization secondary to loss of blood supply.

122. The **anterior compartment** consists of the extensor digitorum longus, extensor hallucis longus, peroneus tertius, and tibialis anterior muscles; the tibial artery; and the deep peroneal nerve. The **lateral compartment** encloses the peroneus longus and brevis muscles and the superficial peroneal nerve. The **superficial posterior compartment** consists of the gastrocnemius and soleus muscles. The **deep posterior compartment** encompasses the tibialis posterior, flexor hallucis longus, and flexor digitorum longus muscles; the tibial nerve; the posterior tibial artery; and the peroneal artery.

123. The most reliable symptom is pain out of proportion to the injury.

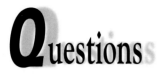

**124.** What is the labeled structure in this anteroposterior radiographic film of an infected tibial nonunion shown in Figure 6-8?

Figure 6-8

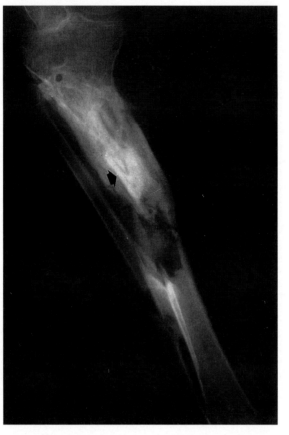

**125.** What are the treatment principles in the surgical management of osteomyelitis?

**126.** Which is the most common type of hip dislocation?

**127.** Describe the mechanism of injury in posterior hip dislocation.

**128.** What is the usual position of the extremity with a posterior hip dislocation?

**129.** Define "hip pointer."

**130.** Evaluation of a 21-year-old man with "hip pain" indicates the following: passive ROM is full and pain-free; he has pain with both resisted hip extension and external rotation; and no other resisted motions cause pain. The problem is most likely with which tissue?

**131.** What is a slipped capital femoral epiphysis?

**132.** Name a test used to evaluate for tightness of the iliotibial band.

**133.** In the athlete who runs frequently and has iliotibial band friction syndrome, where is the common area of pain with palpation?

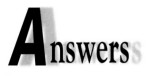

# Answers

124. The labeled structure is a sequestrum. A sequestrum is the hallmark of osteomyelitis; it is necrotic bone and is recognized radiographically as an area of sclerosis surrounded by new bone formation (involucrum).

125. Successful treatment of osteomyelitis depends on adherence to several basic principles: the complete debridement of necrotic and infected tissue, the maintenance or creation of osseous stability, the elimination of dead space, and the provision of durable soft-tissue coverage.

126. Posterior hip dislocations, classified by Epstein on the basis of associated femoral head or acetabular fractures, account for up to 90% of all hip dislocations. Type I is a posterior dislocation with or without an associated minor acetabular rim fracture. Type II has a large posterior acetabular rim fragment. Type III has comminution of the posterior acetabular rim with or without a major fragment. Type IV is a posterior dislocation with a fracture of the acetabular rim and floor. Type V is associated with fractures of the femoral head.

127. Posterior hip dislocations are the result of a force applied to the flexed knee along the axis of the femur.

128. Flexed, adducted, and internally rotated is the usual position.

129. A contusion to the iliac crest.

130. The gluteus maximus muscle. Given that resisted movement caused pain and passive movement was pain-free, most likely the tissue involved is muscle. Given that the action of the gluteus maximus muscle is both hip extension and hip external rotation, the most likely muscle to be involved is the gluteus maximus. If the hamstring muscle were involved, pain with resisted knee flexion would be expected and pain with resisted hip external rotation would not be expected.

131. The head of the femur slips at the epiphyseal plate to become displaced downward and backward on the neck of the femur. This may cause pain in groin or knee. It occurs in children (boys more than girls) 12 to 16 years old, who are often obese. Treatment includes immediate reduction and surgical pinning for acute slips.

132. Ober's test. The patient is side-lying while the examiner passively abducts and extends the patient's upper leg. The examiner slowly lowers the upper leg, but if tightness is present, the leg will remain abducted and not reach the table. If no tightness exists, the leg will passively adduct to the table.

133. The lateral femoral epicondyle. At about 20° knee flexion, the iliotibial band passes over the lateral femoral epicondyle. In a runner with a tight iliotibial band, the repetitive "rubbing" over the epicondyle will cause friction and pain. Treatment includes stretching of the tight iliotibial band.

# Chapter 7

# Foot and Ankle

MICHAEL SHEREFF, MD

TIMOTHY S. LOTH, MD

JAMES SFERRA, MD

GRANT DONA, MD

DEB NAWOCZENSKI, PhD, PT

1. Identify the labeled structures on the lateral view of the ankle and foot in Figure 7-1.

**Figure** 7-1

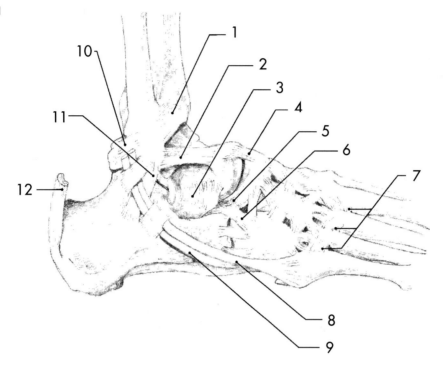

2. The hindfoot comprises what bones?

3. The midfoot comprises what bones?

4. The forefoot comprises what bones?

5. What is the midtarsal joint?

6. Define the clinical condition of hindfoot varus, according to the Orthopedic Foot and Ankle Society guidelines.

7. Define subtalar joint "neutral" and describe the relevance of this measurement.

8. Describe how the position of the subtalar joint (STJ) influences the midtarsal joint (MTJ) during terminal stance of gait and the effect on foot function.

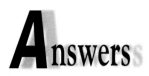

1. (1) Anterior tibiofibular ligament; (2) anterior talofibular ligament; (3) cervical ligament (interosseous talocalcaneal); (4) dorsal talonavicular ligament; (5) calcaneonavicular ligament; (6) dorsal calcaneocuboid ligament; (7) dorsal intermetatarsal ligament; (8) peroneus brevis tendon; (9) peroneus longus tendon; (10) posterior talofibular ligament; (11) calcaneofibular ligament; and (12) tendo Achilles.

2. Calcaneus and talus (see Figure 7-2).

3. Navicular, cuboid, and three cuneiforms (see Figure 7-2).

4. Metatarsals and phalanges (see Figure 7-2).

**Figure** 7-2

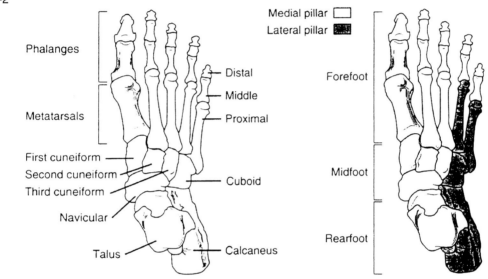

5. The midtarsal (Chopart's, transverse) joint includes the talonavicular and calcaneocuboid articulations. Although the two joints have separate cavities, they move in unison. The midtarsal joint has two independent axes of motion, each of which is oblique to cardinal planes, thus producing triplanar motion.

6. Hindfoot varus can be defined as the frontal (coronal) plane angulation of the central heel line with respect to the midline of the lower leg. (The central heel line is the proximally to distally directed line that bisects the posterior aspect of the calcaneus).

7. Subtalar joint "neutral" is the position of congruency of the talocalcaneal and navicular articulations. It has also been described as the position in which the subtalar joint is neither pronated nor supinated, i.e., a neutral position. This measurement is frequently used as the basis for describing foot alignment and relationships of the hindfoot to the leg and the forefoot to the rearfoot.

8. During terminal stance, the STJ axis and MTJ axis "diverge," locking the transtarsal joint and creating a more rigid foot. This is critical during this phase of gait in order for the foot to become stable in preparation for push off. This STJ/MTJ interaction is in contrast to the events of early stance (initial contact/loading response) when the foot is required to function as a mobile adapter, accommodate changes in terrain, and absorb shock.

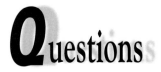

9. What are the four muscular layers of the plantar foot (from superficial to deep)?

10. What is the motor innervation of A in Figure 7-3?

**Figure** 7-3

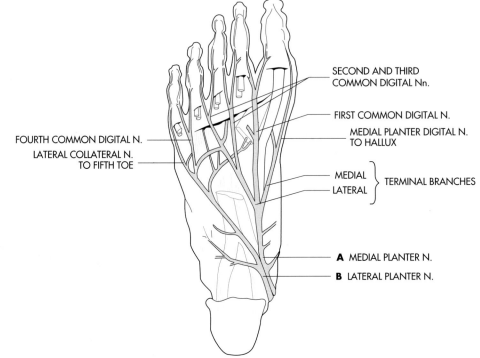

SECOND AND THIRD
COMMON DIGITAL Nn.

FIRST COMMON DIGITAL N.

MEDIAL PLANTER DIGITAL N.
TO HALLUX

FOURTH COMMON DIGITAL N.

LATERAL COLLATERAL N.
TO FIFTH TOE

MEDIAL ⎫
LATERAL ⎭ TERMINAL BRANCHES

**A** MEDIAL PLANTER N.

**B** LATERAL PLANTER N.

11. What is the motor innervation of B in Figure 7-3?

12. Identify the structures on the cross section through the forefoot at the base of the metatarsals in Figure 7-4.

**Figure** 7-4

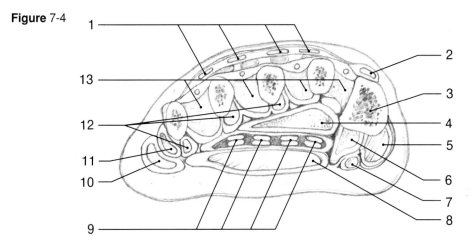

13. How are minimally displaced calcaneal body fractures treated?

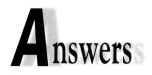

# Answers

9. (1) Abductor digiti minimi, flexor digitorum brevis, abductor hallucis; (2) flexor hallucis longus, flexor digitorum longus, quadratus plantae, lumbricals; (3) flexor digiti minimi, adductor hallucis, flexor hallucis brevis; and (4) interossei, peroneus longus, tibialis posterior.

10. The medial plantar nerve innervates the flexor hallucis brevis (FHB), abductor hallucis, flexor digitorum brevis (FDB), and first lumbrical muscles.

11. The lateral plantar nerve supplies motor innervation to the quadratus plantae, abductor digiti minimi, flexor digiti minimi, adductor hallucis, all plantar and dorsal interossei, and the second through fourth lumbrical muscles.

12. (1) Extensor digitorum longus tendon; (2) extensor hallucis longus tendon; (3) first metatarsal; (4) adductor hallucis muscle; (5) abductor hallucis muscle; (6) flexor hallucis brevis muscle; (7) flexor hallucis longus tendon; (8) flexor digitorum brevis muscle; (9) flexor digitorum longus tendon and lumbrical muscle; (10) abductor digiti minimi muscle; (11) flexor digiti minimi brevis muscle; (12) plantar interosseous muscles; and (13) dorsal interosseous muscles.

13. Elevation and bed rest in a bulky compression dressing for 48 to 72 hours, followed by active range-of-motion (ROM) exercises and touch-down weight-bearing crutch ambulation.

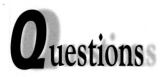

# Questions

14. What other injuries are associated with calcaneal fractures?

15. Which ligament in the ankle prevents ankle inversion in a neutral position?

16. Which ankle ligament prevents excessive inversion in plantar flexion?

17. How are ankle sprains evaluated radiographically?

18. Describe the anterior drawer test of the ankle.

19. Differentiate between grade I, grade II, and grade III ligament sprains.

20. What are initial treatment recommendations for grades I and II ankle sprains?

21. What are appropriate rehabilitation goals following grades I and II ankle sprains?

22. Describe an appropriate *treatment progression* for grades I and II ankle sprains.

23. How are complete tears of the anterior talofibular and calcaneofibular ligaments treated?

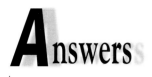

# Answers

14. Thoracolumbar spinal fractures are associated in 10% of calcaneal body fractures. Other injuries of the lower extremity are common. Since bilateral injuries frequently occur, X-ray films of the opposite foot are recommended. Comparison views are useful if no injury is present. Ankle films and thoracolumbar spine films are recommended in all calcaneal fractures.

15. The calcaneofibular ligament.

16. The anterior talofibular ligament.

17. Standard views: AP, lateral, and mortise views. Additional studies: AP view neutral and plantar flexion stress radiographs, lateral anterior drawer, and arthrogram.

18. The ankle is slightly plantar flexed, and the foot is drawn anteriorly from behind the heel by the examiner. With the opposite hand, the examiner holds the tibia fixed and palpates the amount of anterior talar translation in the ankle mortise. This ankle is compared with the opposite ankle. Excessive translation implies injury to the anterior talofibular ligament.

19. Grade I (first degree; mild) sprain is an incomplete tear with no apparent joint instability. A grade II (second degree; moderate) sprain is associated with clinical evidence of joint instability but not complete functional loss. It may describe: (1) a significant, but incomplete tear of the ligament; (2) a complete tear of one structure (e.g., anterior talo-fibular ligament) plus incomplete tears of other structures (calcaneofibular ligament or joint capsule); or (3) partial tears of several structures. A grade III (third degree; severe) sprain disrupts the ligament completely and produces functional instability.

20. For grade I sprains, immediate treatment includes rest (24 to 48 hours), ice, compression, and elevation (RICE). Weight bearing is usually to tolerance for these sprains. The goal of early treatment is edema control through compression. This may be accomplished through use of compression wraps and/or Cryotemp (Jobst® compression pump using cold water). Grade II sprains are also managed using the RICE protocol, but stability is a major concern in these injuries. Weight bearing status, with or without assistive devices, depends on the extent of injury. In addition to edema control, support is a key goal of early treatment for grade II sprains. This may be accomplished through use of taping or ankle orthoses.

21. In addition to the initial goals of edema control and stability, treatment goals include restoration of ROM, strength, and proprioception. In the population of athletes, muscle endurance and power must also be given strong consideration. Ability to function in a work environment and agility are also important goals, particularly for the worker who must return to challenging circumstances.

22. The rehabilitation program should include ROM exercises, heel cord stretching, selective muscle strengthening (e.g., ankle dorsiflexors and evertors), and proprioceptive exercises. Closed kinetic chain activities are an important component of the rehabilitation program and may include use of equipment such as a leg press machine and stair climber. Isokinetic training may assist in meeting the goals of increasing endurance and power. Agility activities should progress from straight plane movement to cariokas, pivoting, and figure-eight skills. Plyometric training may also be helpful in the rehabilitation program. In most circumstances, patients with grade II ankle sprains will progress slower than those who have sustained a grade I injury.

23. This is controversial, but they are often repaired and immobilized in a cast or cast brace for 3 to 4 weeks. Another option is closed treatment in a long leg cast for 6 weeks.

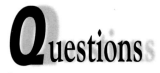

**24.** A 35-year-old man is seen in your office for ankle pain. He reports he "sprained" his ankle 2 months earlier when he tripped going up a flight of stairs. This was treated with a cast for 4 weeks followed by use of a lace-up support. He now notes persistent pain in the lateral ankle area and a painful "popping" sensation when walking. Describe the evaluation and most likely diagnosis.

**25.** A 20-year-old soccer player complains of posteromedial ankle pain, felt most prominently when kicking the ball. Resisted plantar flexion of the great toe is painful. Describe the likely differential diagnosis and further evaluation.

**26.** Describe the treatment of posterior ankle impingement.

**27.** What is the recommended treatment for stress reactions of the foot?

**28.** A 35-year-old runner presents with spontaneous onset of vague pain in the dorsal medial aspect of the foot. The patient noted no injury. Upon physical examination, there is no swelling or discoloration noted. The patient is tender over the navicular. Radiographs of the foot are normal. What is this patient's most likely diagnosis and how should it be confirmed and treated?

**29.** A 22-year-old ROTC cadet returned from his 2-week summer camp with severe bilateral foot pain. Minimal swelling is noted. There is pain over the second and third metatarsals bilaterally. His activity level has been much higher than usual during his training camp, with 20-mile marches and daily 2-mile runs. What tests should be ordered? What is the most likely diagnosis and how should he be treated?

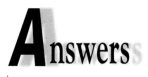

# Answers

24. This history is typical for peroneal tendon subluxation or dislocation. The injury is frequently associated with simultaneous peroneal contractions and ankle dorsiflexion. Upon examination, there is acute tenderness along the posterior margin of the lateral malleolus. The peroneal tendons may at times be palpated over the lateral malleolus or felt to sublux on ankle dorsiflexion. There may be a popping sensation elicited with ankle motion. X-ray films may show a tiny fragment at the lateral malleolus or the calcaneus, avulsed by the peroneal retinaculum. Acute injuries may be managed by immobilization, although some practitioners advocate immediate repair of the retinaculum to the posterior surface of the lateral malleolus. Patients who exhibit persistent pain and recurrent dislocations of the tendons after closed treatment may be managed with operative repair. This repair consists of three main types of surgical intervention: (1) *rerouting procedures* that substitute the calcaneofibular ligament for the incompetent superior peroneal retinaculum; (2) *groove deepening procedures* that either slide bone blocks or decancellation of the posterior surface of the lateral malleolus and recess the cortex in this region; and (3) *soft tissue reconstruction or reinforcements* that may involve direct repair of the retinaculum or may use transplanted or local tissues to reconstruct a new peroneal retinaculum.

25. A number of structures may be impinged between the calcaneus and the posterior tibia. The posterior process may sustain an acute fracture; the os trigonum may become symptomatic (i.e., with or without acute separation at the synchondrosis); or impingement pain may exist secondary to a large posterior process on the talus, to a large or a thickened posterior capsule, or to inflamed adjacent tissues caused by a posterior process on the calcaneus. Patients may complain of posteromedial or posterolateral ankle pain on plantar flexion. Additionally, coexisting flexor hallucis longus (FHL) tendinitis may occur, as evidenced by pain on resisted flexion of the dorsiflexed great toe. The source of impingement may be recognized on a lateral X-ray of the foot. In some cases, a bone scan or computerized tomogram (CT) may be needed to verify the diagnosis.

26. Posterior ankle impingement from whatever cause is generally treated initially nonoperatively by avoidance of full plantar flexion and rest. A short leg cast may be used if an acute fracture is suspected. If nonoperative treatment fails, excision of the offending structures, as well as FHL tenolysis when indicated, may be performed through a posteromedial or posterolateral incision.

27. Stress reactions present with localized pain, swelling, and tenderness secondary to active remodelling of the bone to the newly applied stresses. Radiographs are negative. A bone scan can be positive as early as 2 days after the pain begins. Complete fracture can be avoided by stress protection until symptoms resolve, usually in 1 to 2 weeks.

28. This patient most likely has a stress fracture of the navicular. A bone scan is helpful in identifying this problem as well as tomograms. For nondisplaced fractures, a short leg, non-weight-bearing cast for 6 to 8 weeks is recommended. With displaced fractures, open reduction and internal fixation should be performed.

29. This patient has stress fractures of the metatarsal shafts. They are frequently associated with intensive training, particularly in new military recruits and athletes. Radiographs of the foot—AP, lateral, and oblique—will diagnose stress fractures 10 to 14 days after they have developed. Changes may include a hairline fracture through one cortex, reactive bone or localized periostitis, endosteal thickening, intramedullary sclerosis, and resorption at the fracture line. The patient should be treated based upon the degree of symptomatology. Minimal pain warrants taping and supportive footwear and a decrease in activities. The patient's activities are limited for 4 to 6 weeks until fracture healing is evident on radiograph and clinical examination. A short leg walking cast is used for more symptomatic patients. Serial radiographs will confirm the diagnosis.

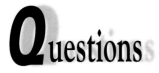

30. What is the keystone of the tarsometatarsal joints?

31. Define forefoot adductus.

32. Describe the deformity present in metatarsus adductus.

33. What are the upper limits of the intermetatarsal and metatarsophalangeal (MTP) angles of the great toe in hallux valgus deformity?

34. What muscle(s) and tendon(s) insert into the first metatarsal head?

35. What accounts for the medial prominence in hallux valgus?

36. What are the clinical manifestations of a mild hallux valgus deformity?

37. What are the clinical and radiographic findings in moderate hallux valgus deformity?

38. Describe the clinical and radiographic appearance of a severe hallux valgus deformity?

39. What three structures are released in the first web space when performing a modified McBride soft tissue release during a hallux valgus procedure?

40. Which toe is most frequently affected by mallet toe deformity?

41. Describe the treatment of mallet toe deformity.

# Answers

30. The second metatarsal base articulation with the second cuneiform. The metatarsal is recessed between the medial and lateral cuneiforms and therefore articulates with all three. It is rare to see tarsometatarsal dislocations without a fracture of the base of the second metatarsal.

31. Forefoot adductus is medial deviation (towards the midline of the body) of the forefoot relative to the midfoot in the transverse plane.

32. Forefoot adduction and slight varus. The lateral border of foot is convex with a dorsal and lateral prominence at the base of the fifth metatarsal and cuboid. Moderate to severe heel valgus is present. No equinus is present. A radiograph shows the first metatarsal to be more sharply angulated than the fifth.

33. An intermetatarsal angle greater than 9° and a MTP angle greater than 15° are considered abnormal.

34. No muscle or tendon inserts into the first metatarsal head.

35. Several factors contribute to this deformity. Displacement of the proximal phalanx in a lateral direction uncovers the medial aspect of the metatarsal head, which makes it appear more prominent. In addition, there is hypertrophy of the soft tissues overlying the medial metatarsal head and the bone here may hypertrophy up to 3 to 5 mm. The medial deviation of the first metatarsal also contributes.

36. There is minimal metatarsus primus varus, the MTP joint is congruent, and there is very little valgus deformity (MTP angle less than 20°). There is, however, a painful, medial prominence of the metatarsal head. The sesamoids are in anatomic position on radiographs.

37. Radiographs demonstrate an MTP angle of 20° to 40° with loss of congruence of the MTP joint. There is nearly complete displacement of the lateral sesamoid from beneath the metatarsal head. The hallux is pronated.

38. Radiographs demonstrate total dislocation of the lateral sesamoid into the intermetatarsal space. The MTP angle is greater than 40°, and there is significant incongruence of the MTP joint. There is marked lateral deviation of the great toe with associated pronation of the hallux. Significant metatarsus primus varus may also be present.

39. (1) The adductor tendon is detached from its insertion into the base of the proximal phalanx and the lateral aspect of the fibular sesamoid. (2) The lateral first MTP joint capsule is perforated and torn. (3) The transverse metatarsal ligament is released with caution as the nerve and blood vessels lie immediately plantar to this structure.

40. Mallet toe is a flexion deformity at the distal interphalangeal joint. It occurs most frequently in the second toe, which is usually the longest of the foot. The cause is pressure against the end of the shoe.

41. For flexible deformities, release of the flexor digitorum longus (FDL) tendon is recommended. For a flexion contracture, however, FDL release as well as a middle phalanx head resection are required.

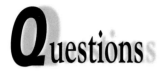

**42.** Identify the labeled structures on the dorsum of the foot and ankle in Figure 7-5.

**Figure** 7-5

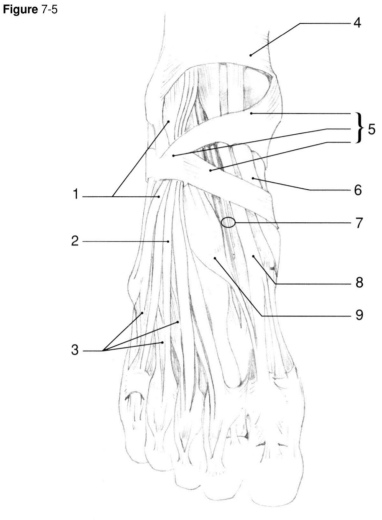

**43.** What function(s) do the interossei and lumbrical muscles perform?

**44.** What is the most common etiology of hammer toe deformity?

**45.** What is a claw toe deformity and how does it differ from a hammer toe?

**46.** A young woman complains of painful corns on the dorsum of her second and third toe PIP joints along with a burning sensation in her forefoot. When standing, hammer toes are present, but when she sits and dangles her feet, no deformity is present. What is the initial treatment for this condition?

**47.** If conservative measures fail, what surgical options are available?

**48.** A 45-year-old obese woman with claw deformity of the toes has metatarsalgia. There are no other significant foot problems noted upon examination. Her neuromuscular exam is likewise normal. Clawing of the toes resolves with ankle plantar flexion. With ankle dorsiflexion, the clawing returns. What are the options for conservative care?

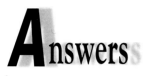

**42.** (1) Peroneus tertius tendon; (2) extensor digitorum longus tendon; (3) extensor digitorum brevis muscle; (4) superior extensor retinaculum; (5) inferior extensor retinaculum (superomedial band); (6) tibialis anterior tendon; (7) neurovascular bundle (dorsalis pedis artery and vein and deep peroneal nerve); (8) extensor hallucis longus tendon; and (9) extensor hallucis brevis muscle.

**43.** The four dorsal interossei are the abductors of the toes, whereas the three plantar interossei are the adductors. They all pass dorsal to the deep transverse intermetatarsal ligament, whereas the lumbricals remain plantar to this ligament. Nevertheless, the interossei and lumbricals pass plantar to the axis of motion at the MTP joint and dorsal to the axis of motion at the proximal interphalangeal (PIP) joint. Thus the interossei and lumbricals plantar flex the MTP joints and cause weak extension at the PIP and distal interphalangeal (DIP) joints.

**44.** Hammer toe deformity can be caused by neuromuscular diseases such as Friedreich ataxia, Charcot-Marie-Tooth disease, cerebral palsy, multiple sclerosis, compartment syndrome of the deep posterior compartment, myelodysplasia, disc disease, diabetes, and leprosy. It is most frequently seen in patients with ill-fitting shoes.

**45.** A claw toe deformity consists of flexion of the interphalangeal joints with hyperextension at the MTP joints. Hammer toe, in contrast, has no involvement of the MTP joints. Causes of claw toe are similar to those of hammer toe.

**46.** The patient has a flexible or dynamic hammer toe deformity. Conservative treatment consists of wearing roomy, well-fitted shoes with increased width and height in the toe box. This treatment helps avoid direct pressure against a hammer toe, the development of plantar callosities, and resulting metatarsalgia. A metatarsal pad with or without a custom insole or local cushioning over the dorsal callosity can also be added.

**47.** This deformity seems to be caused by contracture of the FDL tendon, but mere release of this tendon is not usually sufficient for lasting correction. FDL to extensor digitorum longus (EDL) transfer realigns the toes and enables the FDL to plantar flex the MTP joint and dorsiflex the PIP and DIP joints via the extensor hood. Others prefer to perform a PIP joint arthroplasty in either fixed or flexible hammer toe deformities.

**48.** Conservative care may include use of cushioned insoles inside her shoes, with or without a metatarsal pad. Accommodative footwear with a metatarsal bar or rocker outersole design should also be considered in recalcitrant cases. Asking the patient to walk slower will lessen the loading on the metatarsal heads. A weight-reduction program should also be recommended. A stretching program that focuses on the extrinsic muscles, especially the FDL, may improve this nonfixed deformity.

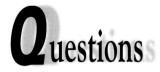

**Questions**

49. What are the surgical options for this patient?

50. What is hallux rigidus and how does it present clinically?

51. A 16-year-old boy has had problems with great toe pain, particularly when running. Upon physical examination, there is swelling about the MTP joint without any angular deformity. Plantar flexion is satisfactory, but he has no dorsiflexion of the toe. Radiographs demonstrate an osteochondritic defect in the metatarsal head. What is this patient's problem and how should it be treated?

52. What is the conservative management for adult hallux rigidus?

53. Describe the detailed anatomic pathology of a grade III "turf toe" sprain in a 22-year-old football player.

54. Where are corns and calluses usually located on the foot?

55. What are calluses?

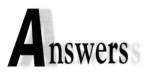

# Answers

49. Surgical options include extensor tenotomies and MTP joint capsulotomies associated with transfer of the FDL to the extensor mechanism, similar to flexible hammer toe correction.

50. Degenerative joint disease of the MTP joint of the great toe. It is usually associated with bony proliferation in the dorsal aspect of the joint. The plantar aspect is usually spared. Patients with hallux rigidus typically have pain in the first MTP joint associated with limitation of dorsiflexion. Also, plantar flexion can cause pain as a result of traction of the extensor hallucis longus (EHL) tendon over the dorsal osteophyte on the metatarsal head. Patients tend to shift their weight away from the hallux and toe off on the lateral metatarsal heads.

51. This patient has a congenital or juvenile hallux rigidus. Conservative care includes rest and immobilization. In the adolescent patient, wedge resection of the dorsal aspect of the proximal phalanx has been shown to be helpful in restoring motion and relieving pain. Excision of the osteochondritic defect may also be considered.

52. Accommodative footwear consisting of a hard-soled or rocker-bottom shoe with an adequate toe box to avoid pressure on the MTP joint of the great toe. Semirigid or rigid orthotic inserts that incorporate a "relief" or cut-out under the first metatarsal head may improve function in this deformity. Nonsteroidal antiinflammatory drugs (NSAIDs), intraarticular steroid injections, and occasionally a short leg walking cast for 1 month may be beneficial.

53. Grade I sprains involve stretching of the capsulo-ligamentous complex about the first MTP. Grade II sprains have a partial tear of this complex. Grade III sprains involve tearing of the plantar plate from its origin on the metatarsal head-neck junction and impaction of the proximal phalanx into the metatarsal head dorsally. There may be a sesamoid fracture or separation of a bipartite sesamoid in this grade.

54. These are usually located over periarticular areas, specifically near condylar prominences. They are rarely seen over the shafts of long bones. They are the result of pressure from the shoe and underlying bone acting upon the skin.

55. These are essentially the same as corns, the only difference being that they occur on the plantar aspect of the foot. Symptomatic plantar calluses are known as intractable plantar keratosis.

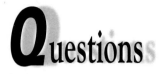

# Questions

56. What should you evaluate when looking at the potential causes of plantar keratoses?

57. Describe the conservative treatment of plantar keratoses.

58. What is the most common cause of intractable plantar keratosis of the great toe MTP joint?

59. What is a "tailor's" bunion?

60. What are the causes of "tailor's" bunions?

61. Describe the treatment of "tailor's" bunions.

62. Where are foot interdigital neuromas most frequently seen?

63. Describe the demographic characteristics of the population with interdigital neuromas.

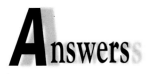
**56.** Hindfoot and forefoot varus or valgus angulation may produce excessive weight bearing on the forefoot, which leads to keratoses. (Figure 7-6, A demonstrates a forefoot varus deformity.)Bony problems such as a plantar-flexed metatarsal (see Figure 7-6, B), enlarged sesamoid, or a particularly long metatarsal may lead to plantar keratoses. Finally, ill-fitting footwear such as high-heeled pointed shoes can produce excessive pressure.

**Figure** 7-6

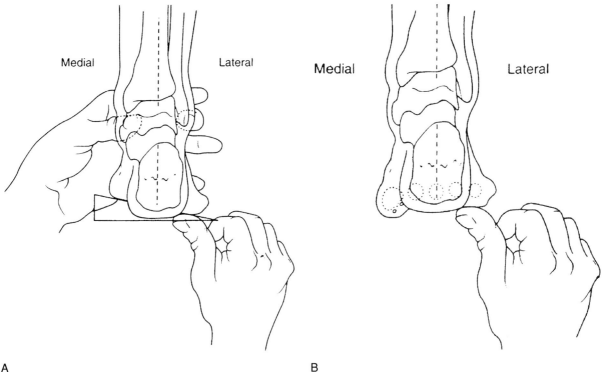

A

B

**57.** Low-heeled accommodative footwear with metatarsal support.

**58.** A localized keratosis most frequently occurs plantar to the medial sesamoid. This can be due to either medial sesamoid enlargement or displacement to a more central position overlying the metatarsal head, thereby producing excessive localized pressure.

**59.** A "tailor's" bunion, also known as a bunionette, develops at the small toe MTP joint. It is similar to classic hallux valgus, except that the bump is on the lateral aspect of the foot, and the phalanges angulate toward the great toe.

**60.** Soft tissue hypertrophy over the lateral aspect of the metatarsal head, congenital enlargement of the metatarsal head, or lateral angulation of the fifth toe metatarsal, singly or in combination.

**61.** Conservative care is appropriate for mild and moderate cases and consists of accommodative footwear. Surgical treatment in severe cases depends upon the cause. If a wide metatarsal head is implicated, then the lateral condyle is excised. If the cause is a laterally deviated plantar-flexed metatarsal, then a fifth toe metatarsal osteotomy should be performed.

**62.** In the third or second intermetatarsal space. Neuromas of the first and fourth spaces are rare.

**63.** These are seen more frequently in women than in men, with a female to male ratio 4:1 to 10:1. Average age of patients is the mid-fifties. Most lesions are unilateral.

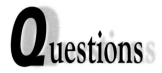
# Questions

**64.** What are the characteristic signs and symptoms of interdigital neuroma?

**65.** What is the differential diagnosis for a suspected interdigital neuroma in a 50-year-old woman?

**66.** Describe conservative treatment for interdigital neuroma of the foot.

**67.** Failing conservative care, what surgery is performed for interdigital neuroma?

**68.** A 35-year-old woman falls after stepping into a hole. She complains of ankle pain with swelling medially and laterally. X-ray films of the ankle reveal a transverse fracture of the medial malleolus. What additional radiographic films, if any, should be obtained and why?

**69.** A 26-year-old woman presents with localized pain and tenderness over the Achilles tendon, just proximal to its insertion into the calcaneus. She reports the onset of symptoms occurred following a recent change in her running workout that now includes "hill" training. What factors may be contributing to this acute inflammatory process of the Achilles tendon?

**70.** What is the treatment approach for a patient who may be in the acute inflammatory stage of Achilles tendinitis?

**71.** While playing racquetball, a 40-year-old man experiences a sharp pain in his posterior ankle area, accompanied by a loud pop. Upon examination, he is able to actively plantar flex, although weakly. The foot does not plantar flex when the calf is squeezed. What is the diagnosis?

**72.** Describe the presentation of posterior tibial tendon insufficiency.

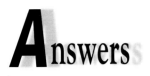

**64.** The primary symptom is pain in the plantar aspect of the foot between the metatarsal heads that is aggravated by activity and relieved by rest. Physical findings consist of plantar tenderness between the metatarsal heads to palpation. Sometimes you can palpate the neuroma. There should be an absence of MTP joint pain with manipulation.

**65.** In all cases of suspected interdigital neuroma, you should consider the possibility of tarsal tunnel syndrome, deficient plantar fat pad, MTP synovitis, subluxation or dislocation, plantar callosity, and lumbar disc disease.

**66.** Sensible footwear: low heels, wide toe box, a comfortable soft-soled shoe. Sometimes a metatarsal pad proximal to the involved site will distribute the weight over a wider area and relieve symptoms.

**67.** Excision of the neuroma.

**68.** A radiographic film of the entire leg should be performed to rule out a proximal fibula fracture, frequently accompanied by a rupture of the syndesmosis interosseous membrane up to the level of the fracture (the Maisonneuve fracture).

**69.** The change in the patient's running program may be directly linked to the onset of symptoms of Achilles tendinitis. "Hill" climbing is associated with increased ankle dorsiflexion that creates greater tensile loading of the gastrocsoleus muscles. Symptoms may be exacerbated by running on roads or sidewalks with a camber. This places one foot in excessive pronation and the opposite foot in (relative) supination. Inappropriate or worn footwear may also create symptoms. Inadequate stabilization from the heel counter of the shoe may allow the foot to pronate excessively, thereby increasing the torque to the tendon. Finally, structural malalignment of the foot resulting in excessive pronation may contribute to Achilles tendon problems.

**70.** The treatment approach should start with a combination of ice massage, active dorsiflexion using low-resistance theraband elastic tubing, gentle stretching of the calf, and eccentric calf exercises. Ultrasound or phonophoresis may be beneficial in pain relief and reduction in local irritation. Temporary heel lifts may be added to shoes to decrease stress on the tendon. The height of the lift should be reduced as pain-free ROM improves. Footwear should be examined and changed if necessary. A biomechanical foot exam should also be performed to rule out structural malalignments that may cause excessive pronation. In some cases, orthotics may be appropriate to control the excessive pronation. For the patient in question 69, the running program should be altered to minimize overuse of the tendon. This would include elimination of "hill" training for this patient.

**71.** The most likely diagnosis is a complete rupture of the Achilles tendon. Although squeezing the calf does not produce plantar flexion (Thompson test), the patient is able to plantar flex by using his tibialis posterior, toe flexors, and possibly the peroneal muscles. This is a common injury in middle-aged athletes.

**72.** Upon first presentation, symptoms may be limited to pain posterior to the medial malleolus or along the course of the posterior tibial tendon. As insufficiency progresses, the heel collapses into valgus, the midfoot becomes pronated with decrease in the height of the longitudinal arch, and the forefoot becomes abducted. From behind, the examiner can visualize more toes on the affected side than are observed on the other limb (i.e., the "too many toes" sign). A single limb heel raise may be painful or impossible.

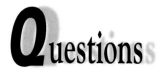

73. What are the gait manifestations of a posterior tibial tendon rupture?

74. A 25-year-old woman complains of frequent ankle sprains and pain beneath the balls of her feet. She recalls that her mother complained of similar symptoms. Examination reveals bilaterally elevated arches, clawing of toes, and mild atrophy of the calves. Describe the most likely diagnosis.

75. A 60-year-old diabetic man complains of spontaneous onset of redness and swelling across his midfoot. He has only mild pain. Describe the likely diagnosis.

76. Describe initial treatment of the condition described in question 75.

77. Differentiate between a dysvascular and a neuropathic foot ulcer.

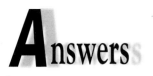

73. The calcaneus will remain everted throughout the midstance and terminal-stance phases of gait (as viewed from the rear). In a "normal" foot, the calcaneus would be vertical to slightly inverted during these phases of terminal stance.

74. Although other conditions may produce a similar scenario, these symptoms likely represent Charcot-Marie-Tooth disease. In this condition, there is a cavus foot with a plantar flexed first ray, contracted plantar fascia, varus hindfoot, and clawing of the toes. The intrinsics and peroneus brevis are commonly the most weakened muscles. The peroneus longus muscle is usually spared until late in the process, accounting for the plantar flexion deformity of the first ray.

75. A diabetic with spontaneous erythema and swelling of the foot may have developed a Charcot foot. The foot may or may not be painful. An important differential diagnosis is infection, and differentiating the two may be difficult. Absence of ulceration, normal white blood cell (WBC) count, no elevation in insulin requirement, or no elevation of serum glucose are helpful indicators. X-ray films may be normal initially, progressing to subluxation and fragmentation of multiple bones. Labeled WBC bone scan may be the only definitive test.

76. Although improved glucose control may occasionally improve neurologic function, Charcot neuropathic changes are generally not reversible. Therapy during the inflammatory stage is primarily directed at prevention of deformity. Total contact casting, orthotic support, or restricted weight-bearing bones are all recommended to reduce development of collapse and deformity.

77. Features of the dysvascular ulcer include: usually painful; irregularly shaped; multifocal; located on toes or other nonplantar areas; lesions tend to be necrotic; and ulcer area is cool and pale.

    Features of the neuropathic ulcer include: lesions are painless, circular in shape, develop over plantar bony areas, associated with callus formation, and tend to be clean. The ulcer area is warm and pink (see Figure 7-7).

**Figure** 7-7

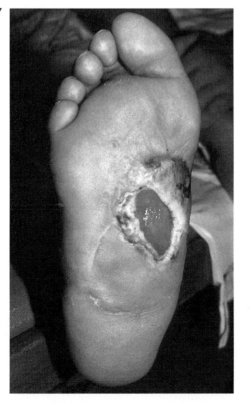

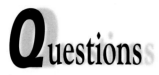

# Questions

78. Identify foot ulcers using the Wagner Classification System.

79. What are viable treatment options for Wagner Grade 1 or 2 neuropathic plantar ulcers?

80. What is the most common deformity following a Chopart-level (midfoot) amputation, and how may this condition be avoided?

81. What is the underlying source of almost all diabetic foot problems?

82. What are the typical complaints of a 50-year-old woman with a 10-year history of insulin-dependent diabetes and a recent onset of neuropathy?

83. At her initial clinic visit, a 40-year-old female diabetic is noted to have lost the ability to feel a 5.07 Semmes-Weinstein monofilament on the plantar aspect of her forefoot. No deformity or ulcers are present, but callus is present beneath her metatarsal heads. How do you approach her problems?

84. Describe the relative benefits and disadvantages of the solid-ankle, cushion-heel (SACH) foot; the single-axis foot; the multiaxis foot; and the flexible-keel, dynamic-response foot prostheses.

# Answers

78. Grade 0—intact skin
    Grade 1—superficial ulcer involving skin only
    Grade 2—deep ulcer involving tendon, bone, ligament, or joint
    Grade 3—deep infection (abscess or osteomyelitis in foot)
    Grade 4—gangrene of forefoot only
    Grade 5—gangrene of majority of foot

79. Total contact cast, posterior-shell walking splint, and prefabricated walking braces with air bladders that will allow graduated pressures are examples of devices used successfully to heal neuropathic plantar ulcers.

80. The most common deformity is equinus deformity. To prevent this, the tibialis anterior tendon should be attached to the talus, and an Achilles tenotomy is commonly performed. This prevents unopposed pull of the Achilles tendon.

81. Neuropathy, especially sensory neuropathy, in combination with pressure over a bony prominence, is the initiating event of almost all ulcerations and most subsequent infections of the feet in diabetic patients. It is a widely held misconception that diabetic ulcers occur primarily because of circulatory impairment; although circulatory impairment coexists and contributes to poor healing, it is not the initiating event.

82. In addition to diminished sensitivity, she describes a burning, searing, tingling, or lancinating dysesthesia, often unrelenting or excruciating in degree. It is often bilateral, symmetric, and worse at night.

83. This condition represents the absence of protective sensation. As a result, she needs to be educated regarding care and daily inspection of her feet. Appropriate footwear should be prescribed with total contact inserts to protect and unweight the high-pressure areas on the plantar surface of her feet.

84. The **SACH foot** is relatively inexpensive, durable, and cosmetic. There is, however, a limited degree of adjustability of resistance to plantar flexion and dorsiflexion. As the heel cushions deteriorate, the prosthesis loses shock absorption.

    The **single-axis foot** provides increased knee stability, but it is bulkier and requires somewhat more maintenance than a SACH foot. It is more commonly used as the prosthetic ankle for an above-knee amputation.

    The **multiaxis foot** provides more motion than any other prosthetic foot. It is useful for patients who must frequently ambulate over uneven terrain. It is, however, heavy and requires more maintenance than a SACH foot or a single-axis foot.

    The **flexible-keel, dynamic-response foot** (Flex-foot, Seattle Foot) allows for not only shock absorption but also some degree of push-off. These prostheses are constructed of extremely lightweight materials. This provides for a more fluid gait and may decrease high activity energy expenditure. The chief disadvantage is their expense. Although these prostheses are best suited for the active, high demand individual with an amputation, they may be equally appropriate for the active geriatric ambulator.

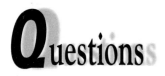

85. Identify structure 1 in Figure 7-8.

86. Identify structure 2 in Figure 7-8.

87. Identify structure 3 in Figure 7-8.

88. Identify structure 4 in Figure 7-8.

89. Identify structure 5 in Figure 7-8.

90. Identify structure 6 in Figure 7-8.

**Figure** 7-8

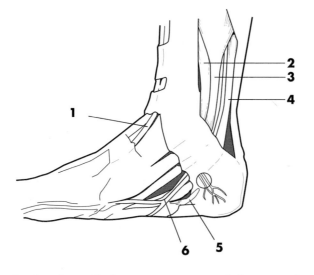

91. Describe the classic findings in a patient with long-standing rheumatoid arthritis of the forefoot.

92. What is the initial management of a rheumatoid patient with metatarsalgia?

93. What is the preferred treatment for monarticular end-stage arthritis of the ankle joint in a 35-year-old laborer?

94. What is the best position for ankle fusion?

95. Describe the gait disturbance associated with an ankle fusion in excessive ankle plantar flexion.

96. What ROM is required at the ankle (talocrural) joint for normal gait?

97. What muscle or muscle groups are primarily responsible for control of the foot between the initial contact and loading response of gait?

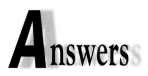
**85.** Tibialis anterior tendon, passing beneath the inferior extensor retinaculum to insert on the base of the first metatarsal and the first cuneiform.

**86.** Tibialis posterior tendon, the most anterior of the tendons in the tarsal tunnel, passing behind the medial malleolus, through the tarsal tunnel, and above the sustentaculum tali to insert on the navicular. It also inserts on the first, second, and third cuneiform; on the cuboid; and, at times, on the base of the fifth metatarsal.

**87.** Flexor digitorum longus, posterior to the tibialis posterior tendon, crossing superficial to the FHL, giving rise to the lumbricals before attaching to the phalanges (2 to 5).

**88.** FHL, the most posterior and lateral of the three tendons, passing inferior to the sustentaculum tali.

**89.** Abductor hallucis, passing superficial to medial and lateral plantar nerves. (The fascia surrounding this muscle can act as a site of impingement to these nerves.)

**90.** Posterior tibial artery and nerve, superficial to the FHL, dividing into medial and lateral plantar branches.

**91.** There is hallux valgus with obvious intraarticular involvement of the MTP joints. The lesser toes drift laterally with dorsal subluxation or dislocation. The metatarsal heads are directed more plantarward, the toes show a hammer toe or claw toe deformity, and the protective plantar fat pad is drawn distally, further exposing the metatarsal heads.

**92.** Metatarsal arch supports and soft-soled or rocker-bottom shoes. If hammer toes are present, then an extradepth shoe with Plastizote lining may be necessary (see Figure 7-9: example of a rocker-bottom shoe with angled [a] or curved [b] design).

**Figure** 7-9

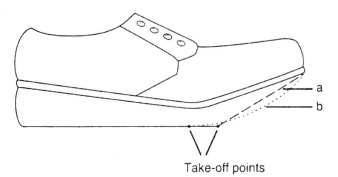

Take-off points

**93.** Tibiotalar arthrodesis.

**94.** Neutral flexion (slight plantar flexion in a woman who wishes to wear heels) in 0° to 5° of valgus and 5° to 10° of external rotation.

**95.** Excessive plantar flexion may cause genu recurvatum at heel strike. Additionally, the extremity may rotate externally in an attempt to avoid passing directly over the plantar flexed foot, leading to laxity of the medial collateral ligament (MCL).

**96.** Range of ankle motion required for normal gait is 10° of dorsiflexion to 20° plantarflexion.

**97.** The pretibial muscles; weakness of this muscle group will cause the patient to have a forefoot initial contact and excessive plantarflexion during loading response. Toe drag may also occur during initial and midswing phases of gait.

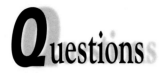

**98.** What is an appropriate orthotic recommendation for a patient whose primary problem is weakness in the pretibial muscles (tibialis anterior, EHL, and EDL) that causes alterations in gait, i.e., foot slap and/or steppage gait, and may potentially affect the patient's endurance and safety?

**99.** What muscles are primarily responsible for control of the tibia during midstance of gait?

**100.** How would you differentiate between structural (bony) and soft tissue restrictions of the ankle joint during a clinical examination?

**101.** A 26-year-old man complains of burning pain at the medial calcaneal tubercle, morning stiffness in the foot when getting out of bed, and pain as he walks on his toes. The patient also presents with an excessively pronated foot. What is the most likely diagnosis?

**102.** What are common radiographic findings with plantar fasciitis?

**103.** What are the treatment goals for plantar fasciitis?

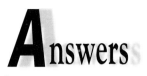

**98.** A lightweight dorsiflexion-assist, polypropylene ankle foot orthosis (AFO) is recommended to assist with foot pick-up, primarily during midswing and terminal swing when ankle dorsiflexion to "neutral" is required for adequate limb clearance. This AFO also assists in maintaining good foot positioning in terminal swing so that a heel-first contact is possible.

**99.** The gastrocsoleus muscle is primarily responsible for controlling the advancement of the tibia over the foot during midstance to terminal stance of gait.

**100.** If there is soft tissue restriction secondary to gastrocnemius tightness, there will be an increase in ankle dorsiflexion when the knee is flexed (compared with the knee extended position). With a bony block, there will be no change in ankle dorsiflexion ROM with a change in knee position.

**101.** Plantar fasciitis is the likely problem. This inflammatory stress syndrome of the plantar fascia is believed to be related to the stress from the forces of impact, combined with weight transfer up onto the toes. This leads to metatarsophalangeal joint extension and a "windlass" effect on the plantar fascia. The plantar fascia is often stressed with excessive foot pronation as the medial longitudinal arch collapses. Injury and stress usually occur at the medial calcaneal tubercle, but may also occur within the midsubstance of the fascia (see Figure 7-10). Plantar fasciitis has also been linked to a pes cavus foot structure .

**Figure** 7-10

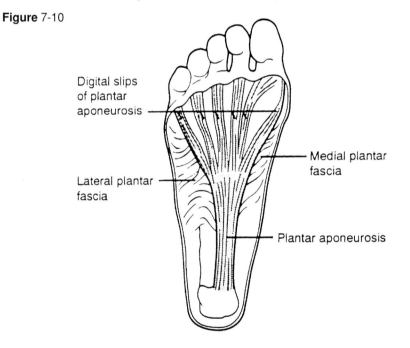

**102.** The periosteal reaction at the origin of the plantar fascia can result in hemorrhage, microtearing, and ultimately a heel spur. In many cases, heel spurs are asymptomatic, but are a sign of stress overload of the plantar fascia. Heel spurs are frequently mistaken as the cause of the problem, rather than the result of abnormal overload to the fascia.

**103.** Treatment is aimed at reducing inflammation, decreasing tension on the plantar fascia, restoring strength and mobility if the problem is related to soft tissue tightness of plantarflexors, and correcting any biomechanical abnormality of the foot.

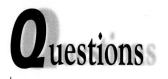
# Questions

**104.** What are the management strategies for plantar fasciitis?

**104.** Inflammation can be controlled with ice and antiinflammatory medication. Physical therapy treatment for acute symptoms of pain and tenderness includes ultrasound/phonophoresis with corticosteroid cream with the fascia held on stretch. Gastrocsoleus muscle stretching is needed to increase dorsiflexion and prevent the foot from excessively pronating in order to compensate for the lack of ankle dorsiflexion. Low Dye modified arch taping may help to hold the foot in a neutral position. In some cases, heel lifts and heel cups provide relief (see Figure 7-11). Low frequency muscle stimulation, massage of the plantar fascia, intrinsic foot muscle exercises and assessment for proper footwear are all important in management of plantar fasciitis. In cases of persistent morning stiffness, use of a night splint to maintain dorsiflexion and stretch of the plantar fascia have been shown to have good results.

**Figure** 7-11

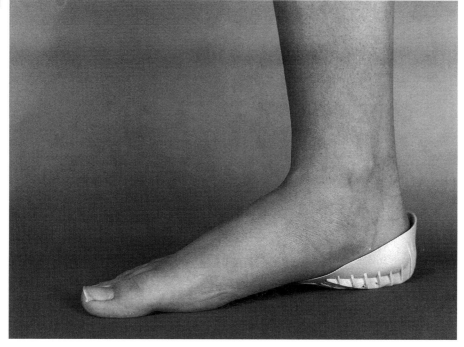

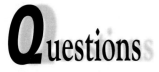

**105.** A biomechanical foot examination is a critical component in the evaluation and treatment of a patient with plantar fasciitis. In the previous patient example, the biomechanical foot exam revealed a (nonrigid) forefoot varus deformity during the non-weight-bearing examination. The patient compensates during weight bearing by excessively pronating. If orthotics are indicated, what would be appropriate recommendations for this patient?

**106.** What would be appropriate footwear recommendations for this patient?

**107.** What is the most commonly seen ankle and foot deformity after cerebral vascular accident (CVA)?

**108.** A 30-year-old man sustains a crush injury to his foot. Fractures of the second and third metatarsal necks are treated by a short leg cast for 6 weeks. When seen 3 months after injury, he complains of persistent burning pain in the foot, and he is unable to bear weight. Radiographic films reveal healing of the fractures but marked osteoporosis of the entire foot. Describe the likely diagnosis, work-up, and treatment.

**109.** Identify the components of the shoe in Figure 7-13.

**Figure** 7-13

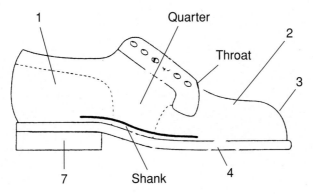

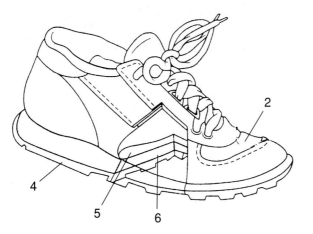

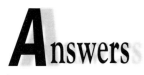

# Answers

**105.** The goal of orthotic intervention is to prevent excessive pronation. Because of this patient's forefoot varus, the orthotics should be "posted" medially at the forefoot location. Depending on the severity of the forefoot varus, rearfoot posting in combination with forefoot posting may be necessary. The activity level of the patient as well as his weight would determine if a soft, semirigid, or rigid orthotic is indicated. If the activity level is fairly light (walking, swimming, sitting throughout the day), and the patient is not heavy, soft or semirigid orthotics are appropriate choices. If greater control of pronation is required, the activity level is more aggressive (running, jumping), or if the patient is heavy, then semirigid or rigid orthotics may be a better choice (see Figure 7-12).

**Figure** 7-12

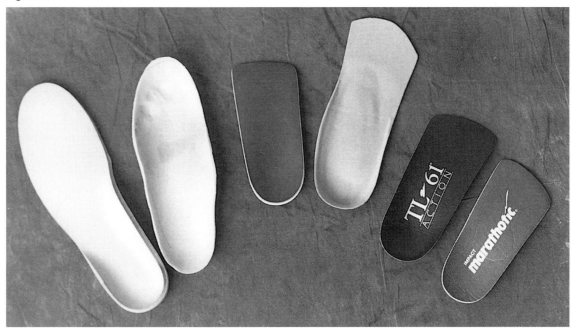

**106.** Shoes should have a shock-absorbing outersole, a firm heel counter, a removable insole (for interchanging with orthotics inside the shoe), and whenever possible, a reinforced midsole on the medial side of the shoe. Many of the athletic shoes on the market today offer features that control excessive pronation and supination and frequently provide the solution to many foot problems.

**107.** An equinovarus deformity, usually with curling of the toes, is the most common deformity that occurs following a CVA.

**108.** Reflex sympathetic dystrophy (RSD) is a poorly understood spectrum of symptoms. Hyperesthesias and pain out of proportion to the injury, particularly if it is diffuse and nonanatomic, is typical but not specific for this syndrome. Vasomotor instability may be evident as discoloration, warmth or coolness in comparison with the opposite side, and edema. Diffuse, patchy osteoporosis may provide radiographic film evidence of RSD. Bone scan may show diffusely increased uptake, particularly in juxtaarticular areas. Other diagnoses, such as infection, tumor, or unrecognized fracture, should be ruled out. Treatment is controversial, but generally it involves some form of sympathetic blockade, as well as physical therapy emphasizing desensitization, motion, and return of function.

**109.** (1) Heel counter; (2) upper; (3) toe box; (4) outersole; (5) insole; (6) midsole; and (7) heel.

Chapter 8

# **O**rthopedic **M**anual **T**herapy

CAROLYN T. WADSWORTH, MS, PT, OCS, CHT

GARVICE NICHOLSON, MS, PT, OCS

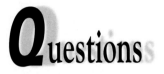

# Questions

1. What is orthopedic manual therapy, and what is its role in orthopedic physical therapy?

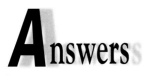

# Answers

1. The broad field of orthopedics encompasses the prevention, diagnosis, and treatment of disorders and injuries of the musculoskeletal system by medical, surgical, and physical means. Within this traditional specialty, a system of patient evaluation and treatment through skillful manual contact has evolved. Known as orthopedic manual therapy (OMT), this method is one component of the nonsurgical management of musculoskeletal dysfunction. It includes a variety of techniques directed toward eliminating pain and improving function. Orthopedic manual therapy incorporates the direct application of physical force at a specific speed and amplitude to selectively stress connective tissues.

   Orthopedic manual therapists apply precise palpatory techniques and passive joint movement in the evaluative process of observation, testing, and interpretation of clinical findings. By physically identifying changes in the status, alignment, and movement of joints and soft tissues, a manual therapist can plan an appropriate treatment strategy. Therapeutic intervention utilizes passive techniques, in addition to exercise and patient education, to restore synovial joint movement.

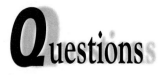
# Questions

2. What are the goals of orthopedic manual therapy?

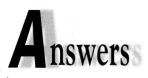nswers

2. The goals of manual therapy should relate to those mutually agreed upon by the patient and therapist. In general they include relieving pain, increasing or decreasing mobility, and maximizing function. Many patients seek treatment because they are in pain. Manual therapy can quickly reduce or alleviate musculoskeletal pain of a mechanical nature. However, the effects will probably be short-lived if other elements of the patient's movement dysfunction are not addressed, e.g., faulty posture or body mechanics, poor conditioning, etc. Patient education and participation in an exercise program are usually essential to achieving the overall goal of enhancing functional mobility. Manual therapy techniques can eliminate compensatory patterns of movement by facilitating specific functions. For example, improving restricted motion at the glenohumeral joint eliminates the need to substitute with excessive scapulothoracic motion during abduction. Figure 8-1 reveals a patient with right glenohumeral joint hypomobility, secondary to adhesive capsulitis, compensating with excessive scapulothoracic motion. By restoring joint play, tissue extensibility, and mechanical balance, manual therapy produces full, pain-free joint function.

**Figure** 8-1

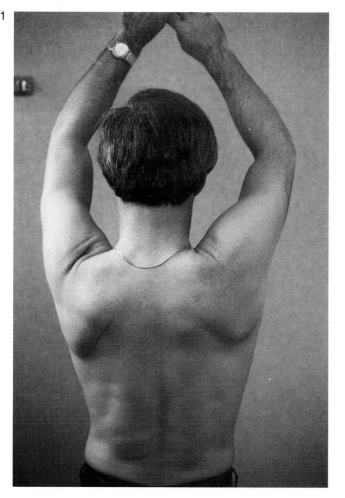

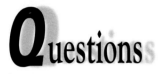
# Questions

3. Classify the synarthrodial and diathrodial joints, and describe the features of the fibrous, cartilaginous, and synovial joint categories.

4. What is synovial fluid, and why is it a good lubricant?

5. How do collagen and articular cartilage respond to immobilization?

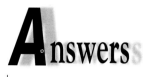

# Answers

3. The two major categories of joints are the synarthrodial, with limited or no movement, and the diarthrodial (synovial), with greater movement. The synarthrodial category includes fibrous and cartilaginous joints. Fibrous joints unite bones through dense connective tissue; examples are the cranial sutures and the distal tibiofibular joint syndesmosis. Cartilaginous joints include synchondroses, temporary unions at epiphyseal plates that eventually fuse, and symphyses, in which fibrocartilage unites hyaline cartilage-lined surfaces. Examples of symphyses are the vertebral interbody joints and the symphysis pubis.

    Diarthrodial joints typically join bones whose articular surfaces are lined by hyaline cartilage. They possess a joint cavity containing synovial fluid and are enclosed by a joint capsule lined with a synovial membrane. Various systems have been described to classify the diarthrodial joints according to their shape and/or movement. MacConaill and Basmajian proposed four classifications based on articular surface configuration: (1) modified ball and socket with spheroid surfaces and 3 degrees of freedom, e.g., hip joint; (2) modified ovoid-ellipsoid and sellar with convex or concave surfaces in all directions and 2 degrees of freedom, e.g., MCP joint; (3) unmodified sellar-saddle with convex and concave surfaces perpendicular to each other and 2 degrees of freedom, e.g., thumb CMC joint; and (4) modified sellar, ginglymus, or trochoid with 1 degree of freedom, e.g., IP joint.

4. Synovial fluid is a clear, pale yellow substance that is similar in composition to blood plasma, but also contains hyaluronic acid. Hyaluronic acid is responsible for the characteristic viscosity (thickness) of the fluid, and its hyaluronate molecules contribute to lubrication of the synovial folds and periarticular tissues. Synovial fluid exhibits non-Newtonian properties, i.e., its viscosity decreases as the rate of fluid shear increases. Therefore when there is little movement, the viscosity is high, permitting improved lubrication under a heavy load. Conversely, as speed increases, the viscosity lessens, reducing the "drag" within the joint.

    The lubricating properties of synovial fluid stem from characteristics of both the fluid and the articular cartilage. Articular cartilage is porous and relatively sponge-like, and is able to absorb and bind synovial fluid. **Hydrodynamic lubrication** occurs during movement because a layer of synovial fluid adheres to, and separates, the joint surfaces. This fluid film reduces irregularities in the articular surfaces and eliminates excessive wear secondary to friction. In addition, static weight bearing squeezes a small amount of fluid from the slightly deformable articular cartilage. The shallow depressions produced by loading the adjacent articular surfaces trap this fluid, producing **hydrostatic (weeping) lubrication**. Deformation of the viscoelastic articular cartilage also increases the effective contact area between adjacent surfaces.

5. Most of the scientific information on the effects of immobilization comes from laboratory experiments on animals. Collagen's tensile strength decreases by about 40% following total body immobilization in plaster for 6 weeks. In addition, loss of connective tissue ground substance (proteoglycan and water) decreases the space between collagen fibers, allowing intermolecular cross-links to form between the fibers. In essence, the tissue becomes stiffer and weaker. Loading and forces that were previously well tolerated may become injurious if they are introduced too soon after immobilization. Immobilization induces the formation of fibrofatty connective tissue within joints that adheres to the articular surfaces; it also leads to thinning of the articular cartilage and pressure necrosis. Although the findings of animal experimentation can be applied in similarly arranged human conditions, e.g., cast immobilization following trauma, they may not be applicable in other instances. Painful conditions and muscle spasm that cause focal areas of relative immobility, e.g., adhesive capsulitis of the shoulder and acute low back pain, may have quite different effects on the respective tissues.

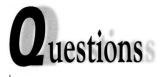

# Questions

6. How does the collagen in dense connective tissue, e.g., tendons and ligaments, respond to progressive loading, and how does this apply to treating contractures?

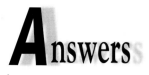

**6.** Mechanical loading, i.e., stress, plays an important role in collagen formation and maintenance. Under normal circumstances, tensile stress stimulates collagen production and influences the alignment of collagen fibers. During healing of traumatized tissue, *controlled* stress applied soon after injury promotes parallel alignment of new collagen, leading to stronger tendon and ligament unions and fewer scar adhesions. On the other hand, inappropriately directed, or lack of, stress is associated with random collagen alignment, tissue shortening, and loss of movement.

Physical therapists commonly treat contractures that develop secondary to trauma and/or immobilization. They generally direct treatment toward increasing range of motion (ROM) by stimulating tissue remodelling or alleviating adhesions by denaturing or rupturing collagen. In situations where adhesions restrict joint motion, rupturing them through joint manipulation can produce a favorable response, if it does not jeopardize joint stability and function. The biggest drawback to this treatment is the ensuing inflammatory reaction with the potential for additional fibrosis. Less traumatic techniques include the application of short-term stress through joint mobilization with the goal of stretching and denaturing collagen while minimizing the inflammatory reaction. Joint mobilization allows a therapist to localize stress to target tissues, but research is lacking on the magnitude and duration of force necessary to produce plastic deformation.

Another technique involves the application of lighter loads for a longer duration to reverse the collagen remodelling that produces the contracture. To be effective, a constant fixed load (traction, splinting, or casting) that elongates collagen 1.5% to 2% must be maintained for more than 1 hour. It causes transient melting of tropocollagen bonds, with eventual denaturing and permanent elongation. Researchers recommend the intermittent application of force, tolerable to the patient, for a total of 11 hours per day. The advantage of this treatment is that it causes less vascular and cellular trauma. The disadvantage is that it may fail to localize stress to target tissues and may adversely stress adjacent normal structures.

Prophylactic treatment to reduce or prevent deep connective tissue contractures is important. Practitioners should implement treatment when appropriate by maintaining tissues in a lengthened position during immobilization, applying stress through isometric contractions during limb immobilization, instituting controlled motion during the healing process, and minimizing the inflammatory response.

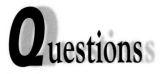

# Questions

7. What are some factors that influence the repair of injured tissues?

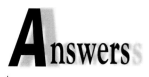

# Answers

7. The goal of repair following injury is a well-healed scar that is functionally strong in the directions of potential stress. Factors that influence the quality of, and time required for, healing are: (1) Age and general health—Absorption of nutrients, tissue vascularity and the ability to remain mobile without reinjury all contribute to healing; these factors decline with age and with the presence of risk factors such as smoking. Connective tissue disorders with accompanying inflammation may weaken tissue or lead to increased fibrosis. Medications that control inflammation, such as corticosteroids, should be used judiciously, as they can mask symptoms or weaken collagen and interrupt the repair process. (2) Forces applied to healing tissues—Although bone requires relative immobilization for healing, controlled forces along normal lines of stress enhance the strength of the repairing fracture site. Likewise, connective tissue (ligament, joint capsule, tendon) healing is enhanced by carefully applied active or passive motion to orient fibrous repair along normal lines of stress. Without movement during the healing process, the collagen is laid down randomly, leading to lack of functional mobility and strength and prolonging the recovery process. Healing of articular cartilage is controversial. Since it is avascular, healing time will be longer and will vary with the severity of the injury. Fibrocartilage, rather than hyaline cartilage, may repair the defect. Compression and distraction forces are essential to create diffusion of nutrients for cartilage healing. However, as with other tissues, the compressive loading must be applied in a controlled way that does not jeopardize tissue healing. (3) Timing of loading—Connective tissue continues to remodel and strengthen for months after injury, requiring both protection and stimulation for proper healing. The ideal progression is far from an exact science, but in addition to the factors above, the clinician should consider the healing time for each tissue in question, along with the individual presentation of each patient.

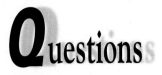

# Questions

8. Contrast osteokinematic (physiological) and arthrokinematic (accessory) synovial joint movements, and discuss their relevance to the treatment of joint dysfunction.

# Answers

8. Osteokinematic joint movement refers to the movement of a bone about an axis and includes spin, swing, and rotation. Traditionally, clinicians describe osteokinematic movement in terms of the limb segment motions (flexion, extension, abduction, adduction, and rotation) using the more distal segment as a point of reference. Arthrokinematic joint movement is the movement that occurs directly between two joint surfaces. It is responsible for the roll, glide (slide), spin, compression, or distraction that is necessary in most joints to accommodate incompatibility in the size, shape, or contour of the joint surfaces. Arthrokinematic movement is produced by the resistance of soft tissues, joint surface configuration, and external forces. It is required for full, pain-free osteokinematic movement, e.g., the humeral head must glide caudally to achieve full arm abduction. (Figure 8-2, A demonstrates decreased caudal glide during abduction.)

Orthopedic manual therapists use exercises such as active and passive ROM to restore osteokinematic joint movement and techniques such as joint mobilization to restore arthrokinematic joint movement. (Figure 8-2, B shows the application of a manual technique to increase humeral caudal glide.)

Joint and soft tissue lesions can affect both osteokinematic and arthrokinematic movement. Since normal joint function depends upon movement, and vice versa, manual therapy is useful in the nonsurgical management of movement disorders.

**Figure** 8-2  A

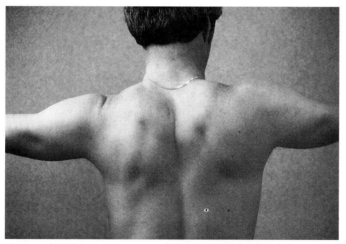

B

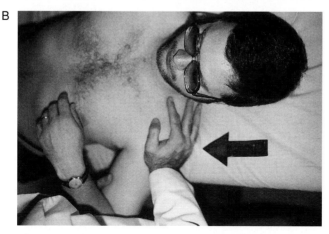

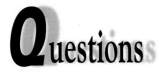

# Questions

9. What is joint play?

10. Define the five grades of joint mobilization and the indications for each.

11. What are the three grades of joint distraction (Kaltenborn) and how does a manual therapist use each of them?

12. Describe open- and closed-pack positions, and discuss their relevance in assessment and treatment of synovial joints.

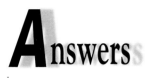

# Answers

9. Joint play is the normal laxity within a joint that allows arthrokinematic movement to occur. A manual therapist uses specific passive techniques to evaluate the existing amount of joint play and related symptoms, then plans treatment accordingly. Treatment incorporates graded mobilizations to restore joint play movement (that a patient cannot perform or isolate actively) and achieve full and painless osteokinematic movement. For example, in the knee, **ventral tibial glide** (an arthrokinematic movement) is necessary to obtain full knee extension (an osteokinematic movement).

10. Grade I involves small amplitude oscillations performed in the beginning of the available range. It is used when pain exists at rest or movement elicits pain or spasm early in the range.

    Grade II involves large amplitude oscillations performed approximately halfway into the available range. It is effective when spasm limits movement from a quick oscillation more than from a slow one, and when the gradual onset of pain limits movement halfway into the range.

    Grade III involves large amplitude oscillations performed between the middle and end of the available range. It is indicated when pain and resistance together limit motion near the end of range.

    Grade IV involves small amplitude oscillations at the end of the available range. It is applied in the absence of pain and spasm.

    Grade V involves a high velocity, small amplitude thrust through the end of the available (restricted, not anatomical) range. It is used when minimal resistance limits the range, but may potentially damage tissue if used indiscriminately. Only highly skilled practitioners should apply this technique.

11. Grade 1 or "piccolo" traction is a very gentle force that only serves to neutralize joint compressive effects. It does not produce separation of the articular surfaces. Grade 2 traction involves taking up the slack in periarticular tissues and only using a small amount of force to move the joint partner as far as the soft tissues allow. Grade 3 traction involves more force and is intended to stretch soft tissues.

12. The open-pack (loose) position refers to a joint position that is relaxed, i.e., the periarticular structures are loose and the congruency between the articular surfaces is minimal. It is a position of rest and/or mobility but not stability. Examples of the open-pack position include a slight amount of flexion, abduction and neutral rotation at the shoulder or 20° to 30° of flexion at the knee. The open-pack position is where the intracapsular volume potential is greatest; in the presence of edema, a patient assumes an open-pack joint position to minimize painful capsular distension forces. The open-pack position is usually the choice for applying mobilization techniques, particularly during the initial sessions.

    The closed-pack position is the opposite of the open-pack position. The joint surfaces are in maximal contact or congruence and the periarticular tissues are tight, e.g., full knee extension or full finger metacarpophalangeal joint flexion. This is the position of maximal stability in a normal joint. It may be necessary to assess or mobilize a joint toward its closed-pack, or end range, position in cases where progress has ceased with treatment in the open-pack position. Also, mobilizing in this position may be indicated with end range motion restrictions, e.g., a lack of 5° of knee extension. Although a minimal restriction, this lack of the terminal 5° can have detrimental functional implications if not resolved.

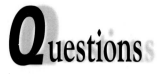

# Questions

13. How does one apply the joint kinematics concepts of convex and concave surface movement during joint mobilization?

14. What is the role of the afferent joint receptors in joint protection and the implication during manual therapy?

# Answers

**13.** MacConaill described the kinematic principles that when a concave surface moves on a convex surface (see Figure 8-3, A), roll and glide occur in the same direction, thus osteokinematic and arthrokinematic joint movements occur in the same direction. Conversely, when a convex surface moves on a concave surface (see Figure 8-3, B), roll and glide occur in opposite directions, thus osteokinematic and arthrokinematic movements occur in opposite directions. To apply these principles to joint mobilization, when moving a concave surface on a convex surface, one should mobilize the joint surface in the same direction as the limb segment movement. When moving a convex surface on a concave surface, one should mobilize the joint surface opposite to the direction of the limb movement. For example, when mobilizing the convex proximal carpal row on the concave radius, perform a dorsal glide to increase wrist flexion.

**Figure** 8-3

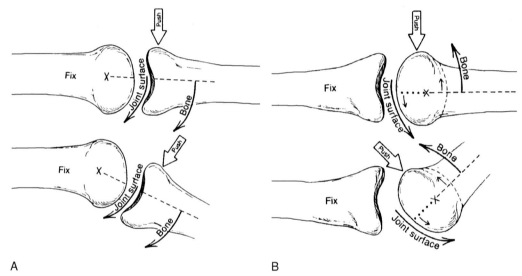

A                                             B

**14.** Joint receptors protect a joint from damage by excessive stretching. They also help regulate the balance between synergistic and antagonistic muscle forces. Type I and type II articular receptors (terminology according to Barry Wyke) are located in the superficial and deep layers of the joint capsule, respectively. They respond to increasing or decreasing tension within the joint, and protect it by regulating the tone of the muscles controlling the joint. Type III receptors, found in the ligaments, fire as excessive tension develops, inhibiting muscle contraction and preventing additional stress on the ligaments. Some authorities report that grades I and II joint mobilization enhance joint mobility by reducing muscle spasm through triggering type III mechanoreceptors.

Type IV receptors represent free nerve endings in the joint capsule, ligaments, fat pads, and blood vessels and mediate a pain response to noxious stimulation. Inactive under normal conditions, type IV receptors respond to forceful stretch, or other noxious mechanical or chemical stimuli, by producing muscle contraction. It is important not to stimulate the type IV receptors, which have a high threshold, through vigorous mobilization. Painful stimulation, in the presence of acute inflammation, will elicit muscle spasm and restrict joint movement, negating the beneficial effects of mobilization.

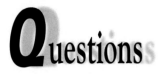

**Questions**

15. What are the mechanical and neurophysiologic effects of passive joint movement (mobilization)?

16. Why are techniques for lengthening muscles important in cases of hypomobility?

17. What are the objectives of a physical therapy examination?

18. When obtaining a patient's history, what information is essential for describing the present illness or episode?

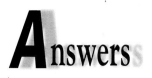

# Answers

15. The mechanical effects include enhancing synovial fluid circulation, stretching and limited rupturing of collagen, and breaking adhesions. Mobilization may increase the extensibility of periarticular structures by influencing collagen alignment and improve collagen fiber gliding by increasing lubrication and breaking cross-links between fibers. By reducing mechanical restrictions, an OMT can restore joint play movement and increase the ROM of synovial joints and the general function of the body segments.

    The proposed neurophysiologic effects include relieving pain, muscle guarding, and spasm. A reflexogenic effect, occurring through the fusimotor-muscle spindle loop systems, may facilitate or inhibit muscle tone and the excitability of stretch reflexes. Also, oscillatory movement may suppress pain through spinal interneurons, which produce presynaptic inhibition of nociceptive afferent activity. Theoretically, stimulating the types II and III receptors that are associated with relatively fast-conducting, larger diameter proprioceptive fibers blocks the transmission of small diameter, pain-conducting fibers (gate control mechanism). Possibly through both mechanical and neurophysiologic mechanisms, joint mobilization can enhance the quality as well as the quantity of movement.

16. Adaptive muscle shortening, related to changes in the number of sarcomeres as well as the connective tissue within the muscle, may have adverse effects on joints, such as restricting motion and altering load distribution. Physical therapists use soft tissue techniques such as massage, stretching, muscle energy, and myofascial manipulation to counteract muscle shortening. While treating soft tissues, however, it is important to minimize procedures that contribute to pain and muscle guarding, thus potentially compromising the desired joint movement.

17. A physical therapist examines a patient to clarify the source and nature of his disorder, with an emphasis on the resulting disability it imposes. The examination should identify events in the patient's history that relate or predispose to his chief complaint. It should determine the patient's physical status, functional capabilities, and the desired outcome of treatment. This information allows the physical therapist to formulate a plan to restore the involved body part to maximal use and the patient to an optimal functional status. Data from the examination also provides a baseline from which clinicians can assess the outcomes of treatment procedures.

18. The present illness or episode generally presents with specific symptoms. A patient should indicate the location of her symptoms, noting the exact areas of pain, paresthesia, and numbness, as well as areas devoid of symptoms. Visual analog scales assist the patient in defining the severity of symptoms. The patient also describes the nature of her symptoms, i.e., aching, burning, stabbing pain, etc. Symptom behavior is very important. The patient should state whether her condition is constant or intermittent and what relieves or aggravates it. She notes specific activities that influence the *severity, intensity,* or *duration* of her symptoms. This information assists the examiner in determining the lesion's irritability, i.e., whether it is easily aggravated or only provoked by an intense stimulus. Also, the fluctuation of symptoms over a 24-hour period may reveal the influence of the patient's job or leisure pursuits. Since most musculoskeletal disorders are aggravated by physical activity and relieved by rest, symptom behavior assists in identifying the system of origin.

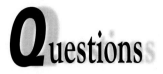

# Questions

19. How are medical screening questionnaires, pain drawings, visual analog scales, and self-report measures beneficial?

20. What information is needed to describe the mechanism of injury?

21. What are some "red flags" that would lead an examiner to suspect serious pathology or medical conditions?

22. What are the crucial elements of a past history and a family history?

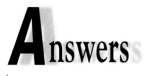
# Answers

19. Medical screening questionnaires allow patients to summarize much of their medical history within a brief format. Practitioners can use this information to plan further questioning and testing. The questionnaire may reveal confounding factors (underlying medical conditions, medications, delayed healing) or it may implicate other potential sources of problems (referred pain from internal organs). A body chart facilitates a patient's description of symptoms, particularly when there is more than one lesion. The patient can detail the exact location of various symptoms on the chart. Visual analog scales, when used in subsequent assessments to plot progression or regression, offer a means of quantifying a patient's complaints. A variety of standardized self-report measures are available, providing reliable and valid means for a patient to rate his capacity to perform household, occupational, and recreational activities. These tools help a therapist determine a patient's level of perceived disability, and follow his clinical course and response to treatment.

20. Traumatic injury often involves a fall, blow, crush, or laceration. If a fall produced the injury, determine the position of the body part that sustained impact. If a blow occurred, identify the site of impact and involved structure(s). For example, a lateral blow to the partially flexed, weight-bearing knee can produce a valgus force sufficient to injure the medial collateral ligament. Following a crush injury, obtain a description of the surfaces and/or moving elements that contacted the involved part. Thermal injury and chemical contamination also influence the type and extent of tissue damage. Although a laceration may be obvious, an examiner should inquire about the circumstances. For example, a laceration in the palm that occurs when grasping a sharp object may produce tendon lacerations at levels different from the skin injuries.

21. "Red flags" that warn of grave conditions: (1) *Pain at rest*, particularly if it awakens the patient at night, may indicate an active disease process such as infection or metastatic cancer. (2) *Unexplained weight loss* of at least 10 pounds in less than 6 months may also indicate cancer or systemic infection. (3) *Bilateral paresthesias in the hands or feet* may indicate CNS pathology or peripheral neuropathy. (4) *Persistent or spiking fever* may indicate an infectious or inflammatory disorder. (5) *Pain not influenced by position or movement* may stem from an internal organ and is not likely to be a musculoskeletal disorder. (6) *Multiple myotomal weakness* suggests a space-occupying lesion compressing the spinal cord, a neurological disease process, or a tumor compressing the brachial or lumbosacral plexi. (7) *Severe pain and an empty end feel with passive hip flexion* (sign of the buttock) may indicate a hip/pelvic fracture, infection, or tumor.

22. A past history should include a description of previous episodes of similar problems, their chronology, and the patient's response if she received treatment. An examiner notes whether a trend in the onset, frequency, or severity of episodes exists, putting the present episode in perspective while helping predict the likelihood of recurrence. Other relevant illnesses or disorders may influence the patient's recovery and treatment options, e.g., peripheral vascular disease can delay revascularization and decrease skin graft survival. Preexisting pain affects a patient psychologically and physically. Joint instability requires modification of rehabilitation protocols, perhaps necessitating orthotics or adaptive devices. A patient's general health may affect the progression of her treatment, and the date that she can resume her job, athletic participation, etc.

   A family history reveals diseases with a familial pattern. High blood pressure and atherosclerosis have hereditary links. Genetics plays a role in determining body structure and bone mass, which can be factors in osteoporosis. A family history of connective tissue disorders increases the risk of developing related conditions. A positive family history alerts an examiner to the potential for congenital or developmental disorders, which frequently affect the musculoskeletal system.

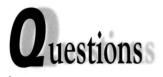

# Questions

23. What are the important aspects of a patient's pain behavior that help an examiner determine the degree of disability and/or impairment that may be present?

24. What medications may influence findings during an examination and/or affect treatment outcomes?

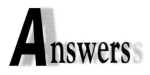

# Answers

23. "Pain behavior" refers to abnormally acting out or behaving in ways that may actually reinforce or prolong illness and disability. Patients may consciously or unconsciously act in this manner. Persons who are injured on a job they dislike may behave in ways to avoid returning to that work, such as exaggerating their symptoms to convince examiners that something is wrong. Addiction to pain medications may be a complicating factor. The longer these behaviors persist, the more difficult they become to resolve. Understanding these behaviors may require a multidisciplinary evaluation that includes medical, psychological, physical therapy, and vocational components.

    There are some examination procedures that assist clinicians in deciphering valid and reliable physical findings. Waddell developed physical examination procedures to identify nonorganic signs in patients with low back pain. These include simulated rotation of the entire body; correlating knee extension and hip flexion, i.e., positive straight leg raising in sitting and supine positions; and simulated axial compression through the neck. Extreme withdrawal to light palpation and "make-and-break" contractions during manual muscle tests are other possible indicators. Experienced clinicians may be able to identify reactivity in patients that exceeds what is typical.

    Caution is necessary, however, because musculoskeletal pain is frequently ambiguous and inconsistent. A therapist should not begin an examination expecting the patient to be untruthful. An environment of trust will yield much more information than one of doubt and distance.

24. Narcotic analgesics may mask pain and reduce the ability to accurately reproduce pain during examination or treatment. Consequently, examination or treatment procedures applied when the normal warning signals are ineffective may exacerbate the condition. Habituation to these drugs may occur rapidly.

    Muscle relaxants can be very effective as an adjunctive treatment in some musculoskeletal pain conditions. These drugs may reduce painful spasm and facilitate rest and sleep needed for recovery. However, they may cause sluggishness and drowsiness, thus interfering with a patient's work or daily activities, or hindering progress in conditions that improve with activity, such as walking for low back pain. They are probably ineffective in treating pain stemming from inflammation.

    Nonsteroidal antiinflammatory drugs (NSAIDs), e.g., ibuprofen, naproxen, piroxicam, and indomethacin, inhibit prostaglandin synthesis and reduce inflammation. Most musculoskeletal conditions have elements of both inflammation and mechanical dysfunction. It is therefore logical to include these drugs along with manual therapy if a significant amount of irritability exists. However, these substances are not without side effects, e.g., GI irritation and renal damage occur with prolonged use. Even though many are now available without prescription, they should not be used without medical supervision if prolonged or higher dosages are necessary. Corticosteriods are powerful antiinflammatory agents, but have significant side effects. They may be administered by local injection or systemically.

    Tricyclic antidepressants (amitryptaline, Nortryptaline) are pharmacologically similar to muscle relaxants. They are used for musculoskeletal conditions such as fibromyalgia and other myofascial syndromes in smaller dosages than used to treat depression. These drugs can be very effective but, like muscle relaxants, can cause drowsiness, sluggishness, poor concentration, and hypotension in some cases.

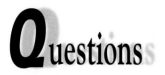

**Questions**

25. What role do radiologic procedures play in an orthopedic physical therapy examination?

26. What is the importance of inspecting body and limb posture and shape during a physical examination?

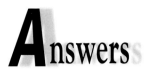

# Answers

25. Radiologic procedures encompass all of the various imaging technologies and are often an integral part of musculoskeletal diagnosis. Although it may be desirable to have radiographs for most patients, they are costly and can expose the patient to unnecessary radiation. In general, radiographs are needed to rule out serious pathology such as fractures, osteolytic defects, or progressive deformities that may not be apparent from a physical examination. Imaging studies are essential after significant trauma or when there is a question about the nature of a patient's problem. An elderly person who has suddenly developed intense back pain would benefit from radiographic evaluation to identify a compression fracture or other lesion. In contrast, a young healthy person with sporadic episodes of back pain may not require radiographic studies unless a practitioner suspects unusual conditions such as spondylolisthesis or a tumor.

Radiographs often identify anomalies such as congenital fusions, lumbarization, cervical ribs, etc., that are important to the OMT. They may reveal changes such as calcific deposits in the subacromial space or lateral humeral epicondyle with important prognostic or diagnostic implications. However, radiographic findings should never be singled out as the only diagnostic criterion. Often, abnormal findings may not be relevant to the individual's clinical presentation. Degenerative changes in the lower cervical and lumbar spine are quite common after age 40. These segments may not be the site of symptom production as identified by careful palpation. Similarly, an X-ray may show degenerative change of the hip, when the iliotibial band and its associated moyfascia are actually the source of pain.

In summary, radiologic procedures often play an important role in orthopedic physical therapy assessment. If studies are available, it would behoove the therapist to review them. Particularly if there is an abnormal bony end feel, an examiner benefits from correlating radiographic and clinical findings. The ultimate decision to request an imaging study should be based on a combination of factors including the patient's age, history, general health, current clinical presentation, and proposed treatment.

26. Body and limb posture may reveal asymmetry, muscle imbalance, deformity, and evidence of neurologic disorders. The resting position of a limb can disclose patterns of muscle weakness, structural abnormalities, and soft tissue contractures that suggest a definitive diagnosis. Disorders including rheumatoid arthritis, muscular dystrophy, spinal cord and peripheral nerve injury, and closed tendon rupture all have characteristic manifestations. Joint trauma and displaced fractures usually produce observable structural changes.

An examiner first performs a cursory screening of the involved part and notes its relation to the rest of the body. Biomechanically-related parts, such as lower extremity alignment in a patient with back pain and vice versa, should also be assessed. The examiner observes whether a patient is overly protective, or ignores, a symptomatic region; then carefully inspects the involved area for edema, nodules, abnormal joint configuration, atrophy, and other clinical signs requiring further investigation.

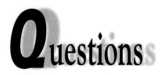

**Questions**

27. Describe the sequence of palpation and associated pathology.

28. List the components of movement assessment, and briefly describe each.

29. What is a painful arc?

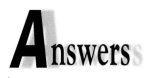

27. Palpation should be performed systematically, as dictated by the results of the patient history and screening. It proceeds from superficial to deep, beginning with the skin and subcutaneous tissue. Redness, warmth, and edema are signs of inflammation. Hyperhydrosis or dryness is associated with nerve regeneration, or loss, respectively, or sympathetic disturbance. Decreased skin mobility may result from scar adhesions. Next, palpating the layers of soft tissues such as muscles and tendons may reveal localized tenderness from strain or excessive tension. The loss of continuity of a muscle or tendon confirms a complete laceration or rupture. Changes in muscle resting length, tone, or bulk occur in various neuromuscular disorders. Palpation may identify decreased tendon excursion secondary to adhesions or swelling within a tendon sheath. Crepitus is a sign of joint inflammation, tendon irritation, or fracture. Palpating or tapping nerves may reveal unusual sensitivity to pressure. A Tinel's sign indicates the level to which a nerve repair has regenerated, or the site of peripheral nerve compression. An examiner checks pulses for evidence of cardiovascular disturbances or decreased arterial perfusion. Deeper palpation may reveal characteristics of bones and joints such as pain, edema, hypermobility, hypomobility, or deformity.

28. Movement assessment commences with a few general activities that are crucial to the function of the involved part. These may include elevating the arm, pinching an object such as a key, or simulating a golf swing. Next, composite motion measurements, e.g., straight leg raising, may reveal active or passive insufficiency. Such findings indicate that a muscle cannot contract or lengthen sufficiently in order that the two or more joints it crosses have full movement simultaneously. Testing gross activities, such as hand grip strength or completing a full squat, also reveals functional ability.

    An examiner follows gross testing with specific evaluations of active, passive, and resistive movements, as indicated by the results of the preceding examination. Active movement shows a patient's willingness and ability to move, but can be influenced by subjective factors. Passive movement primarily assesses the status of inert structures, e.g., the joint capsule and ligaments, although it can also reveal changes in muscle length and mechanical joint restrictions. Both active and passive movement testing will also reveal the quality of movement, e.g., spasm, guarding, etc. While passively moving a joint, an examiner should also assess any associated symptoms, and the end feel present at the joint. Resistive movement requires neuromuscular integration. Isometric strength testing reflects the status of the contractile structures and may elicit pain if there is a musculotendinous lesion. Patterns of weakness may also reveal neurological disorders such as different types of muscular dystrophy, peripheral nerve lesions, etc.

    Arthrokinematic movement assessment indicates the status of the joint surfaces and their movement relative to each other. An examiner also may use special tests to provoke symptoms or isolate specific functions. For example, resisted wrist and middle finger extension produces lateral elbow pain in a patient with tennis elbow, and a positive anterior drawer test implies an anterior cruciate ligament deficiency.

29. Pain produced within a specific part of a joint's ROM. It usually results from impingement of tissue secondary to faulty mechanics or abnormal enlargement of the tissue itself. Examples include the painful arc of subacromial bursitis that occurs between 60° and 120° of GH abduction, and the acromioclavicular painful arc that occurs during the last 30° of GH elevation.

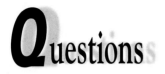

# Questions

30. What are the six types of end feel and the implications of each in the use of joint mobilization?

31. What is a capsular pattern?

32. What are the implications of the sequence of pain and limitation when assessing passive movement?

33. When testing resistive movement, what are the possible combinations of strength and pain, and what do they signify?

# Answers

**30.** According to Dr. James Cyriax, end feel is the quality of resistance to *passive movement* that an examiner feels upon reaching the end of range. **Bony end feel** is an abrupt halt to movement produced by the contact of two hard surfaces. It occurs normally, for example, during full elbow extension. However, if it occurs before reaching the end of range, or in joints without a normal bony block to movement, callous, bone fragments, or malalignment may be interfering with movement. In this situation, joint mobilization is not an effective treatment.

**Capsular end feel** is a firm resistance to movement that permits a slight stretch. It occurs normally during shoulder rotation. If it occurs before reaching the end of range, then capsular tightness or adhesions may be restricting movement. Joint mobilization is indicated in this case.

A **springy block**, or rebound within the range, suggests internal derangement. Skilled clinicians may be able to competently reduce the derangement, although there is a risk of further injury.

**Tissue approximation** represents a gradual, asymptomatic halt to movement as one body part engages another. It occurs during supine hip flexion as the thigh contacts the abdomen. It is a normal variant (except in the case of severe edema) and does not require treatment.

An **empty end feel** occurs when there is no resistance or restraint to movement, e.g., a complete ligament tear. It also occurs when a patient will not permit movement to the end of range due to pain, e.g., an acute or postsurgical condition. Other types of exercise are generally more effective than joint mobilization in treating hypermobility, although mobilization may be effective in relieving associated pain.

**Spasm** occurs when muscle contraction resists movement. It is usually an involuntary response to a painful stimulus. Sometimes a patient is unable to relax or does not want to allow movement, so he resists movement. Joint mobilization in the beginning of range (grades I and II) may effectively reduce pain and spasm.

**31.** **Capsular pattern** is a term described by Cyriax to denote a proportionate pattern of movement restriction produced by joint capsule involvement. A different pattern characterizes each joint. It is quite useful to the clinician to differentiate capsular involvement from other noncontractile or contractile tissue lesions. Upon passive examination, the degree of the capsular pattern of restriction and its associated end feel can vary depending on the degree of inflammation or adaptive tightness that exists. Examples of capsular patterns, listed in the order of most restricted to least, are as follows: (1) shoulder—limitation of external rotation, abduction, and internal rotation; and (2) hip—limitation of internal rotation, flexion, and abduction.

**32.** The sequence of pain and limitation (*passive* resistance to movement) indicates a lesion's level of irritability. The typical presentations include: (1) pain before resistance—demonstrates an acute inflammatory process; treatment should emphasize pain management; stretching is not appropriate; (2) pain coinciding with resistance—signifies a subacute condition that involves an active healing process; treatment includes both pain management and gentle movement; and (3) pain after resistance—indicates a chronic or resolving condition in which contractures are evident; treatment should include stretching that is appropriate for the joint condition.

**33.** According to Cyriax, the five patterns that may emerge are: (1) strong and painful—suggests a minor lesion of a contractile structure; (2) weak and painless—means a complete rupture of a tendon or muscle, or neurologic deficit; (3) weak and painful—reveals a gross lesion of contractile tissue, fracture, or pathology of a more severe or involved nature; (4) strong and painless—indicates a normal status; and (5) painful after repetition—suggests intermittent claudication secondary to a vascular disorder.

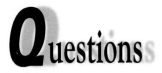

**34.** Describe a grading system for arthrokinematic (accessory) joint movement.

**35.** How are "key" muscles and reflexes used to identify the level of nerve root involvement?

**36.** Identify the dermatomes and cutaneous representation of peripheral nerves shown in Figure 8-4.

**Figure** 8-4

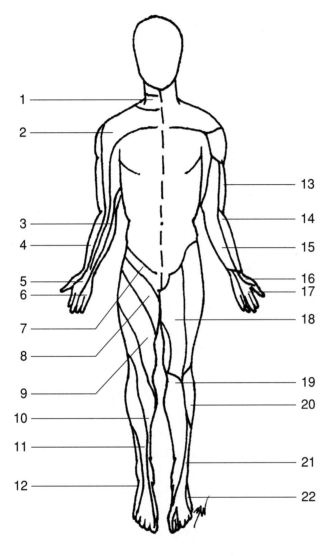

**37.** What characteristics distinguish CNS lesions from PNS lesions?

**38.** What are the signs and symptoms of adverse neural tension (decreased nerve mobility)?

**39.** What are the indications for manual therapy?

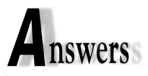
# Answers

**34.** Although several systems exist, examiners commonly grade arthrokinematic movement on a scale of 0 to 6. Zero is ankylosed, 1 is considerably hypomobile, 2 is slightly hypomobile, 3 is normal, 4 is slightly hypermobile, 5 is considerably hypermobile, and 6 is pathologically unstable.

**35.** An examiner can quickly test selected "key" muscles and reflexes representing each cervical and lumbar segmental level to identify the general level of spinal involvement. After this preliminary testing, more specific motor and sensory testing are indicated to better localize the source of a lesion.

**36.** (1) C4; (2) C5; (3) T1; (4) C6; (5) C7; (6) C8; (7) L1; (8) L2; (9) L3; (10) L4; (11) L5; (12) S1; (13) posterior cutaneous; (14) musculocutaneous; (15) medial antebrachial cutaneous; (16) radial; (17) median; (18) anterior femoral cutaneous; (19) saphenous; (20) lateral cutaneous; (21) superficial peroneal; and (22) sural.

**37.** Spinal cord involvement may manifest as abnormal plantar reflexes, e.g., a positive Babinski's sign and ankle clonus. The presence of these signs contraindicates vigorous spinal mobilization. Other signs such as generalized spasticity, clonus, or athetoid movements are indicative of brain or spinal pathology. An examiner should differentiate spasticity from local muscle spasm or guarding. Peripheral nervous system lesions such as nerve root compression can produce either increased irritability, represented by pain and excitable reflexes, or a conduction block, represented by depressed reflexes and pain or numbness. Injuries to peripheral nerves can vary in severity from transient compression to severance, producing corresponding sensory, motor, and sympathetic changes.

**38.** Symptoms of adverse neural tension vary considerably with the particular nerve involved and the area where it is entrapped or restricted. A peripheral nerve may be entrapped, irritated, or compressed as it exits the intervertebral foramen or somewhere along its course through muscles, fascia, or bony canals. Restrictions may also occur centrally in the spinal canal, e.g., central spinal stenosis or arachnoiditis. Often there may be a segmental reference of pain or paresthesia as with classic nerve root syndromes. Extrasegmental reference may occur when the anterior dura mater is irritated. Neurologic signs such as depressed reflexes, hypesthesia, and motor weakness may or may not be present depending on the degree of neural compression or ischemia. What is consistent, however, is reproduction of symptoms and/or movement limitation associated with specific tension-producing movements of the nervous tissue, e.g., straight leg raising with dorsiflexion of the ankle or abduction of the shoulder with elbow and wrist extension.

**39.** Manual therapy is indicated to restore normal, pain-free movement and function. Localized conditions such as adhesions, capsulitis, periarticular adaptive shortening, internal derangement, subluxation, and articular pain have shown favorable responses to manual therapy. Likewise, postural abnormalities, composite motions, and compensatory patterns of movement improve with exercise regimes. Manual therapists use specific oscillatory mobilizations to decrease pain and muscle guarding and to lengthen tissue. Stretching and massage techniques are effective in treating adaptive muscle shortening. Strengthening, endurance, and patient education programs all contribute to promoting health and preventing dysfunction. Other, less conventional methods, i.e., soft tissue procedures, myofascial release, muscle energy ,and craniosacral techniques, also have been proposed to improve functional motion.

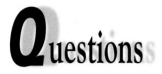

# Questions

**40.** What are the contraindications for manual therapy?

**41.** What are the indications for the use of immobilization, and what are some of the methods that are employed?

**42.** Are exercises indicated in the treatment of symptomatic (painful) hypermobility and instability?

# **A**nswers

**40.** Absolute contraindications include: (1) anticoagulant therapy; (2) prolonged corticosteroid use (weakens collagen); (3) metabolic bone disease (Paget's disease, osteoporosis); (4) vertebral artery symptoms (dizziness, blurring of vision, tinnitus) if treating the cervical spine; (5) bowel or bladder incontinence if treating the lumbosacral region; (6) CA involving the skeleton or specific structures being treated; (7) septic arthritis in the joint being treated; (8) RA or advanced degenerative joint disease in the joint being treated; (9) spondylolisthesis or scoliosis in the area being treated; (10) CNS signs; and (11) unhealed, unstable fractures.

This list includes situations that imply fragility of tissue, risk of iatrogenic injury, or conditions that may rapidly deteriorate without appropriate medical intervention. There are also relative contraindications that may depend on the severity of the condition and the knowledge and skill of the therapist. For example, using manual therapy in a patient with a connective tissue disorder, or who is pregnant, requires selective judgement. The advantage in using manual therapy techniques is that they include a broad spectrum of procedures that allow their potential application in otherwise risky situations. Grade I or grade II oscillations may be perfectly safe in the presence of osteoporosis, whereas high velocity thrusts may cause a fracture.

**41.** Immobilization is used in soft tissue injuries demonstrating hypermobility or instability, or for support in an acutely painful condition. Examples for spinal conditions include soft or hard collars for cervical injuries and corsets or more rigid braces for thoracic or lumbar conditions. It is not possible to completely immobilize the spine, so the goal is to limit motion sufficiently to allow healing and prevent reinjury.

In the extremities, immobilization may range from rigid plaster or plastic to flexible splints for protection. Knee bracing has become quite sophisticated in an attempt to limit excessive mobility during competitive sports or daily activities. Braces or orthoses are sometimes used as substitutes for reconstructive surgery or as adjunctive measures during the recovery process. Taping is still a popular choice for ankle sprains, however, severe ligamentous injuries may require splinting or casting. Immobilization may be used as a protective measure with certain overuse injuries, e.g., wrist and hand splints for carpal tunnel sydrome or for deQuervain's tenosynovitis. Splints are also used extensively to protect healing tissues, e.g., tendon repair.

**42.** Although hypermobility falls at one end of the normal mobility spectrum, it becomes pathologic when its presence produces musculoskeletal signs and symptoms. Examples include postural imbalance, abnormal translation in a joint with insufficient supportive tissue, compensation for adjacent hypomobile joints, and motor performance abnormalities. Therapeutic exercises that increase muscle strength, coordination, and endurance are indicated to enhance joint support and mechanics. Exercises that facilitate co-contraction of muscle groups that serve as dynamic joint restraints in the presence of damaged primary restraints may enhance stability and prevent reinjury.

A patient should begin with low speed, high repetition exercises of local and regional muscles, then progress to submaximal resistance. The focus should be on developing endurance and movement efficiency, rather than strength alone. Exercises should be performed in the inner-to-middle ranges to minimize the risk of stretching into the hypermobile range. Patients with spinal instability should learn to actively stabilize the involved spinal segments. By strengthening the small intervertebral muscles, particularly the multifidi, a patient can fixate hypermobile segments during trunk movements and help protect joints from degenerative changes.

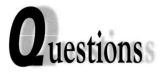
# Questions

43. Define the osteopathic term **somatic dysfunction**. What are the criteria for the diagnosis of somatic dysfunction?

44. What are the criteria for a manipulable lesion, i.e., a condition for which manual therapy is indicated?

45. Discuss Fryette's Laws of Spinal Mechanics.

46. How are Fryette's Laws applied in manual treatment?

47. Contrast the osteopathic term **restrictive barrier** with Cyriax's term **end feel**.

48. What does direct versus indirect treatment mean?

49. Contrast positional diagnosis with diagnosis of restricted movement.

50. What are muscle energy techniques?

51. A 35-year-old woman reports low back pain. Her active movements reveal painful restrictions of extension and left lateral flexion. Upon palpation and passive movement examination, the L4 transverse process is posterior on the right and becomes more asymmetric in the extended prone-on-elbows position. What are the positional and movement restriction diagnoses?

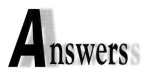

# Answers

43. Somatic dysfunction is impaired or altered function of the somatic system and its related vascular and neural components. Diagnostic criteria include: (1) asymmetry of position, e.g., a vertebral segment that is positionally rotated to the right; (2) ROM abnormality, e.g., decreased or increased mobility at a joint; and (3) tissue texture abnormality, e.g., muscular hypertonus or ligamentous thickening.

44. The criteria for somatic dysfunction (question 43) also identify a manipulable lesion. An additional criterion is a favorable response from the patient following treatment as determined by careful assessment.

45. Fryette's Laws include: (1) In the thoracic and lumbar spine in a neutral position, sidebending and rotation are coupled motions that occur in opposite directions. (2) In positions of extreme flexion or extension, sidebending and rotation occur in the same direction. (3) The introduction of motion in one plane reduces the available motion in other planes. (4) In the cervical spine, the facet joint orientation does not allow for neutral mechanics; sidebending and rotation couple in the same direction.

46. Spinal dysfunction may occur as a nonneutral, single segment dysfunction or a group dysfunction involving three or more vertebral segments. Generally, corrective treatment involves moving the patient in the direction of the restricted motion. In group dysfunction, lateral flexion and/or rotation are usually localized at the apex of the convexity in the neutral position, based on their mechanics. In single segment dysfunction, these segments may require localization also toward the flexion or extension restriction.

47. The two terms are synonymous. Both imply the feeling imparted to an examiner's hands during passive ROM examination. The quality of the resistance, location within the range, and its relationship to pain are important in determining treatment goals.

48. Direct means moving directly in the restricted direction for treatment. For example, a patient with limited left rotation in the lumbar spine would be moved in this same direction with a direct approach. An indirect approach actually involves movement away from the restrictive barrier. Indirect techniques may be useful in cases of extreme irritability when pain or spasm may prevent direct treatment.

49. The positional diagnosis is based on the static position that a body part assumes relative to the rest of the body, e.g., an innominate with the ASIS inferior and anterior and the PSIS superior and anterior could be positionally anteriorly rotated relative to the left side; a posterior transverse process on the right may imply a right rotated vertebral segment. The diagnosis of the movement restriction would be the opposite of these positional findings. The innominate movement limitation would be in the direction of posterior rotation at the sacroiliac joint. The right vertebral segment would be limited in left rotation.

50. These are manipulative techniques developed by an osteopath, Fred Mitchell, Sr., that involve active muscle contraction by the patient while the therapist precisely localizes the restrictive barrier. Usually, the contractions are done in a hold-relax, submaximal manner against an unyielding counterforce provided by the therapist. These techniques may be used in the spine or extremities.

51. L4 is flexed, right rotated, and right laterally flexed. The movement restriction is extension, left rotation and left lateral flexion.

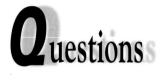 

**52.** Describe an appropriate treatment for the patient in question 51.

**53.** How would you assess the results of the chosen treatment in question 52?

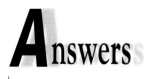

52. The therapist positions the patient on her right side with her lower leg extended and left hip and knee flexed to localize movement to the L4-5 interspace. He then moves the left shoulder girdle and trunk in a posterior direction to create left rotation and extension. He may apply passive stretch, graded oscillations, or hold-relax techniques, depending on the patient's tolerance and response. Alternatively, the therapist may passively raise the patient's legs to move the lumbar spine in left lateral flexion, using his left thumb to stabilize the L4 segment (see Figure 8-5).

**Figure** 8-5

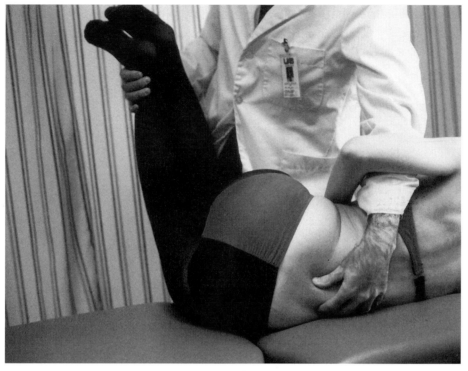

53. By observing the active movements that were painfully restricted and palpating for changes in the asymmetry and available passive movement.

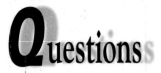

54. A 32-year-old man presents with left nontraumatic shoulder pain of 5½ weeks duration. An arthrogram is consistent with frozen shoulder. His active and passive ROM are limited to 50° external rotation, 100° flexion, and 60° internal rotation. He experiences pain before you detect resistance during manual testing. What treatment would you recommend at this stage?

55. What role do the shoulder rotator cuff muscles play in osteokinematic movement, arthrokinematic movement, and dynamic stabilization of the GH joint?

56. A 19-year-old volleyball player seeks treatment for shoulder pain that has been slowly increasing for 6 months. Her AROM is full but painful in abduction. What additional information from her history is essential in defining her problem?

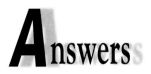
# Answers

54. Because the patient experiences pain before resistance, his symptoms are in an acute stage with pain and muscle guarding limiting motion. High voltage, pulsed galvanic stimulation, and NSAIDs followed by grades I and II joint mobilizations are appropriate treatments at this time. Figure 8-6 demonstrates a posterior glide being performed in a neutral position. As pain diminishes, and fibrosis of the glenohumeral (GH) joint capsule becomes the limiting factor, grades III and IV mobilization and physiologic stretching should be implemented.

**Figure** 8-6

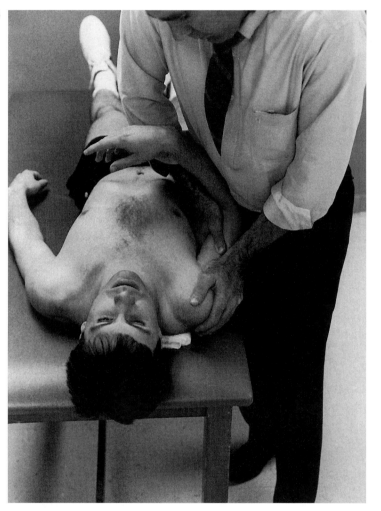

55. In osteokinematic movement, the infraspinatus, teres minor, and subscapularis muscles are the prime movers in GH joint rotation, and the supraspinatus muscle participates in a force couple with the deltoid muscle to produce abduction. The infraspinatus and teres minor muscles also serve as decelerators during throwing. In arthrokinematic movement, all of the rotator cuff muscles depress and stabilize the humeral head in the glenoid fossa during abduction. The rotator cuff also imparts stability by resisting traumatic dislocating forces.

56. Identify the precise location and nature of her pain and her level of disability. Determine if her symptoms are constant or intermittent and what movements and/or positions affect them. Lastly, inquire about the previous status of her shoulder—any past history of similar episodes or injury, if she had received treatment, and how she responded.

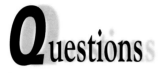

57. Physical examination of the patient in question 56 revealed no changes upon inspection, pain with passive abduction from 60° to 120°, all static resistive movements (with her arm at her side) were strong and painless, and negative neurologic tests. What is her problem?

58. A 38-year-old woman complains of localized lateral shoulder pain of insidious onset. After performing a thorough palpation and movement assessment of the GH joint, you are unable to reproduce her symptoms. What would you do next?

59. A 15-year-old boy was referred to you 1 month following a posterior elbow dislocation. He was immobilized for a week at 90°, then allowed to perform functional activities as tolerated. He now presents with anterior elbow pain and passive ROM from 35° to 145°. What tests would you perform to identify the source of his problem?

60. If further testing of the patient in question 59 revealed that passive extension and resistive elbow flexion reproduced his pain, what is the source of his symptoms?

61. After assessment, you elect to treat a patient's wrist with a grade III volar glide joint mobilization. What is your interpretation of the problem and rationale for treatment?

62. A 27-year-old patient complains of palmar pain near his index finger MCP joint, following a vigorous game of handball 24 hours ago. His hand was asymptomatic prior to this episode. Inspection reveals no structural changes, but the involved palm appears redder than the uninvolved palm. He is tender to palpation over the MCP joint. You can reproduce his symptoms by extending the MCP joint, but it is stable when stressed. His differential diagnosis includes injury to the volar plate or lumbrical muscle. What clinical tests could you perform to identify the lesion?

63. For the patient in question 62, if you determined that the injury involved a partial tear of the lumbrical muscle, how would you position the finger in a splint to relieve tension on the healing tissue? If the lumbrical muscle were stiff after 10 days of immobilization, how would you position the finger to stretch it?

64. You are asked to consult regarding treatment of a 14-year-old girl with complaints of bilateral knee pain. She started track team practice 2 months ago and has experienced gradually worsening symptoms that have prevented her from competing during the past week. She does not recall a specific traumatic incident, nor has she had knee problems in the past. What findings would lead you to suspect chondromalacia patella?

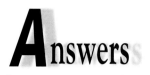 **nswers**

57. This patient has impingement syndrome, with compression of the subdeltoid bursa, supraspinatous tendon, and/or LHB tendon between the acromion and humerus. Because she has full AROM, and resisted movements are strong and painless (when performed in the beginning of range before impingement occurs), it is unlikely that she has a tendon tear or tendinitis. Bursitis is probably producing her symptoms.

58. Evaluate her cervical spine and acromioclavicular joint.

59. Inspect the area for structural changes and signs of inflammation. Palpate to localize tenderness, and identify abnormalities such as hard masses in the bracialis muscle or anterior capsule. Perform selective tissue tension testing to identify an inert versus contractile lesion. Assess A-P and lateral stability of the elbow joint.

60. Contractile tissue, i.e., the biceps brachii or brachialis muscle, is the likely source of symptoms.

61. The patient has a hypomobile joint in which there is minimal irritability and stiffness limits wrist extension near the end of range.

62. Either active or passive extension would stress the MCP joint volar plate—an inert tissue. However, active *flexion* and passive *extension* would stress the lumbrical muscle, a contractile tissue. Therefore, the lesioned tissue can be identified by noting which *combination* of movements reproduces pain.

63. The finger should be splinted with the MP joint in 90° flexion and the IP joints in extension to relieve tension. To stretch the lumbrical muscle, passively hold the MP joint in extension and flex the IP joints.

64. Her pain is deep to, or over, the medial border of the patellae. It is an aching type of pain that is increased by running, squatting, prolonged sitting with bent knees, and descending stairs. Passive patellar movement with compression is painful. Resisted knee extension is also painful and accompanied by crepitus. She has had a few episodes of "giving way" sensations when she makes medial cuts during running. Her Q angle is greater than 20°. Her lateral femoral condyles are less prominent than normal, and she has bilateral patella alta.

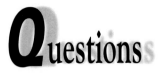

# Questions

65. A 16-year-old female gymnast suffered a traumatic patellar dislocation 5 weeks ago. She required manual reduction, after which she was placed in a knee immobilizer for 3 weeks. She now complains of a low-grade ache, stiffness, and decreased function due to fear of instability. Radiographs are negative. Outline a treatment program, prioritizing three primary areas of concern.

66. You are the physical therapist consultant to the Davis Cup Team for the United States. During a final tennis match, you observe your player falling on the court with a possible ankle or leg injury. You have only 5 minutes to determine whether the athlete will be able to return to participation. Describe the priorities of your on-court examination.

67. What two findings would warrant ending participation?

68. If you isometrically resist a patient's plantar flexion and find it to be weak and painless, what type of disorder is he likely to have?

69. Two significant contraindications for manual therapy treatment of the cervical spine include vertebral artery insufficiency and C1-2 instability. What are medical conditions that may predispose to these conditions?

70. A patient describes the recent onset of pain that extends from his left buttock down to his posterior thigh and calf, heel, and lateral foot. He has difficulty completing 10 toe raises on the left. His ankle jerk reflex is slightly depressed as compared with his right, uninvolved side. He has paresthesias over the posterior aspect of his left calf and lateral foot. Of these signs and symptoms, which *one* merits the greatest attention in supporting a diagnosis of acute nerve root involvement?

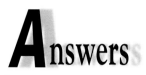

**65.** The pain and discomfort should be treated with NSAIDs, modalities, and grades I and II patello-femoral joint mobilization. Begin quadraceps muscle sets to prevent atrophy, and perform ROM in a pain-free range. After her pain subsides, progress treatment to grades III and IV joint mobilization, protecting against excessive lateral patellar gliding, as shown in Figure 8-7. Begin strengthening in a pain-free range as soon as possible, and SLR, hip abduction, and toe raises to maintain the surrounding tissues. When she regains close to full, pain-free ROM, she can begin strengthening and sport specific training exercises. Education regarding the mechanics and prevention of dislocation and maintenance of quadraceps muscle strength should be emphasized.

**Figure** 8-7

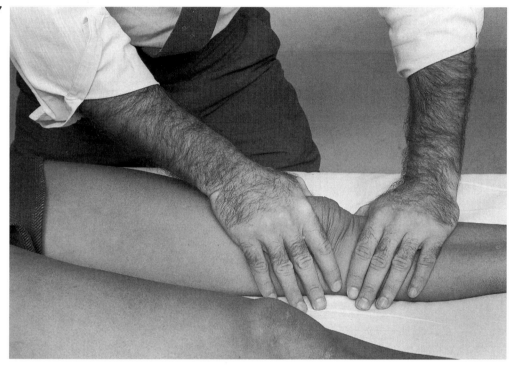

**66.** Perform a brief initial survey to assess the athlete's breathing, circulation, and level of consciousness. Question him regarding the mechanism of injury and his perception of what the injury involves. Localize his pain and inspect for obvious deformities or loss of bone or tendon continuity. Palpate for changes in shape, pulses, and mobility. If not contraindicated, perform gross movement and joint stability assessment. Determine weight-bearing status, and if possible, functional agility. Perform a neurological assessment if indicated by weakness or numbness.

**67.** A medical risk or functional inadequacy would warrant ending participation.

**68.** These findings are indicative of a complete Achilles tendon rupture or a neurologic lesion.

**69.** Degenerative joint disease with associated spurring and osteophytes may narrow the transverse foramina. Rheumatoid arthritis, Down's syndrome, or fractures may produce upper cervical instability. Severe atherosclerosis may compromise the vertebral artery.

**70.** Muscle weakness is a direct sign of nerve root compression. Pain, paresthesias, and abnormal reflexes can result from nerve root compression, but also stem from irritation of other pain-sensitive structures such as the lumbar ligaments, facet joints, or cutaneous nerves.

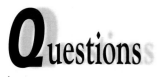

# Questions

71. A 35-year-old man began experiencing pain 2 days ago when lifting groceries from the trunk of his car. He felt an immediate twinge across his lower back that persisted as a mild ache for several hours. His pain became severe in the evening while sitting and continued to worsen over the next 24 hours, with symptoms becoming concentrated over his right lumbosacral and buttock region. His sitting tolerance was limited to 3 minutes, he could tolerate walking, and he was most comfortable lying down. The patient said that his general health had been good with no weight loss or change in excretory function.

   Objective examination revealed a posture of left lumbar sidebending. Palpation identified paravertebral muscle spasm. Central grade II pressure over the L5 spinous process reproduced symptoms. Trunk ROM was forward bending 20° and painful (repeated motions were deferred due to the acuteness of his condition), backward bending 0° and painful, left sidebending WNL, and right sidebending 0° and painful. Straight leg raising was painful at 30° on the right, but WNL on the left. Neurologic testing was WNL. What is this patient's likely diagnosis and what treatment is appropriate during this acute stage?

72. What other treatment options are appropriate for the patient in question 71 as the pain and irritability decrease?

73. A 27-year-old graduate student presents with a 4-year history of recurrent headaches and neck stiffness made worse with school work. She experiences pain along the right side of her occiput with an ache that spreads across the top of her head, and sometimes an ache and/or stiffness occur across the top of both shoulders. Aggravating behavior includes desk work after about 1 hour. Lying down relieves the neck pain and headache after about 2 hours. She is able to sleep satisfactorily.

   Physical examination reveals poor posture with a forward head. Her head and neck are laterally flexed slightly to the right when in the neutral position. Active movements are: flexion is 40° with tightness, extension is WNL, right rotation is 75° with no pain, left rotation is 65° with mild pain in the upper cervical area, right lateral flexion is 35° with no pain, and left lateral flexion is 25° with pulling in the right paracervical musculature. Cervical resisted tests reveal normal strength with mild pain with resisted right rotation. Neurological examination is WNL. Passive accessory movements produce muscle guarding and tenderness with right unilateral grade II pressures (P-A movement) over C2 and C3. Palpation reveals an extremely tender area in the right suboccipital region. Deeper palpation reproduces some of the referred symptoms to the head. What is the likely source of symptoms? What interventions are indicated?

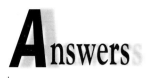

# Answers

71. The patient has strong mechanical evidence of a disc problem. The gradual increase in pain associated with high intradiscal pressure positions is probably due to inflammation and associated swelling within the annulus fibrosis. There is most likely a right posterolateral protrusion. Patient education about avoidance of high intradiscal pressure positions or movements is critical to allow the inflammation to subside and to prevent progression of the lesion. The patient should avoid sitting or forward bending. Brief bed rest for 2 to 3 days and NSAIDs/muscle relaxants may help. Brief periods of walking should be initiated as soon as tolerable. Massage and electrotherapy may be helpful for pain and spasm, but should not be done at the expense of a long car trip.

72. Exercise to modulate pain and improve mobility may be in order. The left lateral shift should be corrected when tolerable to prevent excessive muscular adaptation. A thorough examination of repeated movements in various positions is indicated, noting the effect on the symptoms to clarify which exercises are indicated. Segmental mobility testing and passive mobilization techniques may be necessary to facilitate restoration of functional mobility. Exercise to improve any length/strength imbalances in the trunk and lower extremities should be done along with any needed functional retraining to prevent reinjury.

73. Symptoms appear to be emanating from the suboccipital muscles and the right C2 and C3 zygapophyseal joints. This is a moderately irritable condition that should respond well to soft tissue mobilization of the right suboccipital muscles and mobilization of the C2 and C3 segments. Inhibitive pressure, massage, or hold/relax techniques could be used to treat the tight and tender muscles. Then C2 and C3 could be mobilized with accessory movements, i.e., right unilateral pressures starting with grade II. Exercises are indicated to maintain the mobility gained and to improve her posture. Specifically, left rotation and left lateral flexion movements are indicated. Postural correction may include thoracic extension, O-A flexion, dorsal glide of the head and neck, pectoral muscle stretching, and trapezius muscle strengthening.

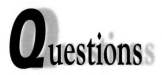

74. A 25-year-old woman fell on her buttocks 2 weeks ago. She developed immediate pain in the right sacral and buttock regions that is now intermittent, but occurs when she walks for more than one block. The pain subsides within 5 minutes when she sits or lies down. Physical examination reveals: (1) higher right iliac crest, higher right PSIS, lower right ASIS; (2) active trunk movements are full, but lateral flexion produces pain; and (3) positive standing flexion test on the right. What is her likely diagnosis? What treatment is indicated?

74. The patient's age and gender, and the mechanism of injury and clinical findings suggest an iliosacral dysfunction, i.e., an anteriorly rotated innominate. The pelvis may be manually corrected by directly contacting the right ischial tuberosity and ASIS and rotating the innominate posteriorly. Isometric hamstring contraction in a prone position with the hip flexed, as demonstrated in Figure 8-8, will also facilitate posterior innominate rotation. Length/strength imbalances must be addressed to prevent recurrence, e.g., tightness in the hip flexor muscles would continually pull the innominate anteriorly. Sacral belts may be necessary in the presence of hypermobility.

**Figure** 8-8

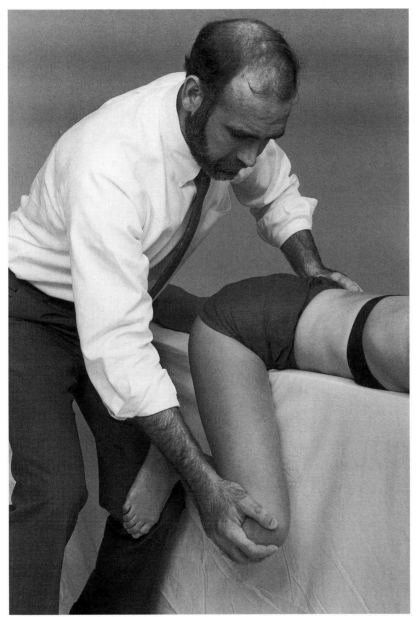

# Figure Credits

## Chapter 1

1-1 Salter R: *Textbook of disorders and injuries of the musculoskeletal system*, ed 2, 434–435, figure 16.12–16.16, Baltimore, MD, 1983, Williams and Wilkins. Copyright holder Robert Salter OC MD.

## Chapter 2

2-1 Canale ST, Beaty JH: *Operative pediatric orthopaedics*, ed 1, St. Louis, 1990, Mosby.

2-2 Canale ST, Beaty JH: *Operative pediatric orthopaedics*, ed 1, St. Louis, 1990, Mosby.

## Chapter 3

3-1 Reckling FW: *Orthopaedic anatomy and surgical approaches*, ed 1, St. Louis, 1990, Mosby.

3-2 Reckling FW: *Orthopaedic anatomy and surgical approaches*, ed 1, St. Louis, 1990, Mosby.

3-3 Saunders HD: *Evaluation, treatment and prevention of musculoskeletal disorders*, 1985, The Saunders Group, p. 108.

3-4 McCulloch JA, McNab I: *Backache*, 1977, Waverly.

3-14 Reckling FW: *Orthopaedic anatomy and surgical approaches*, ed 1, St. Louis, 1990, Mosby.

## Chapter 4

4-1 Saidoff DC, McDonough AL: *Critical pathways in therapeutic intervention: Upper extremity*, ed 1, St. Louis, 1997, Mosby.

4-2 Deltoff MN, Kogon PL: *The portable skeletal x-ray library*, St. Louis, 1998, Mosby.

4-4 Morrey BF: *The elbow and its disorders*, ed 2, Philadelphia, PA, 1993, W.B. Saunders and Co.

4-5 Morrey BF: *The elbow and its disorders*, ed 2, Philadelphia, PA, 1993, W.B. Saunders and Co.

4-6 Bonney G: *Brain* 77: 588–609, figure 19-11, 1954, Oxford University Press.

4-7 Sanders RJ, Roos DB: *Contemporary Surgery* 35: 11–16, 1989, Bobit Publishing Co.

4-8 Reckling FW: *Orthopaedic anatomy and surgical approaches*, ed 1, St. Louis, 1990, Mosby.

4-21 Redrawn from Reckling FW: *Orthopaedic anatomy and surgical approaches*, ed 1, St. Louis, 1990, Mosby.

## Chapter 5

5-1 Smith RJ: *Clinical Orthopedics and Related Research* 104: 95, 1974, Lippincott-Raven.

5-8 Malone TR, Nitz AJ: *Orthopedic and sports physical therapy*, ed 3, St. Louis, 1997, Mosby.

5-10 Reckling FW: *Orthopaedic anatomy and surgical approaches*, ed 1, St. Louis, 1990, Mosby.

5-11 Schneider LH: *Flexor tendon injuries*, 1985, Little Brown and Co.

5-12 Malone TR, Nitz AJ: *Orthopedic and sports physical therapy*, ed 3, St. Louis, 1997, Mosby.

5-14 Jupiter JB: *Flynn's hand surgery*, ed 4, Baltimore, MD, 1991, Williams and Wilkins.

5-23 Hunter JM, Mackin EJ, Callahan AD: *Rehabilitation of the hand: Surgery and Therapy*, ed 4, vol 1, St. Louis, 1995, Mosby.

## Chapter 6

6-1 Reckling FW: *Orthopaedic anatomy and surgical approaches*, ed 1, St. Louis, 1990, Mosby.

6-2 Reckling FW: *Orthopaedic anatomy and surgical approaches*, ed 1, St. Louis, 1990, Mosby.

6-3 Reckling FW: *Orthopaedic anatomy and surgical approaches*, ed 1, St. Louis, 1990, Mosby.

6-4 Reckling FW: *Orthopaedic anatomy and surgical approaches*, ed 1, St. Louis, 1990, Mosby.

6-5 Kapandji IA: *The physiology of the joints: Annotated diagrams of the mechanics of the human joints: lower limb*, vol II, ed 5, New York, 1987, Churchill-Livingstone..

## Chapter 7

7-1 Reckling FW: *Orthopaedic anatomy and surgical approaches*, ed 1, St. Louis, 1990, Mosby.

7-3 Redrawn from Reckling FW: *Orthopaedic anatomy and surgical approaches*, ed 1, St. Louis, 1990, Mosby.

7-4 Reckling FW: *Orthopaedic anatomy and surgical approaches*, ed 1, St. Louis, 1990, Mosby.

7-5 Reckling FW: *Orthopaedic anatomy and surgical approaches*, ed 1, St. Louis, 1990, Mosby.

7-8 Redrawn from Reckling FW: *Orthopaedic anatomy and surgical approaches*, ed 1, St. Louis, 1990, Mosby.

## Chapter 8

8-3 Malone TR, Nitz AJ: *Orthopedic and sports physical therapy*, ed 3, St. Louis, 1997, Mosby.

All other figures are either original or from the following:

Loth TS: *Orthopedic boards review*, ed 1, St. Louis, 1993, Mosby.

Loth TS: *Orthopedic boards review II: A case study approach*, ed 1, St. Louis, 1996, Mosby.

# References and Suggested Readings

## Chapter 1

Blauvelt CT, Nelson FRT: *A manual of orthopaedic terminology*, ed 5, St. Louis, MO, 1993, Mosby.

Bowker JH, Michael JW, editors: *Atlas of limb prosthetics: Surgical, prosthetic, and rehabilitation principles*, St. Louis, MO, 1992, Mosby.

Brotzman SB: *Clinical orthopaedic rehabilitation: A practical approach*, St. Louis, MO, 1995, Mosby.

Canale ST, editor: *Campbell's operative orthopaedics*, ed 9, St. Louis, MO, 1997, Mosby.

Chapman MW, Madison MM, editors: *Operative orthopaedics*, ed 2, Philadelphia, PA, 1993, Lippincott-Raven.

Gartland JJ: *Fundamentals of orthopaedics*, ed 4, Philadelphia, PA, 1987, W.B. Saunders Co.

May BJ: *Amputations and prosthetics: A case study approach*, Philadelphia, PA, 1996, F.A. Davis Co.

Miller MD: *Review of orthopaedics*, Philadelphia, PA, 1992, W.B. Saunders Co.

O'Sullivan SB, Schmitz TJ: *Physical rehabilitation: Assessment and treatment*, ed 3, Philadelphia, PA, 1994, F.A. Davis Co.

Salter RB: *Textbook of disorders and injuries of the musculoskeletal system*, ed 2, Baltimore, MD, 1983, Williams and Wilkins.

Sanders GT: *Lower limb amputations: A guide to rehabilitation*, Philadelphia, PA, 1986, F.A. Davis Co.

Schultz RJ: *The language of fractures*, ed 2, Baltimore, MD, 1990, Williams and Wilkins.

Shurr DG, Cook TM: *Prosthetics and orthotics*, Norwalk, CT, 1990, Appleton & Lange.

Weinstein SL, Buckwalter JA: *Turek's orthopaedics: Principles and their application*, ed 5, Philadelphia, PA, 1994, Lippincott-Raven.

Wilson, Jr. AB: *Limb prosthetics*, ed 6, New York, 1989, Demos Publications.

## Chapter 2

Beaty JH, Canale ST: Orthopaedic aspects of myelomeningocele, *J Bone Joint Surg* 72A: 626–630, 1990.

Bleck EE: Management of the lower extremities in children who have cerebral palsy, *J Bone Joint Surg* 72A: 140–144, 1990.

Bleck EE, editor: Orthopaedic management in cerebral palsy, *Clinics in developmental medicine*, London, England, MacKeith Press, vol 99/100, 187, pp 1–485.

Crawford AH, Gabriel KR: Foot and ankle problems, *Orthop Clin North Am* 18(4): 649–666, 1987.

Goldberg, MJ: Spine instability and the Special Olympics, *Clin Sports Med* 12: 507–515, 1993.

Herring JA: The treatment of Legg-Calve-Perthes disease: A critical review of the literature, *J Bone Joint Surg* 76A: 448–458, 1994.

Moseley CF: General features of fractures in children, Eilert RE, editor: *Instruction course lectures XLI*, 1992, American Academy of Orthopaedic Surgeons, p. 337–346, 1992.

Mubarak SJ, Garfin S, Vance R, McKinnon B, Sutherland D: Pitfalls of the Pavlik harness in the management of congenital dysplasia, subluxation or dislocation of the hip, *J Bone Joint Surg* 63A: 1239–1248, 1981.

Paley D, Tetsworth K, editors: Malalignment and realignment of the lower extremity, *Orthop Clin North Am*, 25, 1994.

Rang M, editor: *Children's fractures*, ed 2, 1983, JB Lippincott Co.

Staheli LT, editor: *Fundamentals of pediatric orthopedics*, 1993, Raven Press, Ltd.

Staheli LT, Chew DE, Corbett M: The longitudinal arch: A survey of eight hundred and eighty-two feet in normal children and adults, *J Bone Joint Surg* 69A: 426–428, 1987.

Staheli LT, Corbett B, Wyss C, King H: Lower-extremity rotational problems in children, *J Bone Surg* 67A: 39–47, 1985.

Wenger D, Rang M, editors: *The art and practice of children's orthopaedics*, 1993, Raven Press, Ltd.

## Chapter 3

Andersson GBJ, Chaffin DB, Pope MA: Occupational biomechanics of the lumbar spine, *Occupational low back pain: Assessment, treatment, and prevention*, Pope MA, Andersson GBJ, Frymoyer JW, Chaffin DB, editors, St. Louis, MO, 1991, Mosby.

Beattie P: The relationship between symptoms and abnormal magnetic resonance images of lumbar intervertebral discs, *Physical Therapy* 76: 601–608, 1996.

Beattie P, Brooks W, Rothstein J, et al: Effect of lordosis on the position of the nucleus pulposis in supine subjects, *Spine* 19: 2096–2102, 1994.

Beattie P, Maher C: The role of functional status questionnaires for low back pain, *Australian Physiotherapy* 43: 29–38, 1997.

Bogduk N, Twomey LT: *Clinical anatomy of the lumbar spine*, New York, 1987, Churchill-Livingstone, pp. 11–24, 130–138.

Cavanaugh JM: Neural mechanisms of lumbar pain, *Spine* 20: 1804–1809, 1995.

Deyo RA, Rainville J, Dent DL: What can the history and physical examination tell us about low back pain? JAMA 268: 6 760–765.

Feuerstein M, Beattie P: Biobehavioral factors affecting pain and disability in low back pain, *Physical Therapy* 75: 267–280, 1995.

Goodman CG, Synder TE: Systemic origins of musculoskeletal pain: Associated signs and symptoms, *Differential diagnosis in physical therapy*, Philadelphia, PA, 1990, W.B. Saunders Co., p. 327–366.

Grieve G: *Common vertebral joint problems*, New York, 1981, Churchill-Livingstone.

McCombe PF: Reproducibility of physical signs in low-back pain, *Spine* 14: 908–918, 1989.

McKenzie R: *The lumbar spine: Mechanical diagnosis and therapy*, 1981, Spinal Publications.

McNab I, McCulloch JA: *Backache*, ed 2, Los Angeles, CA, 1990, Williams and Wilkins.

Porterfield J, DeRosa C: *Mechanical low back pain: Perspectives in functional anatomy*, Philadelphia, PA, 1991, W.B. Saunders Co.

Reckling FW, Reckling JB, Mohn MP: *Orthopaedic anatomy and surgical approaches*, St. Louis, MO, 1990, Mosby.

Siddall P, Cousins M: Spine update: Spinal pain mechanisms, *Spine* 22: 98–104, 1997.

Twomey L: A Rationale for the treatment of back pain and joint pain by manual therapy, *Physical Therapy* 72: 885–892, 1992.

vanTulder M, Assendelft W, Koes B, et al: Spinal radiographic findings and nonspecific low back pain, *Spine* 22: 427–434, 1997.

Waddell G: Chronic low back pain, psychological distress and illness behavior, *Spine* 9: 209–213, 1984.

Waddell G, Newton M, Somerville D, et al: A fear-avoidance beliefs questionnaire and the role of fear-avoidance beliefs in chronic low back pain and disability, *Pain* 52: 157–168, 1993.

Waddell G, Somerville D, Henderson I, et al: Objective clinical evaluation of physical impairment in chronic low back pain, *Spine* 17: 617–628, 1992.

## Chapter 4

Altchek DW, editor: Shoulder instability, *Clin in Sports Med* 14(4), Philadelphia, PA, 1995, W.B. Saunders Co.

Browner BD, Jupiter JB, Levine AM, et al, editors: *Skeletal trauma*, Philadelphia, PA, 1992, W.B. Saunders Co.

Cailliet R: *Shoulder pain*, ed 3, Philadelphia, PA, 1991, F.A. Davis Co.

Donatelli RA, editor: *Physical therapy of the shoulder*, ed 2, New York, 1991, Churchill-Livingstone.

Esch J: *Arthroscopic surgery: The shoulder and elbow*, Philadelphia, PA, 1993, JB Lippincott Co.

Jackson DW: *Techniques in orthopaedics: Shoulder surgery in the athlete*, Vol 4, Rockmiller, MD, 1985, Aspen.

Kelley MJ, Clark WA: *Orthopedic therapy of the shoulder*, Philadelphia, PA, 1995, Lippincott-Raven.

Morrey BF: *The elbow and its disorders*, ed 2, Philadelphia, PA, 1993, W.B. Saunders Co.

Nicholas JA, Hershman EB, Posner MA: *The upper extremity in sports medicine*, St. Louis, MO, 1990, Mosby.

Paulos LE, Tibone JE, editors: *Operative techniques in shoulder surgery*, Gaithersburg, MD, 1991, Aspen.

Plancher KD, editor: The athletic elbow and wrist, Part I, *Clin in Sports Med* 14(2), Philadelphia, PA, 1995, W.B. Saunders Co.

Plancher KD, editor: The athletic elbow and wrist, Part II, *Clin in Sports Med* 15(2), Philadelphia, PA, 1996, W.B. Saunders Co.

Post M: *The shoulder: Surgical and nonsurgical management*, ed 2, Philadelphia, PA, 1988, Lea and Febiger.

Rockwood, Jr CA, Matsen III, FA: *The shoulder*, Philadelphia, PA, 1990, W.B. Saunders Co.

Saidoff DC, McDonough AL: *Critical pathways in therapeutic intervention; upper extremity*, St. Louis, MO, 1997, Mosby.

## Chapter 5

Blair, WF, editor: *Techniques in hand surgery*, Baltimore, MD, 1996, Williams and Wilkins.

Brand PW, Hollister A: *Clinical mechanics of the hand*, ed 2, St. Louis, MO, 1993, Mosby.

Clark GL, Wilgis EFS, Aiello B, Eckhaus D, Valdata-Eddington L, editors: *Hand rehabilitation*, ed 2, New York, 1997, Chuchill-Livingstone.

Cooney WP, Linscheid RL, Dobyns JH, editors: *The wrist: Diagnosis and operative treatment*, St. Louis, MO, 1997, Mosby.

Gelberman RH: *The wrist*, Philadelphia, PA, 1994, Lippincott-Raven.

Green DP, Hotchkiss RN, editors: *Operative hand surgery*, ed 3, New York, 1993, Churchill-Livingstone.

Hunter JM, Mackin EJ, Callahan AD, editors: *Rehabilitation of the hand: Surgery and therapy*, ed 4, St. Louis, MO, 1995, Mosby.

Lichtman DM: *The wrists and its disorders*, Philadelphia, PA, 1988, W.B. Saunders Co.

Smith RJ: Balance and kinetics of the fingers under normal and pathological conditions, *Clin Ortho and Rel Res.* 104: 92–111, 1974.

Stanley BG, Tribuzi SM: *Concepts in hand rehabilitation*, Philadelphia, PA, 1992, F.A. Davis Co.

Strickland JW, Rettig AC, editors: *Hand injuries in athletes*, Philadelphia, PA, 1992, W.B. Saunders Co.

Taleisnik J: *The wrist*, New York, 1985, Churchill-Livingstone.

Tubiana R, Thomin J, Mackin E, editors: *Examination of the hand and wrist*, ed 2, St. Louis, MO, 1996, Mosby.

## Chapter 6

Hunter-Griffin LY: *Athletic training and sports medicine*, ed 2, 1991, American Academy of Orthopaedic Surgeons.

Magee DJ: *Orthopedic physical assessment*, ed 2, Philadelphia, PA, 1992, W.B. Saunders.

Malone TR, McPoil T, Nitz AJ: *Orthopedic and sports physical therapy*, ed 3, St. Louis, MO, 1997, Mosby.

Nicholas JA, Hershman EB: *The lower extremity and spine in sports medicine*, ed 2, St. Louis, MO, 1995, Mosby.

Saunders HD: *Evaluation, treatment and prevention of musculoskeletal disorders*, 1994, The Saunders Group.

Zachazewski JE, Magee DJ, Quillen WS: *Athletic injuries and rehabilitation*, Philadelphia, PA, 1996, W.B. Saunders.

## Chapter 7

Carter TR, Fowler PJ, Blokker C: Functional postoperative treatment of Achilles tendon repair, *Am J Sports Med* 20: 459–464, 1992.

Donatelli R, editor: *The biomechanics of the foot and ankle*, Philadelphia, PA, 1990, F.A. Davis Company.

Drennan JC, editor: *The child's foot and ankle*, New York, 1992, Raven Press.

Hicks J: The mechanics of the foot, I. The joints, *Journal of Anatomy* 87: 345–357, 1953.

Hunt GC, McPoil TG, editors: *Clinics in physical therapy: Physical therapy of the foot and ankle*, ed 2, New York, 1995, Churchill-Livingstone.

Levin ME, O'Neal LW, Bouker JH, editors: *The diabetic foot*, ed 5, St. Louis, MO, 1993, Mosby.

Lundberg A, Svensson O, Bylund C, Goldie I, Selvik G: Kinematics of the ankle/foot complex, Part 2: Pronation and supination, *Foot Ankle* 9: 248–253, 1989.

Lundberg A, Svensson I, Bylund C, Selvick G: Kinematics of the ankle/foot complex, Part 3: Influence of leg rotation, *Foot Ankle* 9: 304–309, 1989.

Magee DJ: *Orthopedic physical assessment*, Philadelphia, PA, 1997, W.B. Saunders Co.

McPoil T, Cornwall MW: Relationship between neutral subtalar position of rearfoot motion during walking, *Foot Ankle* 141–145, 1994.

Michaud TC: *Foot orthoses and other forms of conservative foot care*, Baltimore, MD, 1993, Williams and Wilkins.

Nawoczenski DA, Cook TM, Saltzman CL: The effect of foot orthotics on three-dimensional kinematics of the leg and rearfoot during running, *J Orthop Sports Phys Ther* 21(6): 317–327, 1995.

Nigg B, editor: *Biomechanics of running shoes*, Champaign, IL, 1986, Human Kinetics Books, pp. 139–159.

Nigg B, Segesser B: Biomechanical and orthopedic concepts in sport shoe construction, *Medicine and Science in Sports and Exercise* 24: 595–602, 1992.

Perry J: *Gait analysis: Normal and pathological function*, Thorofare, NJ, 1992, Slack Inc.

Root M, Orien W, Weed J: *Normal and abnormal function of the foot*, Los Angeles, CA, 1977, Clinical Biomechanics, pp. 29–33.

Saltzman CL, Nawoczenski DA, Talbot KD: Measurement of the medial longitudinal arch, *Arch Phys Med Rehabil* 76: 45–49, 1995.

Sammarco GS: *Foot and ankle manual*, 1991, Malvern, Lea and Febriger.

Sims DS, Cavanagh PR, Ulbrecht JS: Risk factors in the diabetic foot, Recognition and management, *Phys Ther* 68: 1887–1902, 1988.

Stiehl J, editor: *Inman's joints of the ankle*, Baltimore, MD, 1991, Williams and Wilkins.

Weissman SD: *Radiology of the Foot*, Baltimore, MD, 1989, Williams and Wilkins.

Winter DA, Eng JJ, Ishac MG: *A review of kinetic parameters in human walking*, St. Louis, MO, 1995, Mosby.

Wright DG, Desai SM, Henderson WH: Action of the subtalar and ankle-joint complex during the stance phase of walking, *J Bone Joint Surg* 46A(2): 361–382, 1964.

Zachazewski JE, Magee DJ, Quillen WS: *Athletic injuries and rehabilitation*, Philadelphia, PA, 1996, W.B. Saunders Co.

## Chapter 8

Currier DP, Nelson RM: *Dynamics of human biologic tissues*, Philadelphia, PA, 1992, F.A. Davis Co.

Cyriax J: *Textbook of orthopaedic medicine, Vol 1*, ed 8, Philadelphia, PA, 1982, W.B. Saunders Co.

Donatelli R, Wooden MJ: *Orthopaedic physical therapy*, New York, 1989, Churchill-Livingstone.

Gross K, Fetto K, Rosen E: *Musculoskeletal examination*, Cambridge, MA, 1996, Blackwell Science, Inc.

Hertling D, Kessler R: *Management of common musculoskeletal disorders: Physical therapy principles and methods*, ed 3, Philadelphia, PA, 1991, Lippincott-Raven.

Kaltenborn FM: *Manual mobilization of the extremity joints: Basic examination and treatment techniques*, ed 4, 1989, Orthopedic Physical Therapy Products.

Lippert FG III, Teitz CC: *Diagnosing musculoskeletal problems: A practical guide*, Baltimore, MD, 1987, Williams and Wilkins.

Magee DJ: *Orthopedic physical assessment*, ed 3, Philadelphia, PA, 1997, W.B. Saunders Co.

Maitland GD: *Peripheral manipulation*, ed 3, 1991, Butterworth-Heinemann.

Maitland GD: *Vertebral manipulation*, ed 5, 1986, Butterworth-Heinemann.

Malone TR, McPoil TG, Nitz AJ, editors: *Orthopedic and sports physical therapy*, ed 3, St. Louis, MO, 1997, Mosby.

Richardson JK, Iglarsh ZA: *Clinical orthopaedic physical therapy*, Philadelphia, PA, 1994, W.B. Saunders Co.

Saunders, HD: *Evaluation, treatment, and prevention of musculoskeletal disorders*, Minneapolis, MN, 1985, Viking Press.

White AA: *Clinical biomechanics of the spine*, ed 2, Philadelphia, PA, 1990, Lippincott-Raven.

# Index

Page numbers in italics indicate illustrations.